Fix IT

See and solve the problems
of digital healthcare

HAROLD THIMBLEBY

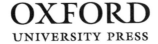

OXFORD
UNIVERSITY PRESS

OXFORD
UNIVERSITY PRESS

Great Clarendon Street, Oxford, OX2 6DP,
United Kingdom

Oxford University Press is a department of the University of Oxford.
It furthers the University's objective of excellence in research, scholarship,
and education by publishing worldwide. Oxford is a registered trade mark of
Oxford University Press in the UK and in certain other countries

First Edition published in 2021

Impression: 1

Published in the United States of America by Oxford University Press
198 Madison Avenue, New York, NY 10016, United States of America

British Library Cataloguing in Publication Data
Data available

Library of Congress Control Number: 2021934818

ISBN 978-0-19-886127-0

DOI: 10.1093/oso/9780198861270.001.0001

Printed and bound in the UK by
TJ Books Limited

Fix IT

The real data of safety are stories.

— James Reason

The most powerful person in the world is the storyteller. The storyteller sets the vision, values, and agenda of an entire generation that is to come.

— Steve Jobs

The Corporation's galaxy-wide success is founded on their systems' fundamental flaws being completely hidden by their superficial design flaws.

— Douglas Adams

The problems of the real world are primarily those you are left with when you refuse to apply their effective solutions.

— Edsger Dijkstra

... and now [1977] when the computer people move in and the non-medical people move in, they can hardly believe what they see. And there is a crisis of major proportions.

— Larry Weed

Digital healthcare is much riskier than we think, but it can be made far more effective and much safer. This book splits up the action into stories of problems, the solutions, and then the better future we can reach.

1

How to read this book

Healthcare has been around for thousands of years, certainly since long before the Hippocratic Oath to do no harm (figure 1.1). In comparison, digital is very new, hardly a blink of an eye. Unsurprisingly, healthcare and digital technology haven't yet had the time to work out how to work well *together*.

Fix IT: See and solve the problems of digital healthcare is a book about digital healthcare and how it has an impact on all of us, both patients and healthcare professionals. The unique contribution of the book *Fix IT* is to show, with lots of powerful stories, how surprisingly risky digital healthcare is. Once we start to be shocked by its problems, it's easy to see how digital healthcare can be made *much* safer for everyone's benefit, for patients and their families, as well as for staff. Digital technologies can certainly be improved to make healthcare more effective, but so, too, could healthcare change to make it easier for digital to help it. It should be a collaboration, not a one-way street.

Fix IT is divided into three parts:

Part 1 ◇ **Diagnosis** ◇ **Riskier than you think** — I want you to see the unnoticed risks of digital healthcare, and the serious problems that arise when digital is misunderstood and misapplied.

Part 2 ◇ **Treatment** ◇ **Finding solutions** — I want you to see that digital healthcare's problems are fixable. The real solutions aren't just about getting newer or more exciting stuff; the solutions are about thinking more clearly to understand what we need, and how to innovate, design, and implement digital healthcare more reliably.

Part 3 ◇ **Prognosis** ◇ **A better future** — there is a possible, much better, safer, and far more effective digital healthcare for all of us. The final part of the book sketches the real digital promise.

Fix It: See and solve the problems of digital healthcare. Harold Thimbleby,
Oxford University Press. © Harold Thimbleby 2021.
DOI: 10.1093/oso/9780198861270.003.0001

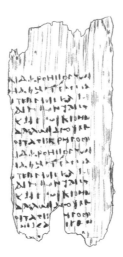

Figure 1.1. Healthcare is as old as humanity, but thinking clearly about health-care came later. Some of the earliest "modern" writing on healthcare was by Hippocrates.[1] Although Hippocrates lived around 400 BC, this is the oldest surviving Hippocratic Oath, written on a fragment of the Papyrus Oxyrhynchus dating from around 300 AD. Thinking clearly about digital healthcare is already long overdue.

All chapters in *Fix IT* have stories that'll be of interest to patients and to healthcare professionals. All the material used in this book is either in the public domain (and fully cited in the book's notes) or has permission from the people involved. This open approach is essential to the integrity of *Fix IT*, and the reasoning behind this openness is discussed later in the book.[a]

The digital in digital healthcare cannot be avoided. There are, therefore, a few slightly technical chapters in this book, which will be of special interest to programmers, developers, and regulators — this book will become a useful reference for them. These chapters are highlighted with a 1960s computer chip (a modern one would be smaller and harder to see), both in the table of contents and in the margins of the chapters themselves, drawn like this:

There's a lot of jargon both in healthcare and in digital technology, often making things harder to understand. Sometimes it's hard to know when what appears to be an ordinary everyday phrase has a specialist meaning. So, when I introduce a specialist term, it's been highlighted in **bold** to avoid any confusion.

---

[a] See Chapter 35: Healthcare openness and acknowledgments, page 553 →

Contents

Part II
Treatment ◇ Finding solutions

Part III
Prognosis ◇ A better future

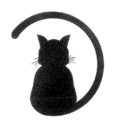

Boxes

For thousands of years, healthcare was held back because we couldn't see and didn't understand the germs making us ill. Today, healthcare is being held back because we don't see computer bugs, and we don't understand the risks caused by them.

2

We don't know what we don't know

Working in Vienna General Hospital, back in the 1840s, Ignaz Semmelweis noticed that two maternity clinics had very different death rates: one death rate was double the other, and his, unfortunately, was the worse one.[2]

Semmelweis started to study everything to try and work out what the reasons were. Many mothers were dying of the horrible and usually fatal puerperal fever.[3] He discovered that there were lower death rates in the summer. Then he noticed the student doctors went downtown in the summer — but in winter they preferred to stay in the warm hospital. Then he noticed that when the students were in the hospital they attended post-mortems.

He gradually came to the conclusion that things, which he tentatively called "cadaverous particles," were being carried by the student doctors from the post-mortems around the hospital. The student doctors examined diseased bodies in the morgue and then walked over to see patients on the wards. Today, we would call that process cross-infection, but Semmelweis had no such modern concepts to understand what was going on. Nevertheless, he instituted handwashing to stop the particles getting around (figure 2.1). The death rate duly rate went down.

Before handwashing, the maternal death rate had averaged about 10% (deaths per births), and was sometimes over 30% in winter months. After instituting handwashing, Semmelweis eventually got the death rate down to zero for a couple of months, despite having 537 births in the same period.

Unfortunately Semmelweis lost his job — his colleagues found him irritating. The success did not continue, and death rates rose again. Semmelweis finally died in ignominy. Today, however, he is a hero, especially in midwifery and statistics. It's interesting that his very early use of statistics in healthcare uncovered the cause of a problem and helped find a solution, yet without his ever understanding the invisible microbes behind his discovery.

Fix It: See and solve the problems of digital healthcare. Harold Thimbleby,
Oxford University Press. © Harold Thimbleby 2021.
DOI: 10.1093/oso/9780198861270.003.0002

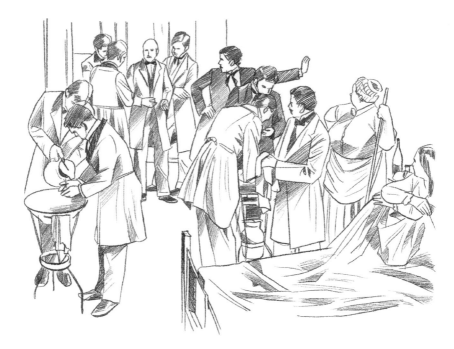

Figure 2.1. A romanticized picture of Ignaz Semmelweis overseeing handwashing in his hospital ward, some time around 1840.

All credit to him, Semmelweis's obstetrician colleague, Bernhard Seyfert, decided to do an experiment too. Seyfert found that when he got his staff to wash their hands, the frequency and severity of disease did not improve.

Why?

Seyfert's doctors were only going through the motions: they were only dipping their fingers in the water. But, crucially, they had all been washing their hands in *the same water* — and after a few days of use it had become opaque! We now understand Seyfert's problem easily: as much as he might have thought his doctors were washing their hands, they were actually cross-infecting everyone. Even the doctors who didn't go to post-mortems were now getting infected, probably through hand contact with those who did "wash" their hands, or with things that were already contaminated.

Today, we take clean water, sinks, taps, and washing hands for granted. We take cleaning surfaces for granted. But Seyfert didn't even have running tap water. Seyfert's original hygiene must have been dreadful, seeing as his experiment apparently didn't increase death rates.

Semmelweis had shown that there was a *rigorous intervention* that saved lives, based on evidence. It was only later, with the development of Louis Pasteur's **germ theory**, that there was a good *explanation* for why the intervention worked. Germs, whether bacteria or viruses, cause diseases, but if you don't know about bugs, then the interventions don't make sense.

We are still making progress with more cures for bugs, and we are starting to realize the problems of over-prescribing antibiotics, which cause bacteria to evolve and get harder to treat. Of course, nearly two hundred years later, handwashing is one of the first lines of defense against spreading the COVID-19 pandemic.

In this, the twenty-first century, we are starting to see that there are *other* invisible bugs that also affect health. We don't understand computer bugs, let alone their cures, and people are being harmed and some are dying unnecessarily.

A bit like Semmelweis's well-meaning colleagues, we tend to hang on to our love of the old ways rather than face up to the fact that maybe we could be doing better. We need to recognize the fact that digital healthcare has bugs, and these digital bugs make healthcare risky *in new ways*. Digital is everywhere; digital bugs are everywhere.

Until we grasp that, and take a more mature approach to managing "digital hygiene" we are as good as washing our buggy hands in the same water as everyone else and just making things worse.

———————◼————————

Some people get fussy over what a computer bug is, and say programs are only buggy when they fail to do what was specified. In this light, bugs are programming errors — we knew what we were supposed to do, but somehow things went awry. In this book I want to take a broader view. When computers do the wrong things, we call those things **bugs**. Strictly, the bugs are the errors that make the computer do the wrong things. The wrong things themselves are the symptoms of the bugs, but it's straightforward to call them bugs too.

Imagine a digital device, like your phone or a drug infusion pump or your laptop computer, and it just stops working and becomes unresponsive. It looks like it's crashed.

This is clearly a bug. Often if you switch it on, or off and on again, it'll reset itself and you can carry on. Resetting it clears the device's memory, and hopefully removes whatever problems the bug caused or was confused about.

Or maybe it's stopped working because it has a flat battery. Is that a bug? Did it warn you the battery was low so you had a chance to fix the problem? It was a bug if it didn't warn you, especially if you were likely to lose work from the problem.

Let's say you recharge the battery, but the device has still lost your work. Your work was probably stored in volatile memory, which is lost when there is no power. A different engineering design choice would have had everything stored in non-volatile memory (like a disk) so it should never disappear.

If you meet the programmers, they say they did exactly what they were told to do — they say they correctly implemented the specification. So if you've got a problem, it's not with them or the program but with the specification, and that's not their fault. They'd argue that since they were supposed to program it, if it works as they thought it should, then it can't be a bug!

So although we can think of lots of different explanations, the end result is a bug. If the user can't tell the difference, or can't work out the cause, whether it's a design fault or a software fault, let's call it a bug. It should not have happened, and the user is inconvenienced.

A special case of bug is not a mistake but is a *deliberate* deception. Like any other bug, the manufacturer hopes nobody notices, but there is some advantage for the manufacturer (or for someone who works there). An example of this is Practice Fusion's system. They have been fined $145 million because they designed in features into their system so it increased prescriptions for addictive opioid drugs, even though over-prescriptions of opioids is a well-known public-health disaster. Pop-ups that supposedly provided objective clinical advice were designed to nudge doctors into prescribing specific drugs: they were designed as subliminal adverts, not for giving professional clinical advice. It is estimated that the Practice Fusion system deceptively boosted opioid sales for one drug company by $11.3 million.[4]

The Practice Fusion system was used by tens of thousands of doctors. From the doctors' point of view, this subtle manipulation is a totally unwanted feature — a bug — that they had no idea about when the Practice Fusion system was acquired. Jamie Weisman had used it for five years but doesn't recall noticing the manipulative alerts. She was reported as saying:

> It's evil. There's really no other word for it. But if you want to model electronic health records as a for-profit system and not regulate them as such and force doctors to be on them, it's almost inevitable that they're going to be manipulated.[4]

Then there are **malware** systems, which are buggy systems designed by criminal hackers for deliberate sabotage, to cause chaos, blackmail, or to steal information. The hackers may work for the manufacturer, but more often the hackers work far away to take advantage of the internet to hack through into hospital systems — see box 2.1. Criminal hackers almost always get malware into your systems by exploiting bugs, though sometimes they trick users into taking a few steps for them, like using their password, which then allows the malware to run. We'll talk about some examples — like WannaCry, a huge malware attack that affected many hospitals worldwide[a] — later in the book.

For this book I'm not going to be pedantic. Bugs are the bits of digital systems doing the wrong things, and we aren't going to worry where these things go wrong, because wherever bugs happen in healthcare they need fixing. This is a more relaxed definition of bug than many people might like,

---

[a] See Chapter 17: The WannaCry attack, page 211 →

> **Box 2.1.** Malware, Trojans, Bugs, Viruses ...
>
> Bugs are unintentional problems with digital systems, but **malware** are deliberate problems, specifically designed to cause you or others problems.
>
> **Trojans**, named after the deceptive Trojan Horse of Greek story fame, are malware that pretend to be something you want, but then cause problems. You get an apparently helpful email, respond to it, and before you know it your computer has been taken over by something nasty. Or, worse, the thing is so nasty you don't realize it's taken over your computer and it just hijacks it to use your identity to do nasty things — like stealing your money, blackmailing you, and so on. Anything is possible.
>
> Like biological bugs, digital malware may infect your systems and lie dormant, symptomless, for a while, giving you a false sense of security.
>
> **Viruses** are a contagious form of bug. They are designed to spread from one system to another. Typically, once you are infected with a virus (generally thanks to a Trojan bringing it in), it then spreads to everything in your organization. Like biological viruses, typically computer viruses only infect specific sorts of computer, so a good protection is to have a variety of computers so it can't infect everything.
>
> Since the basic aim of hackers making malware is to make money, make a political statement, or just cause disruption, they don't have to obey any rules. It follows that it's a bit pointless worrying whether an attack is a virus, Trojan or whatever, since the whole point is to circumvent your defenses.

but since it's increasingly hard to tell the difference between hardware and software, I think people who want different definitions ought to suggest some different words to help us all be more precise. Meanwhile, "bug" will do for us.

———————■———————

The National Health Service, the NHS, is the world's largest healthcare institution, and is the pride and joy of the UK, so let's start, then, with a major digital project in the NHS that went wrong ...

We think that hospitals need *newer* computers. Certainly, a lot of computers in hospitals are not very modern, and it would be exciting to update them. In the UK, back in the early 2000s, the English NHS's National Programme for IT (NPfIT) was a huge investment in modernizing digital hospital computers. It was intended to be a digital transformation into modern healthcare, but it was an expensive flop, costing maybe £30 billion.[5] That huge sum is only counting the main costs, excluding training and lots of other things.

I was part of a group of professors of Computer Science that publicly offered to help, but ended up strongly criticizing NPfIT.[6] NPfIT failed for lots of reasons, but I'd highlight its emphasis on commercial confidentiality, which stopped it accepting help, and its techno-centric assumption that technical solutions could "just" sort out the NHS, and that companies could "just" implement things, and it'd all be fine. In my opinion, *what* to implement should first have been a major research project — preferably done by several independent teams over a period of years, carefully assessing alternatives. Nobody had ever done anything like NPfIT before, and unfortunately mistakes were made in the initial planning. Then it got stuck in its own politics.

Of course, today, computers are more advanced than they were back in 2000, and surely everything has changed? So we just need to invest in *newer* computers. But what have we learned from the expensive National Programme flop? Has our attitude to digital excitement really changed, and why would the results of rushing in with today's new digital dreams be any better? Everybody is more excited by apps, certainly, but I don't think that the quality of healthcare programming has improved much — if anything, more unqualified programmers are doing their things — and so computer *dependability* has not improved enough. In my view, much of what we need to digitize in healthcare won't be helped much by apps, or any other exciting innovations, until the risks and solutions are much more well-known and are universally acknowledged.

The reasons the National Programme failed are still with us. For instance, in 2020 we've "only just realized" that computer system log ins are a serious problem,[7] even though slow and complex logging-in was a recognized problem long before NPfIT.

The main reason for NPfIT's failure, in my opinion, was that NPfIT was not seen as fundamentally a *hard digital-medical co-design* problem which would require a huge investment in multi-disciplinary expertise, but as a routine, if wide-ranging, modernization problem. Digital stuff got updated, but not fundamentally improved. Likewise, the problem with today's log-ins isn't a log-in problem as such, but it's a symptom of the chaotic and uncoordinated systems *behind* the log-ins. People are starting to call out that little was learned from the NPfIT fiasco, and we're just carrying on wasting more money (and more lives)[8] — I hope my book will help change things, not just by lamenting the problems but by providing insights and solutions.

———————————————— ■ ————————————————

A provocative analogy with digital healthcare is blood-letting.[9] Blood-letting is one of the oldest medical interventions, with a history going back at least 3,000 years to the Ancient Egyptians. Blood-letting means draining blood from patients to cure diseases, justified by all sorts of strange beliefs, including that disease originates in imbalances in our four "humors": blood, yellow bile, black bile, and phlegm (which now has a very different meaning).

Blood-letting was very popular, possibly because it made quite a drama that doctors could play on. Many wise, sensible people believed in it. The first US President, General George Washington (1732–1799), who had a

---

Box 2.2. Fix IT — the big picture

From time to time, we all suffer IT and other digital problems. In healthcare these problems can cause serious issues, from overwork to harming patients. IT needs fixing.

What's the message of this book? What should we do?

- ◗ We could just carry on suffering with poor IT. Missed appointments, slow log ins, lots of passwords, lost data, incompatible systems, old equipment; this is how it works. This is unacceptable.

- ◗ We could just update to newer, better IT. This is a very popular choice, especially as there's always an obvious gap between our existing stuff, like our mobile phones and all their apps, and newer, fancier ones. Why not just bring healthcare up-to-date?

- ◗ But what if the problem is deeper than just bringing in more modern IT? We should get better-thought-out and better-developed IT. The case for this is argued throughout this book. The problems with IT are *preventable*.

- ◗ We could change and improve what healthcare is doing. Sometimes the "problems" with IT are actually just exposing underlying structural problems with healthcare.

- ◗ We should do all of the above, but with a conscious and effective strategy to improve. In particular, until the digital regulatory structures are brought up-to-date — they currently permit the mess — improvement on the ground is going to be very hard.

---

throat infection, was bled, losing — as it's now estimated — between five to nine pints of his blood in a matter of hours. Few people could survive that even if they weren't ill to start with. George Washington died that evening.

When blood-letting was popular, the doctors often claimed that the patient would have survived *if only* they had been able to take *more* blood from them. Perversely, this sort of thinking reinforces the belief in the crazy idea.

Most practitioners in George Washington's day ignored the insights of scientists like William Harvey (of blood circulation fame) and Louis Pasteur (of germ fame), until the *visible* success of blood transfusions in World War I and the arrival of antibiotics challenged the blood-letting ignorance. The enthusiasm for blood-letting only faded when there were treatments that clearly worked better.

Many people have the same style of "blood-letting thinking" with digital; that is, if something digital doesn't work well enough, well, we just need newer digital. Going digital with the very latest tech is like blood-letting despite persistent misunderstandings; just being more enthusiastic doesn't make it work better.

Part I ◇ Diagnosis ◇ Riskier than you think

"Let's have the latest digital" brings to mind Einstein's famous dictum:

> The definition of insanity is doing the same thing over and over again, but expecting different results.

Digital plays to this tune with its continual reinvention: what was a good digital intervention in the 2000s is quite passé today, so now we need a more modern intervention. It seems obvious, but until we understand bugs, it is still doing the same thing over again, just with different problems. Actually, what we now need is clear, well-informed digital thinking to work out how to do better, not a mere modernization of something that hasn't been working too well. Digital means bugs; if we get new digital without ensuring we have fewer bugs, all that we'll achieve is having different bugs. Digital healthcare will be unnecessarily risky until it's fixed.

Healthcare has political problems, like how health in the US costs the nation per person *much* more than it does in Iceland or in the UK, but in principle modern healthcare is wonderful, and its failings — although always high-profile — are rare and unusual. On balance, we are better off using computers than not, but we could be much better off if we understood them and started to improve them.

Going back to medicine ... We now understand disease, we have eliminated smallpox completely, we've invented antibiotics, and we can look forward to healthier futures where millions of lives are saved. The Bill & Melinda Gates Foundation,[10] has set a goal of ridding the world of malaria, a really worthwhile thing to do, which will save hundreds of millions of lives. With what we now know about science and medicine, this is an eminently achievable goal: we are well beyond the days of magical thinking about disease.

We should now be setting goals of using our knowledge about computers to rid the world of magical thinking about digital. We need to get rid of computer bugs along with all the damage and chaos they cause. It's really worth doing, certainly once we realize it's such a serious problem. That's what this book is all about.

Part I ◇ Diagnosis ◇ Riskier than you think

Cat Thinking explains our love of all things digital. Our hormone-driven love of technology overrides objective thinking. Thinking that computers are wonderful, we feel we don't need to worry about looking for rigorous evidence that they are safe and effective.

3

Cat Thinking

I've been wondering why we do not think clearly about digital healthcare. I've developed an idea I call **Cat Thinking**.

Let me explain.

I have a cat called Po. He's named after Master Po Ping, the black-and-white Kung Fu Panda.[11] Po came to us as a little kitten. Kittens haven't been inoculated, and until they are, they should live inside so they don't catch unnecessary infections — we live in a house with a garden and woods, so it was natural to want Po to roam outside. So when Po first arrived, he had to use an indoor litter tray.

So, one day, we're sitting down eating a meal at the kitchen table, and we can hear Po scrabbling around in his litter tray, scattering litter to try to cover his poo. Then he walks into the kitchen and jumps up on our table.

Po is an infection risk! His feet have been paddling in feces, and now he is walking around on the kitchen table. "Get off!" we shout at him!

Po rolls onto his back, and he purrs loudly. As if on command, we tickle his tummy. Aaaaah. He's *so* sweet ...

In less than a second, we have gone from being sensible people, thinking about infection risks and healthy-eating hygiene, and have turned into mindless people totally seduced by a furry, purring animal. We aren't thinking about hygiene, he's so cute. Our brains aren't big enough to think "cute" *and* "infection risk" at the same time. "Cute" wins hands down.

Underneath our rapid *volte face* is a cocktail of hormones: endorphins, dopamine, oxytocin, norepinephrine, and prolactin are all released as we stroke and pet the cat. Overwhelmed by hormones, we don't have any choice but to feel good. The world is a happy place, and Po purrs at the center of totally uncritical appreciation.

Here's the insight. The same effect occurs when we buy the latest technology, mobile phone, or any other attractive thing. Naturally, the same happens with digital healthcare.

Fix It: See and solve the problems of digital healthcare. Harold Thimbleby, Oxford University Press. © Harold Thimbleby 2021.
DOI: 10.1093/oso/9780198861270.003.0003

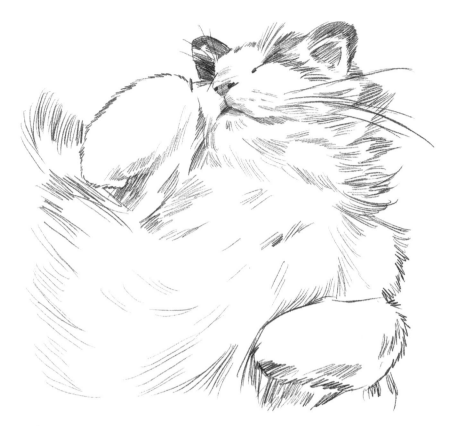

Figure 3.1. Po the cat — rolling onto his back and purring after being told off.

To spell it out a bit more, the following chain of thought takes over:

🐾 Digital healthcare is wonderful — purrfect, in fact — and our hormones make sure we feel good about this.

🐾 We *know* digital healthcare is wonderful. We have no need to question this because our hormones are silently convincing us.

🐾 Nevertheless, bad things like errors will still eventually happen. There are plenty of stories about digital errors later in this book.

🐾 But because we are so happy with digital technology, the errors *must* be the nurses' or the doctors' fault, as we can't see any fault with the purrfect digital stuff.

In short: we're so attracted to the excitement of digital innovation that we're blind to its risks. That's **Cat Thinking**.

The logic of Cat Thinking may sound trivial, even childish, but its consequences can be very serious. Later in this book, we'll see investigations into the causes of serious patient harm and deaths often follow the faulty patterns of Cat Thinking, as outlined above (the story about Lisa Norris is one of many examples[a]). A patient dies from an overdose, and the investigators say the technology worked as designed, they may not actually say it purred, but therefore any problems *must* have been caused by its users. Sack, discipline, or imprison the users (often nurses) and your problem is solved — except it's a misunderstood problem.

Let's make an analogy, one we'll explore at greater length later:[b] in the 1960s many people thought cars were wonderful and exciting. So when a car accident happened, it *must* have been the driver's fault because the car worked as designed. If you are excited by cars, lulled into a gentle hormonal haze, you are unlikely to wonder whether they could be at fault if you feel so happy with them. As we'll see, it took Ralph Nader's insights to expose the flaws in blaming the driver: in fact, many cars were intrinsically unsafe, so their poor *designs* accounted for many accidents.

———————————————————

I am not denying the benefits of good computers, but Cat Thinking explains how we all very easily get uncritically over-enthusiastic about computers. Here's an example of this uncritical enthusiasm as it misleads healthcare:

> [...] the goal should be no errors that reach the patient [...]
> Computerized approaches are ideal for this because reliability
> can approach 100%, while methods that rely on human
> inspection will always miss some errors.

This is a quote taken from a 1995 paper published in the mainstream *Journal of the American Medical Association*.[12] Somehow the paper's authors seem to have overlooked that computers themselves rely on human methods for their design and programming, so they can't be immune to error any more than humans can be.

It is, of course, cynical to point out that enthusiasm for computers is good for digital business. It's just good business to intentionally promote our enthusiasm in a cycle of mutual reinforcement.[13] It would be even more cynical for me to suggest that the main people promoting digital technology, and certainly those with any resources to advertise it and to influence us, have, just maybe, a small conflict of interest.

Cat Thinking does not mean computers are all bad. Computers can be wonderful. How better to show off their stunning power than with a CAT (short for Computerized Axial Tomography) scan as in figure 3.2? In a CAT

---

[a] See Chapter 7: The Lisa Norris incident, page 69 →
[b] See Chapter 11: Cars are safer, page 137 →

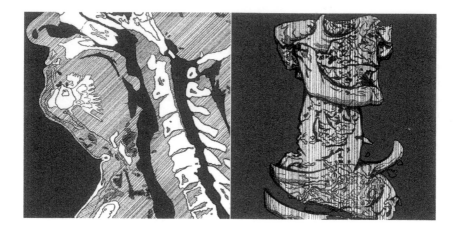

Figure 3.2. Amazing CAT scans of a human head. Not so long ago, even in science fiction, seeing inside a living human with this level of detail would have been implausible.

scan, a computer cleverly combines many X-ray images taken of the head into a solid model of it, which can then be represented and interactively manipulated on screen in various ways. CAT scans can be used for diagnosing problems, such as cancer, as well as for guiding surgery. CAT scanners can be made portable and small enough to be used in ambulances, where they are particularly useful for assessing head injuries.

A twist to Cat Thinking is that because we all think technology is wonderful, we also over-rate our own knowledge about it. If I believe my gadget is wonderful (even if I think I know this only because of a rush of hormones) and I believe I am rational, then I'll have to invent a *reason* to rationalize my love of my gadget. If I don't, I'll have to face up to the depressing fact that I'm not rational. This rationalization is a well-known cognitive mechanism called **cognitive dissonance**.[14] Ah, I know, I am clever, and so I must know a lot about this stuff to have such strong feelings. Then we've made our hormone-driven feelings make sense.

Daniel Kahneman's excellent book *Thinking, Fast and Slow*, speaks directly to this.[15] When we are faced with a complicated problem — like understanding some digital technology — we do what's called **attribute substitution**. Digital is too hard to understand, so we flip to "thinking fast" — we pick up some idea or attribute we *do* understand, and then follow our immediate impression rather than putting lots of effort into thinking slowly and carefully about the issue. Thinking slowly, as Kahneman calls it, is really hard work, but quick impressions are easy. And of course, with a dose of dopamine to encourage us, we get excited and hence very certain about our fast thinking, certain about our first impressions *even if they are wrong*.

Box 3.1. Success bias

The facts seem to speak for themselves: computers make companies successful, and some companies are astonishingly successful. Amazon, Apple, Facebook are multi-billion[5] dollar corporations that owe their existence to computers.

Therefore, computers will make healthcare successful!

Unfortunately, there's a fallacy with this thinking, called **success bias**.

There are millions of companies that use computers that have failed, and some never even got so far as to see the light of day. Here are a few I can remember: Acorn Computers, Ashton-Tate, Commodore, Control Data Corporation (CDC), Digital Equipment Corporation (DEC), Elliott Brothers, International Computers Limited (ICL), Wang, and many others. We could make a similar long list of digital healthcare companies and products that have failed.

The point is, if we think about digital systems today, necessarily the only ones we can see are the successful ones. We can't see the ones that have gone bust, and we can't see the start-ups that just failed to get going, and we can't see the software products that have been ditched. Success bias, then, is our reasonable tendency to believe ideas will work because that's the only evidence we can see.

There are a whole range of similar problems.[16] Successful companies have huge resources; competing with them, even with better ideas, is almost impossible. A typical medical app start-up has one or two programmers, yet they are motivated by the success of apps that, say, Apple might be making, with thousands of programmers and thousands of quality control people. Another problem is that successful companies obviously survived the **innovator's dilemma**,[17] but any start-up has to overcome it — and successful innovation is not as easy as the successful companies seem to make out it is.

Successful digital healthcare is not as easy as success bias makes it look.

However sensible all of us are, the marketing folk have got us to believe that new digital stuff is *really* exciting. The big companies would go out of business if they were not successful at this. There's a consulting company called Dopamine Labs, now renamed Boundless Mind, specifically to do this: Dopamine Labs combine using Artificial Intelligence (AI) with increasing your desire to use systems.[18]

They do research to find out how best to stimulate our dopamine levels: once hormones start flowing, we feel happy and stop thinking about details like how much things cost or how hard they may be to learn to use, or even whether we are adding to the tons of landfill of obsolete electronics e-waste. If something feels so good, surely it *is* good? We willingly go along with this hormonal deception. We all want new stuff, we want the latest stuff. I want a new phone. The new one will be faster, thinner, have a better battery, and it'll purr.

Digital is exciting, and the adverts give us lots of persuasive stories that convince us we are leaders, innovative, and clever to want to buy new stuff. The adverts and popular media images are part of a culture of adoption.

That's when we stop thinking.

It does not follow that an exciting thing for me, like a new phone — or any other shiny new digital idea, however exciting it seems, is good enough for a hospital, or better than older things in the hospital. Or, much harder to get our minds around, it may be better, but not as better as it could have been. So many new and exciting things just have new bugs in them, and will need new updates, and more support, and other new problems we didn't anticipate. It is easy to gloss over how risky new digital innovations may be and how much more work needs doing on them first. We can't help inhabiting a happy, Cat Thinking, consumer culture of wanting the latest technical solutions before we've even worked out what the problems we are trying to solve are.

That's a clue to one of the surest defenses against Cat Thinking. Somebody must ask for a **safety case**. A safety case is a reasoned document that *rigorously* explores the benefits and risks and how safety is impacted.[19] Don't just buy a new digital system; first write a safety case — this engages your slow thinking, isolates you from dopamine, and gets you to systematically explore issues. Safety cases encourage informed innovation; at the other end of the timeline — say, when there is a court case about some digital system that's gone wrong (usually the court case is about a nurse caught up in some digital mess) — the cross-examination should ask, "Where is the safety case?" For without a safety case, there is no reason to think the system is safe, and therefore every reason to think the nurse or doctor is innocent; in fact, every reason to think somebody has succumbed to Cat Thinking.

Digital makes many persuasive promises, but it's sometimes — much more often than we care to admit — making healthcare *less* safe, or at least making it a lot less safe than it needs to be. It needn't be like that, but the culture that has embraced digital as an automatic solution is pervasive.

I'll explore the problems and solutions with stories and examples throughout this book. I hope my stories give us pause (paws?) to think, and some powerful and effective ideas to start improving. We need to.

Look carefully for them, and you'll uncover lots of stories of digital healthcare bugs. This chapter has lots of examples of buggy digital health.

4

Dogs dancing

It is amazing when a dog dances. It is amazing that computers do their magic. But dogs don't dance very well, and nobody dare say so, in case they upset the circus.

In 2000, incorrect Down syndrome test results were given to 158 mothers in England, with tragic consequences. Let's see how this happened.

One of the best-known computer bugs is the Millennium Bug, which is also known as the Y2K bug. Unlike most bugs, the Millennium Bug is very easy to understand. We'll first explore what the bug was, then show how it caused incorrect Down syndrome test results.

When digital computers started to get popular, around the 1950s, nobody thought about the end of the millennium: it was still a lifetime away. Computers in those days were slow and expensive, and what programmers worried about was saving time and money. It was natural, then, to write dates in a cost-saving shorthand. Instead of writing years in full, like 1950, 1960, or 1967, they were programmed in a much tighter form using only the last two digits, like 50, 60, or 67. The two digits of the year use only half the space, and can be processed twice as fast. If you were storing the birth dates of, say, thousands of patients, the savings would have been worthwhile. Everybody — and every computer — benefited from the efficiency gains.

Computers very soon became smaller, faster, and *enormously* popular. They started to be used everywhere. People started to lose track of them: they were used in lifts, in microwave cookers, ticket machines, airplanes, nuclear power stations ... they were in everything.

I was born in 1955, so in 1956 I had my first birthday. If a computer treated my date of birth as 55, and treated the year 1956 as 56, then it would have done the quick calculation "56 minus 55" and, of course, got the right age: I'd have been one year old in 1956.[20]

I grew up through the 60s, 70s, and 80s, and I didn't see the problem coming. Nor did a lot of other people.

Fix It: See and solve the problems of digital healthcare. Harold Thimbleby,
Oxford University Press. © Harold Thimbleby 2021.
DOI: 10.1093/oso/9780198861270.003.0004

A computer could work out my age whenever it was needed. So, over the last few years of the millennium — 1995 to 1999 — my age would of course have been 40, 41, 42, 43, 44 in each successive year. In each year, the computer would have done the sum $95 - 55 = 40$, or $96 - 55 = 41$, and so on. But in 2000 the computer would calculate my age not as 45, but as *minus* 55! My age would have been calculated by doing the sum $00 - 55$, getting the nonsense negative age of *minus* 55. That's the Y2K bug in a nutshell.

The Y2K bug potentially affected every computer in the world and almost everything they did. When people realized the scale of the Y2K problem an international effort rapidly got underway to fix it. The huge amount of work, and the very short time left to do it in before 2000, created enormous pressure. In the UK, even prisoners helped out as they ran out of programmers.

Fortunately, most of the bugs were fixed in time, but unfortunately some were missed.[21]

Here's a tragic story of a missed and misunderstood Y2K bug.

The chances of giving birth to a Down syndrome baby increase with age, and many mothers opt to have a Down syndrome test. In 2000, incorrect Down test results were given to 158 women in England, thanks to a missed Y2K bug that had been overlooked. Tragically, some terminations were carried out as a result, and some Down syndrome babies were born to mothers who had been told their tests put them at low risk.

The Down syndrome test relies on lots of measurements, including blood tests, number of weeks into pregnancy (based on ultrasound measurements), and the mother's age and weight. The test mixes these measurements in a complex formula to estimate the risk of Down syndrome. Thanks to the Y2K bug in the program, any pregnant mother tested in 2000 would have seemed to have a negative age, which would inevitably mess up the calculations.

The incident has now had an inquiry, and there is a long report on it.[22] The report presents a catalog of chaos, under-staffing, under-resourcing, lack of digital skills, and lack of awareness of the need for digital competence.

It's curious that the report's authors and consultants had no digital qualifications themselves. The report did not explicitly see the test's Y2K problems as a symptom of digital incompetence — lack of training, skills, and supervision — and therefore it contributed no useful learning to improve digital healthcare after the experience. They saw it as a one-off problem.[23]

The Down testing service had been running successfully for ten years, and the hospitals using it had become over-confident; what could possibly go wrong with such a reliable service? When midwives first noticed that some test results looked strange, the hospitals thought they were just different women. Not a bug, let alone a systematic bug. Midwives started to raise the alarm, and the bug was finally identified as such in May 2000.

Responsibility for the program had ended up with a single, self-taught hospital IT specialist, an anonymized "Mr W," who was unsupported and out of their depth. The entire line management was clearly out of its depth, too, as this critical role was not properly supported or supervised.[24] The NHS, rightly, ended up with a huge compensation bill.[25]

This *easily* avoidable bug,[a] combined with a failure to regulate digital healthcare to avoid bugs, and develop and manage digital systems professionally, turned into a disaster for mothers and babies.

The story is typical.

First, everyone thinks developing a digital healthcare system is easy. Initially, using the system seems absolutely fine, but then something happens that the system can't cope with. Things go wrong, and patients are harmed. Unfortunately, it is very hard to notice when things go wrong like this; you need a level of suspicion, critical thinking, and technical knowledge of how digital systems can fail. With the Down Y2K bug, some patients were harmed before the midwives had noticed there was a systematic problem.

There must be competent external oversight, because you can't know what you don't know — somebody else needs to look. Of course, there's no reason why healthcare professionals should be expected to have the highly technical skills to spot, let alone avoid, the problems that arise; healthcare needs more competent digital experts. Indeed, even the investigation team for the Down Y2K bug had inadequate computing expertise to interpret the digital evidence so there could be useful, wider learning.[23]

The Down tragedy shows the importance of routinely monitoring everything for unusual activity — ironically, this is one thing computers are very good at. Many people, though, think the important lesson to learn from this story is that healthcare has a skills problem: there should be more formally qualified IT staff.[26] Given the poor quality of digital systems, better qualified staff would certainly help, but, really, the true cause of the problem is the low quality of digital systems in the first place.

———————————————■———————————————

In 2002, a car knocked my student Nick Fine off his motorbike. Nick was taken to hospital, and he was hooked up to various drugs to help him recover. Being a hemophiliac, he was given a clotting factor through a syringe driver.

Syringe drivers have a motor in them that pushes a syringe, which squeezes the drug down a tube which is usually inserted into a vein in the patient's arm. The syringe driver has a little computer in it to control the motor and how fast it runs. It also does important things like sensing whether the syringe is jammed, as might happen if the tube is kinked and blocked.

Nick's syringe driver had a large paper notice stuck on it, warning staff not to touch any of its buttons.

If you need to stick such notices on hospital equipment, there's probably something wrong with the design.

---

[a] See Chapter 21: Avoiding the Down test bug, page 286 →

Part I ◇ Diagnosis ◇ Riskier than you think

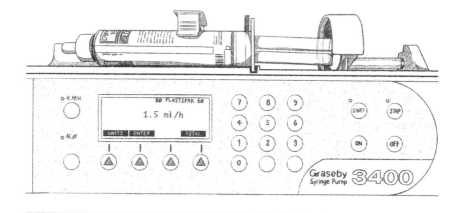

Figure 4.1. My computer simulation of the Graseby 3400 syringe driver. In my simulation, as you press the buttons (or click on them with a mouse) the lights and screen change exactly as on a real, working Graseby syringe driver.

Why didn't the manufacturers of the syringe driver, Graseby, find out how their product would be used, and build in features so that it was easier and safer to use? Why does anyone need to rely on labels that may fall off?

So, sensing a story, I bought myself a Graseby syringe driver like Nick's to see how it worked.

To help me really understand the Graseby syringe driver, I built a computer simulation of it and made some videos that you can watch.[27]

It was while building this simulation that I discovered a **timeout** issue — I was spending too long trying to understand it, and it went and timed out on me. I was trying to understand how entering drug doses worked, and as I tried to enter 0.5 mL per hour, I paused just after pressing the decimal point (so I could make sure my simulation worked exactly the same way), and the thing got bored waiting for me and timed out. It also zeroed the number I was entering. I'd found out that if you entered a number slowly for any reason, the number you actually entered could change — sometimes in surprisingly complicated ways. For example, if you enter 0. (that is, zero followed by a decimal point) it might get changed to 0 (with no decimal point), so entering 0.5 mL per hour slowly could end up as 5 mL per hour, which is ten times higher than you intended. If you are doing a complex job — like paying attention to a patient — you may never notice.

A ten-times overdose could be very serious, so I wondered why the syringe driver had been designed the way it had. Was the timeout there because it somehow helped how the thing was used in hospitals? I realized I didn't know enough. At this stage, I didn't know whether this "problem" was my lack of understanding of how the device was supposed to work, or whether it was some genuine problem in the design that might trip up users of it. I would soon find out.

So I met up with an anesthesiologist, and scrubbed up to join in some operations. I took a low profile, did what I was told, and generally kept out of the way. I just watched what happened.

A patient was wheeled up for our first operation. He had been in a fight and had had his jaw broken. The anesthesiologist set up the equipment so that the patient could be anesthetized.

The anesthesiologist started talking with the patient to find out things like how much he drank, as that would affect how much anesthetic he might need. The anesthesiologist entered the patient's weight and then the right dose rate of the drug (fentanyl in this case) into the syringe driver. Several times the anesthesiologist got a bit flustered and, as he was also talking to me, he said he didn't really understand the syringe driver. He got it sorted out eventually, and the patient went under, and we took him into the operating room.

While the surgeon was putting wires in the patient's jaw, I asked the anesthesiologist about the Graseby syringe driver he'd been using, so I could try to figure out what had caused all his problems with it. What we worked out was because the patient had come to theater with a broken jaw, he was having difficulty talking, so the anesthesiologist had taken "too long" to enter the drug dose. The syringe driver had silently timed out, making a mess of things. So the anesthesiologist had to try again and again as the problem kept repeating.

Fortunately, anesthesiologists pay close attention to what's happening to the patient, and nothing went wrong for them — this time. I was interested that the anesthesiologist blamed himself for not properly understanding the syringe driver, when the reality was that *it* didn't understand how to be safe in a real, demanding operating room. More to the point, its designers hadn't understood.

This is just one example where the digital system — here a syringe driver — is critical in achieving the clinical effectiveness of a drug. The drug itself has to pass very stringent regulations, to ensure it's safe and effective, but the syringe driver has very little regulation, beyond having to be electrically and mechanically safe.

The next operation I attended, the ventilator crashed.

When you are anesthetized and given a muscle relaxant (so your body does not twitch when it is operated on) you can't breathe unaided, so the ventilator is programmed to pump gases into your lungs at the appropriate rate, taking so many breaths per minute. So when the ventilator screen announced that the ventilator's computer had crashed, the error message it displayed proved it had not been designed for safe use in healthcare (figure 4.2). That is, the error message came from the operating system; the ventilator itself had crashed without *it* being prepared for the bug that crashed it.

Part I ◇ Diagnosis ◇ Riskier than you think

Abort, Retry, Fail? _

Figure 4.2. A ventilator has crashed, but there is no explanation of the problem, and the choices "Abort" and "Fail" don't help get the ventilator working, and the choice "Retry" is futile unless the program has sorted out the bug that caused the failure. The only sensible option — which is not stated — is to switch the ventilator off and on again, so it reboots and hopefully sorts itself out in the process. This error message appearing on a ventilator proves the system was not designed for safe use in healthcare.

The anesthesiologist quickly got up and rebooted the ventilator, and then had to re-enter all the patient data (lung capacity, and so on) and restart it, which took a while. "You'll report it?" I said. The anesthesiologist said nothing had happened to the patient, so no, he wouldn't report it. I said if the surgeon had stood on one of your lines or there had been another problem at the same time, would that have been OK? Probably not.

I and the anesthesiologist may have had a slight misunderstanding. Since nothing happened to the patient, there was no adverse event that required reporting as a *clinical* problem, but there was a device malfunction that should have been reported as a *device* problem. By not reporting the device crashing, nobody will learn that the ventilator has a bug, and nobody will look into it and fix it. One day it may happen again at a more critical moment.

———————————■———————————

In an ideal world, medical devices — and especially digital medical devices — support the needs of the doctors and nurses, and ultimately support the needs of the patients and their treatment. But go into many hospitals, and sticky notes and other workarounds are visible everywhere (figure 4.3). You can argue that this is staff breaking **standard operating procedures** (SOPs), and they should be reported, or that this is an indication that the digital devices are inadequately designed and that the local staff are trying to improve patient safety — in which case, the device designs should be improved. Sometimes both.

Are they notes from one nurse to the next to help make handover more reliable? If a sticky note is saying, "Don't give more than 10 mLs," why doesn't the device keep track of that and make sure no such error happens? If a note is saying, "This is insulin," why doesn't the device itself help keep track of that and make sure it really is insulin? If a note is saying, "Refill at 10 pm," why doesn't the device keep track of that and make sure it is refilled?

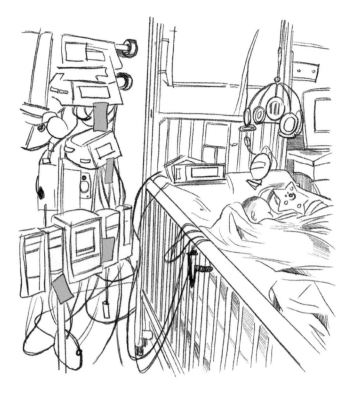

Figure 4.3. A poorly baby in a US hospital bed. Sticky notes attached to digital devices are workarounds showing that the devices (in the picture, syringe drivers and infusion pumps) are not adequately designed to support the needs of the health-care professionals using them. What happens if any sticky note falls off? Or, worse, if any sticky note is put on the wrong device?

If a note falls off and something terrible happens, will the nurse go to prison? Did the sticky note postpone things going wrong earlier or did it contribute to the problem? Isn't it time to design more safely?

There is similar practice in low-income countries, too (figure 4.4): in these places, there is no alternative to post-it or other notes to help manage patients lying spread out on the floor along hospital corridors.

Yet, in all countries, why don't digital devices themselves help keep track of the details that nurses so clearly *need*? Why aren't manufacturers making devices that support the needs of patient care; for instance, nurses' notes could be saved and shown on each device, managed by computer and (in principle) made much more helpful — and there need be no possibility of the notes for one device being mixed up with another device's notes.

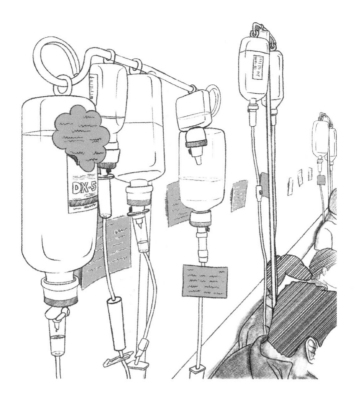

Figure 4.4. Patients lying along a corridor in a Mexico City hospital. Sticky notes are being used to keep track of vital information on drips. There are no digital devices, unlike in figure 4.3 — though even there sticky notes were still needed.

The Children's Hospital, Pittsburgh, USA, brought in a new system called PowerOrders, and got it installed in just six days. PowerOrders is for organizing orders, such as admitting patients and ordering treatments; PowerOrders was developed by Cerner as part of their PowerChart system.

The hospital wanted to know how the implementation of the new system affected deaths among children who were transferred (e.g., in ambulances) between hospitals into their specialized care.

I've drawn a bar chart (figure 4.5) based on their paper.[28]

What the chart shows, and what the paper argues at greater length, is that death rates more than doubled after their new computer system was installed. Each bar in the graph shows the children's mortality over each quarter, covering the 18-month period of their survey. The stepped line running across the graph shows the average mortality before and after the new system was implemented. So in the first year, the average mortality was 2.8%, as 39 out of 1,394 children admitted over that year died — remember that these are sick children, and, as a specialized facility, the Children's Hospital would

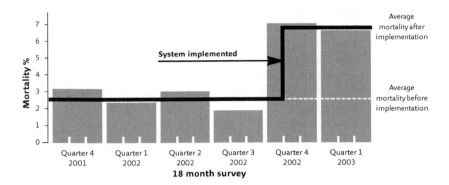

Figure 4.5. Death rates of transfered children on a pediatric ward in a US hospital, before and after a new computer system was installed.[28]

expect to get very sick children that other hospitals had transferred to them for better treatment, including better end-of-life treatment.

The hospital ran Cerner Millennium, and this new PowerOrders system was installed as an "add-in" module to Millennium towards the end of month 13 of their survey. You can see the jump in mortality rate occurs at the same time, sometime during the fifth quarter in the bar chart. The average more than doubles.

Naturally the Cerner Millennium paper is controversial as many people want to disagree with its findings. It's not only an old survey, but maybe the doubling of the death rate happened because of something else? The trouble with powerful stories is that you do not know how representative they are of the rest of the world. You can't tell if the lessons from the story are about *this* ward, *this* hospital, *this* new computer system as implemented in *this* hospital, or are about something more general and we should all take notice. A stronger criticism liked by traditionalists is that the study wasn't a **Randomized Controlled Trial** — an experimental method designed to address such concerns, which I'll discuss later.[b]

Despite the age of the paper, the Cerner Millenium type of problems are still around. When an Epic system — like Cerner Millennium, another well-established digital healthcare system — was implemented at a leading UK hospital, Addenbrooke's Hospital, in 2014, they had a large drop in Accident and Emergency performance, among other problems, and Epic became un-stable. A "major incident" was declared, and ambulances had to be re-routed to other hospitals.[29] The details may change but the big picture hasn't.[30]

But if you want to dismiss the paper, you should worry that doing and publishing this sort of research work is heavily constrained by **gag clauses**, whereby the manufacturers and vendors of systems systematically under-

[b] See Chapter 28: Randomized Controlled Trials, page 393 →

mine good research.[31] For example, hospitals have to sign contracts with suppliers — to be permitted to use the systems — which then stop them sharing anything about them, particularly pictures such as screenshots, even if there are incidents causing patient harm. This means that other hospitals will be unable to learn from problems, and the research community will not be able to find solutions. On the other hand, it means the manufacturer's reputation is protected.

> ☝ The gag clause problem, combined with hospitals' reasonable concerns about patient confidentiality, is why this book doesn't discuss hospital systems as much as medical devices. Fortunately, small devices like apps and infusion pumps are also much easier to access and are much easier to describe in detail without getting too boring. You can also acquire them easily (you can easily buy all of those discussed in this book), and check my claims if you want to; in contrast, confidentiality and gag clauses would severely restrict your access to hospital systems.

Whatever the Pittsburgh study's shortcomings, it's surprising that an established computer system such as the one they installed — not a brand new, experimental one — had such problems. I don't know details of the contracts, but perhaps there should have been precautions; maybe the hospital should have contracted that the manufacturers must ensure the systems work reliably, and that until it's shown to be an actual improvement, they wouldn't be paid in full. After all, that's what happens with new buildings: there is a period of "snagging" when the architect and client go round the building pointing out and getting the builders to fix the remaining problems.

Manufacturers might argue that this idea isn't workable. For too long, digital businesses have got used to rapid and easy turnaround — and by Cat Thinking,[c] so has everyone else — but this is not how to develop safe and reliable digital solutions for complex systems like healthcare.

The Pittsburgh paper[28] discusses some of the reasons for the jump in the fatality rate. One was that before the system was installed, when a child was picked up by ambulance, the paramedics at the scene could call the hospital by radio and ask them to get ready for the patient. The hospital would prepare the necessary medications.

Now, with the newly installed PowerOrders system, the hospital can't get things ready until the child is fully registered with the system, so there is a delay because they have to wait until the child arrives at the hospital. Another reason was that, although the new system promised increased productivity, in practice it required someone to actually use the computer. That, in itself, took those clinicians away from directly looking after patients — the paper says that, previously, a paper form might be filled out in a "few seconds," but

---

[c] See Chapter 3: Cat Thinking, page 25 ←

the computer form takes ten clicks and several minutes.

The computer system delayed treatment and reduced the effective number of staff available for patient contact. Sometimes the computer required the full attention of a doctor for 15 minutes to an hour, as other clinicians tried to stabilize the patient.

Other times, the Wi-Fi system got overloaded and the computer systems would freeze during heavy periods, and then nothing could be done. If a pharmacist accessed the system to prepare some drugs, the nurses in the ward were locked out of the system, because the system could not cope with two people looking at the same information. Why isn't it obvious that to be of benefit, a new system must be an improvement over and beyond any inefficiencies or problems it introduces.

No doubt the hospital has started to sort out these problems, but it's important to remember that this was not a totally new system where any of these problems could have been excused as a surprise. It had been used elsewhere, and the manufacturer, Cerner, had years of experience behind it. Yet the death rate doubled.

Six years after the Pittsburgh Children's Hospital paper was published, Dr Hadiza Bawa-Garba, together with nurses Isabel Amaro and Theresa Taylor, was working in the Leicester Royal Infirmary in an under-staffed ward when Jack Adcock, a poorly six-year-old child with Down syndrome, was admitted. Bawa-Garba ordered blood tests, but the computer system, iLab, was down. A junior doctor spent most of the day on the phone trying to get the results — the IT failure exacerbated the staff shortage, and increased everyone's workload:

> A failure in the hospital's electronic computer system that day meant that although she had ordered blood tests at about 10.45am, Bawa-Garba did not receive them until about 4.15pm. It also meant her senior house office was unavailable.[32]

> Provision of care was dogged by the break down in IT facilities for the whole hospital, meaning that the team were constantly phoning to try to get results. Even when back on line, the flag system for abnormal results was down. The nursing staff were hard pressed, with staffing and equipment shortages logged. [...] Due to hospital IT failure the Senior House Officer was delegated to phone for results from noon until 4pm. [...] Therefore on this day Dr Bawa-Garba did the work of three doctors including her own duties all day and in the afternoon the work of four doctors.[33]

At the end of the day, sadly Jack died of sepsis.

The clinicians were indicted for gross negligence manslaughter. Theresa Taylor was cleared, but both Hadiza Bawa-Garba and Isabel Amaro were convicted, and struck off the General Medical Council (GMC) register and the Nursing & Midwifery Council register, respectively.

Thousands of Bawa-Garba's colleagues signed a letter of support, stating the case would "lessen our chances of preventing a similar death."[34] So far as I know, no comparable campaign has been made on Isabel's behalf, though the case made against her would have been different.

A tribunal of judges at the Court of Appeal said in August 2018 that Bawa-Garba's actions were neither deliberate nor reckless, and that she does not pose a continuing risk to patients. But she remained suspended for a year.

In the mass of discussion about this controversial case, I haven't found any mention of improving the hospital IT systems[35] — yet everybody in the hospital depends on reliable digital systems, and when they fail so badly that they contribute to manslaughter, one would expect some public acknowledgment and serious effort to improve them.

I wonder why such unreliable digital systems are used, and why hospitals put up with them, and why criminal investigations pay so little attention to the system failures. Perhaps it's because blaming the doctors and nurses seems to solve the problem. If nothing else, the problem becomes a whole lot simpler: you don't have to understand any complicated systems, you just focus your sense of betrayal against a person who, you're saying, let the patient down. Telling somebody off, retraining them, disciplining them, or sacking them, is cheaper and will appear to be doing something; hospitals even have standard processes that can swing seamlessly into action to start formal procedures to do this.

Once there is a scapegoat, everybody feels getting rid of the scapegoat takes away the problem — but the systems are left unchanged. To change the systems would mean admitting that the hospital and, in their turn, the IT developers and suppliers, had made mistakes, which is a harder problem to admit, let alone understand. It's also far more costly to fix.

So, unfortunately, the next doctor or nurse will face the same problems. Ultimately, this will create a climate of fear where clinicians do not want to speak up. It then gets worse: if there is a culture where nobody is speaking up, certainly nobody wants to be the first person to confess to an error, which itself further reinforces the culture. The system will then believe "everything is fine" and "errors don't happen here," and the culture of denial gets entrenched right across the organization.

Healthcare is supposed to have a **just culture**,[36] which includes the idea of the **substitution rule**. The idea of the rule is that if anybody else (with similar role and qualifications) would have been caught up in a similar incident under the same circumstances, then the individual should not be blamed because the problem is the system. The system has failed.

Blaming Bawa-Garba and the nurses is unjust by this rule, a point taken up by Rachel Clarke, blogging in the *British Medical Journal*: as she put it,

> **Box 4.1.** Bugs are often obvious in manuals
>
> Often training material and documentation helps users understand design problems with systems. For example, the manual notes for Cerner PowerOrders says (with my *italic* emphasis):[37]
>
>> Large PowerPlans may take a few seconds longer to process, and if the As Of button is clicked before the plan has completed processing it will cause the plan to revert back to the Planned Pending stage and *could potentially create duplicate orders outside of the plan.*
>
> This is not only useful advice to help users avoid problems, but it also shows clear descriptions of unnecessary bugs that should be fixed. Nobody wants duplicate orders. By putting this comment in the manual, Cerner has turned the bug into the user's problem. I'm also surprised that large plans may "take a few seconds longer to process": that's something else that needs fixing. It all begs questions about how PowerOrders is implemented.
>
> Instead, such descriptions in user manuals should be seen, not as bugs to explain, but as bugs *to fix.* Then the manuals can be revised and become simpler. Fixing most bugs would be quicker than explaining them and how to manage the problems they cause!

Hadiza Bawa-Garba could have been any member of frontline staff.[38] Moreover, blaming Bawa-Garba and the nurses does not help improve the system, nor does it help anyone else — not even patients. In fact, the hospital lost several people in the fallout from the incident.

Ten years later, Dr Hadiza Bawa-Garba returned to medical practice — after having to crowd-fund around £350,000 for her legal case.

As Jenny Vaughan, chair of the Doctors' Association UK and lead for the Learn Not Blame campaign, says,

> Healthcare desperately needs an open, transparent, learning culture, where harm is minimised by learning from error and failings. Scandals such as Mid-Staffordshire,[39] Gosport,[d] and Morecambe Bay[e] repeatedly demonstrate how a culture of defensiveness and denial can escalate into widespread cover-up, leaving families fighting for answers.
>
> The climate of fear among the medical profession created by the GMC's actions over Bawa-Garba only makes it more likely that this will happen again. Jack Adcock should have received better care, and his tragic death was the result of systems failure.[40]

---

[d] See Chapter 8: Gosport War Memorial Hospital tragedy, page 84 →
[e] See Chapter 33: Morcambe Bay NHS Trust and Joshua's Story, page 476 →

Dr Marie Moe is a well-known international medical cybersecurity researcher.[41] She has a heart pacemaker.

Visiting London in 2011, Marie traveled on the London Underground (metro) to Covent Garden, where she climbed up the stairs from the depths of the station. She lost her breath and was struggling. She didn't know there were 177 steps! But something was wrong.

She'd been living perfectly well for a few weeks since having had the pacemaker, but climbing the stairs at Covent Garden was the first time she'd done any real exercise since the surgery when it had been fitted.

As Marie climbed the staircase at Covent Garden, her heart rate climbed. Her heart rate soon reached 160 beats per minute maximum, as fixed by her pacemaker. Her pacemaker then hit a problem, and went into a "2:1 atrioventricular block (AV block)," a sort of "safe" mode, which means your heart gets forced down to half the pulse rate,[42] so she went from 160 to 80; it's a really horrible feeling, as you need a higher rate and you aren't getting enough oxygen. This rate was hardly enough for the demands she was putting on her body! She collapsed and, fortunately, slowly recovered.

Each patient's pacemaker is programmed specially for that patient. Most patients with pacemakers are old, so the default setting for the maximum heart rate for Marie's type of pacemaker is only 160 beats per minute. But Marie is fit and young, and quite able to exercise and put higher demands on her heart. She should have had a much higher rate preset. The default rate had not been corrected when her pacemaker was first programmed.

The sort of pacemaker programming device Marie needs looks like a large laptop computer (figure 4.6). Marie is a computer scientist, so she tracked down the problems. The user interface of Marie's pacemaker programming device got the numbers wrong, and the nurse setting up her pacemaker did not know she was making a mistake because the user interface design had a bug that misled her. It was a bug that led to the wrong maximum being set. (It's also strange that the pacemaker programming device does not alert the user to confirm all settings have actually been correctly set for a new patient.) In other words, a bug in the pacemaker programming device caused the incorrect maximum heart rate setting.

The good news is that Marie persevered and got her pacemaker's problems fixed. She is still alive and well. Another patient, less technically savvy, might have been forced to live a quiet life at a reduced speed just to avoid the problems. We'll meet Marie a few more times again in this book, with a few more of her stories.[f,g]

To put the examples of this chapter into perspective, the US Food and

---

[f] See Chapter 19: Marie Moe's pacemaker and cosmic rays, page 248 →
[g] See Chapter 30: Marie Moe runs New York Marathon, page 427 →

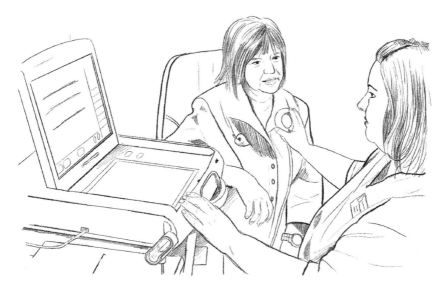

Figure 4.6. Checking and reprogramming a patient's pacemaker. The circle on the patient's chest uses Wi-Fi (or similar) to connect to the implanted pacemaker, letting the nurse look at the pacemaker's settings on her laptop-like pacemaker programming device. The good news is that the pacemaker can be configured wirelessly without needing an operation to open up the patient's chest; the bad news is the pacemaker programming device and the pacemaker itself may have bugs.

Drug Administration, the FDA, formally records over 140 medical device recalls per year due to user interface software problems — and they know there is a lot of under-reporting.[43] The true figures are higher. Those are medical devices recalled within the US, and, as I've shown above, there are many faulty devices that nobody is realizing are inadequate. If nurses, doctors, and patients were more safety-conscious, more aware of the value of reporting digital problems, the recall figures would be higher, probably much higher.

When a nurse or doctor gets caught up in an error, they are probably stressed and focused on the patient's needs, so carefully diagnosing and accurately reporting technical details of any problems will be the last thing on their mind. The patient in front of them is, rightly, far more important. This means there is little drive to improve the systems, yet future patients will rely on the systems being safer to avoid or block the same errors occurring again.

It's amazing what computers can do. It's amazing when a dog dances; but dogs don't dance very well, and nobody dare say so in case they upset the circus.

Denise Melanson died after a calculation error that led to a drug overdose. What can we learn from the incident?

5

🐈 🐈 🐈 🐈 🐈

Fatal overdose

Denise Melanson was being treated at the Cross Cancer Institute in Alberta, Canada. She had throat cancer and was being treated with chemotherapy. The dose in chemo is critical: too little and the cancer is not treated, or too much and other organs and tissues get damaged by the chemo. Even with a correct dose, chemo usually has side effects like losing your hair, but an overdose is dangerous. Many chemo drugs don't have antidotes if there is an overdose.

Denise was on a regular dose of fluorouracil, one of the most commonly used drugs to treat cancer. She was getting her fluorouracil from an Abbott AIM[44] Plus infusion pump that, very conveniently, she was able to carry around with her.

When her bag of fluorouracil ran out, Denise would go back to the Alberta Cancer Care Centre and get some more. Her bag would be replaced, and nurses would press buttons on her infusion pump to set the rate of the new drug infusion correctly.

Normally two nurses are involved in the calculation. The idea is that if one of them makes a mistake, the other nurse will notice. Unfortunately, on one day in 2006, the two nurses both made the same mistake. Together they agreed to program the infusion pump with a dose that they didn't realize was 24 times too high.[45] There are 24 hours in a day, and the correct calculation involves 24 hours. Unfortunately, both nurses, by chance, omitted to divide by 24 in their calculations. They agreed their answers, but they were wrong.

Denise Melanson later died from the overdose.

The two nurses had to do a calculation. The picture (figure 5.1) is taken from the official report,[46] hence the doctor's names and a few other details have been anonymized, as in the report itself.

The drug bag is filled and labeled by the pharmacy in the hospital. The nurses' job is to read the prescriptions, check the labels, connect the drug supplies to the infusion pump, check or connect the lines to the patient, work

Fix It: See and solve the problems of digital healthcare. Harold Thimbleby, Oxford University Press. © Harold Thimbleby 2021. DOI: 10.1093/oso/9780198861270.003.0005

Part I ◇ Diagnosis ◇ Riskier than you think

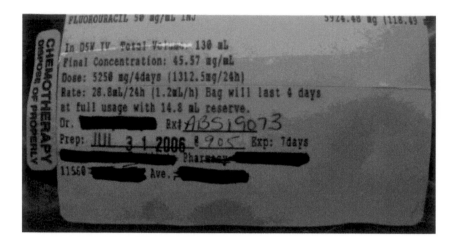

Figure 5.1. Original fluorouracil drug bag label for Denise Melanson. Black pen marks anonymize names, as in the original report.[46]

out what dose is required, prime the infusion pump, and then program[45] it to deliver the required dose. It's a lot of work, and, in particular, the drug dose calculation is rarely easy.

Curiously, the pharmacy had already done the correct calculation (which is 1.2 mL per hour), but they — or, rather, their digital printing system — had buried it in the mass of other numbers on the drug bag, as can be seen (figure 5.1). It seems strange that nurses are asked to do the calculation again. It risks making errors. Years ago, before computers, it might have made sense for the nurses to check the calculation, but now that computers are better than people at doing calculations, it's counter-productive.

Another curious feature of this sad story is it begs the question why can't nurses easily tell an infusion pump to deliver the same rate as it was doing a moment ago? In the cases here, the infusion pump "knows" that 1.2 mL per hour has already kept a patient alive up until this moment in time, so why not let the nurse just carry on with the same rate? If a different rate is entered (as happened here), the infusion pump should check if the nurse is sure and prompt them to confirm the change to the new dose rate.

Here's another critical problem: calculators have *no idea* what you are trying to do. So if you make any mistakes, you just get the wrong answer with no warning. If, for instance, a nurse misses out keying in the ▣ 24 bit, the calculator will be perfectly happy. If both nurses miss it out — remember that part of the calculation was especially tricky to follow — then both nurses will agree what the answer is, but they'll both be mistaken, though in exactly the same way. They'll both get 28.8 mL per hour, and as the drug bag also has that figure on it, it seems to confirm they're both right: 28.8 is the first

Part I ◇ Diagnosis ◇ Riskier than you think

Box 5.1. Using a calculator

Denise Melanson's two nurses used a calculator and mental calculation, but let's see how calculators would work out her chemotherapy dose.

The drug bag's label gives us about 15 numbers, depending on what you want to count as a number. The nurses have to select the right ones to do their calculation. To cut the story short, here is the correct calculation. The dose is given as "5250 mg/4days (1312.5mg/24h)" on the label, but to program the infusion pump we need a dose per hour, so $5,250$ needs dividing by 4×24 (or $1,312.5$ needs dividing by 24). We also need the dose rate to be in milliliters per hour, so we must divide the milligram rate by the concentration, which is given as "45.57 mg/mL." In all, the nurses need to do this:

$$\left(\frac{5,250}{4 \times 24}\right) \div 45.57, \text{ which will be in mL per hour}$$

We need to translate this into calculator-speak. Here's how it has to be done on the popular Casio HS-8V calculator:

AC 5250 ÷ 4 ÷ 24 ÷ 45.57 =

It's difficult to check this going to do exactly what you want. For example, I used the fact that dividing by dividing is the same as dividing by multiplying — that is, $a \div b \div c = a \div (b \times c)$ — a fact that isn't very obvious, and you cannot be sure will work on your calculator until you test it.[47] Indeed, as many "arithmetic laws" do not work on calculators you may be better off using paper, or at least using it to help check your results, because you can't rely on any laws until you've checked your calculator obeys them.

General-purpose calculators (almost all handheld calculators, mobile phone calculators, desktop calculators, and more) are a mess, and should never be allowed in hospitals to do critical calculations.

---

number on the line. It's prominent and not in brackets; it's a contrast to the correct rate ("1.2mL/h"), which is shown just after it in brackets — which seems to make it less important.

In fact, the bag confusingly says "28.8mL/24h," which is the rate per day, that is per 24 hours, not per hour. We don't know whether the nurses thought the 28.8 was a rate per hour or that they accidentally missed out the division by 24.[48]

The drug was given 24 times too fast. Denise Melanson got a 24-times overdose, and died as a result.

Why is a drug bag printed with a numerical dose 24 times too high? Did it act as **confirmation bias**, a widely understood problem affecting everybody,[a] and encourage the nurses to think the wrong dose was correct? Why

[a] See Chapter 20: Confirmation bias, page 269 →

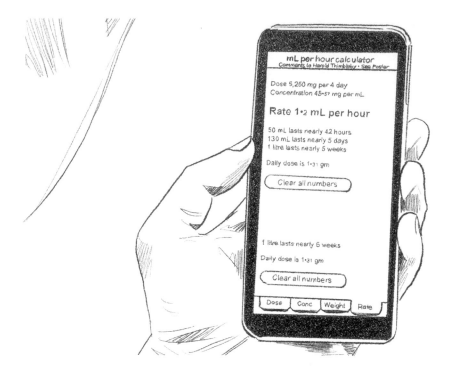

Figure 5.2. A typical screenshot from my app for calculating drug doses; as shown, the screen is green and it's displaying the result of its calculation. (Notice the large decimal point and using smaller decimal digits to make the value easier to read correctly.) The app beeps and the screen will go red and explain errors if there is any problem with the calculation, such as the user omitting details of the drug concentration — tapping the tabs at the bottom allows the user to revise any input. What you can't see is that the code was formally developed and tested.

isn't the pharmacy, which prints the drug details, better informed about the actual infusion pumps in use? They should only have printed the correct dose for the pump in use.

It would be a bit of extra effort for the developers to improve drug bag labels, and make them easier to read. Given that millions of labels are used worldwide every day, improving them even a little bit would save lives.

I was so alarmed by discovering so many problems with these drug dose calculations and with calculators more generally that I programmed my own app to do them more safely (figure 5.2). My app can still be downloaded if you want to try it.[49]

It's hard to remove the possibility of error, but it is easy to design systems to detect error, and hence reduce the chances of patient harm. My calculator can report 35 different error messages to the user to block and help them recover from mistakes, compared to a standard calculator that can only say "Error," and only does so when there is a major problem (such as dividing by zero). *Unnoticed errors* are the critical thing here. If you or the calculator notices any errors, you can correct them (or try to correct them), but unnoticed errors by definition don't get noticed and therefore don't get corrected. In the worst case after an error, harm happens to the patient, and when the harm is noticed, it will be far too late to correct the calculation error.

I used Formal Methods[b] to design the calculator, and I paid close attention to good screen design — for instance, notice the easily visible large decimal point shown in the screenshot.[50] My calculator also explains how long different volumes of drugs will last at this rate, which is **redundancy** (additional information presented in a different way) that helps users themselves notice and manage errors. It would be worth doing **longitudinal experiments** — experiments over the long term — because it's likely that detecting more errors, as my calculator does (in fact, as any well-designed digital healthcare system could), will help make users aware of their errors, and in the long run you'd expect them to improve, as the calculator gives them helpful feedback on their performance that no other calculators do.

Reducing the number of errors is important, but more important is reducing *the impact* of errors on the results. To reduce patient harm, the magnitude of the errors in the final result needs to be reduced, not just how often errors occur. Research suggests that the error-blocking techniques used by my calculator can *halve* the number of significant drug dose errors that will reach the patient.[51]

Even better, of course, would be to get the pharmacy computer to print a drug bag label that had already done the calculation, and so save the nurses all the work and risk of error. It's easy to improve the design for a drug bag label (figure 5.3). Or, rather, it's easy to *think* you've improved something; after all, we've got rid of lots of problems. But we don't actually know how this drug label will work in practice. We are thinking about the design while sitting in a nice calm office, and that's a very different environment from where it will be used. We *must* do some experiments and evaluation before adopting any new design. We won't know until the design is tested, and tested it must be (it's called **User Centered Design** or UCD,[c] which includes Human Factors and other ideas I'll cover later in this book).

Put positively, once you start thinking about making hospitals safer, coming up with ideas like simplified drug bag labels is very easy. But you'd want to trial your ideas to see if they *really* make things safer. For example, I think the QR code in my label design would help — it means nurses can easily scan it, rather than read it, and have to write something down by hand. That sounds easier, but perhaps it would only confuse, or perhaps the wrong QR

---

[b] See Chapter 27: Formal Methods, page 379 →
[c] See Chapter 22: User Centered Design, page 301 →

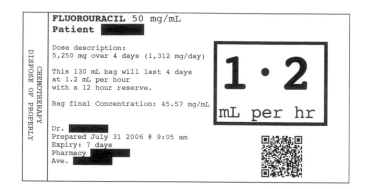

Figure 5.3. My proposal for an improved drug bag label. The idea still needs some further development and testing in real environments to improve it further. (The black blobs in this picture anonymize names not disclosed in the original report.[46])

code might get scanned. Or perhaps by the time we try a new design, RFID tags would be a better idea than QR codes, or, seeing as technology is continually improving, there will be other ideas to try that I haven't thought of.

When the new design is trialed, we can find out lots of other improvements, such as deciding exactly what information on the drug bag helps people. Too much will certainly confuse, but presumably a lot of the detail was necessary — but we don't know whether it *really* is necessary. We may also find out other problems in the trials; for instance, the pharmacy has no idea what infusion pumps are being used, which would sort-of excuse their uncertainty of whether to say milliliters per hour or per day. So our trial starts to have a wider impact, helping improve things across the hospital.

Then why do the nurses have to do anything? Why can't all infusion pumps be developed to read QR codes (or RFID tags) that link through to unique codes that identify the device (they've already been invented: they're called UDIs, or unique device indicators)?[d] Why doesn't the prescribing doctor record the drug dose on the hospital computer system, and then the computer itself tell the infusion pump directly? Why involve people and introduce more sources of error when the whole thing can be automated?

———————————————

Let's return to the specifics of Denise Melanson's case. Not only did the nurses have to calculate the drug dose, they had to program Denise's infusion pump to deliver that rate over the next few days. The drug should have lasted 4 days, but because the drug dose was wrong, the entire dose was delivered 24 times too fast, over just 4 hours.

Denise was using an Abbott AIM Plus infusion pump, which is an am-

———————————————

[d] See Chapter 29: Unique device identifiers, page 404 →

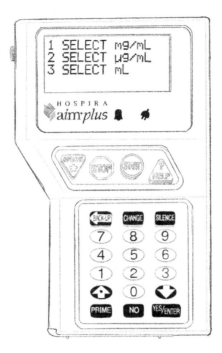

Figure 5.4. Denise Melanson was treated with an Abbott AIM Plus infusion pump. The drawing above shows the Hospira-branded AIM Plus infusion pump I bought from eBay to explore its behavior (Abbott split off Hospira in 2004). In some modes, there are more than three options. The extra options are accessed directly by entering the numbers 4, 5, 6, ... — which means the user will not know what features they are selecting.[52]

bulatory pump, meaning she could walk around using it. This is very convenient and improves your quality of life enormously: you can have continual drug treatment without being stuck in one place.

In the drawing (figure 5.4), you can see the AIM Plus pump is offering three options. If you press 1, 2, or 3, you select one of those options. You can also press 4, 5, 6 ... and you will select other options, but you can't see what they will do or even whether they exist.

You can also see option 2 is to choose μg/mL, meaning micrograms per milliliter.

Canada's Institute for Safe Medication Practices (ISMP) warns not to use μ because doing so can cause serious errors. The ISMP has an important list of rules covering similar avoidable problems:[53]

➊ The Greek letter μ (pronounced "mu") means micro or one millionth; so μg means a microgram, that is, a millionth of a gram. The problem is that a handwritten μ can easily look like an *m* (figure 5.5), and

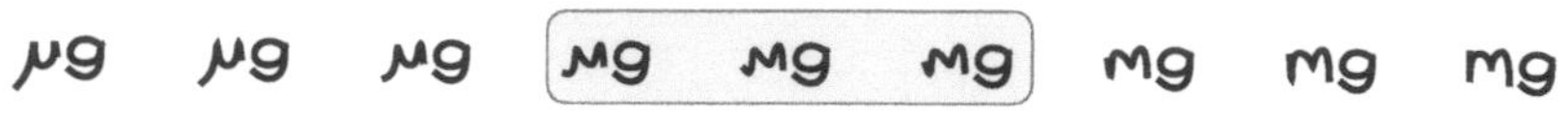

μg　μg　μg　｜ᴍg　ᴍg　ᴍg｜　mg　mg　mg

Figure 5.5. Can computers help eliminate wobbly writing? At the far left, the handwritten unit is clearly μg: the Greek letter μ followed by g — a millionth of a gram. At the far right, the unit is clearly mg: the letter m then g — a thousandth of a gram. In the middle, how people often write less carefully, it could be either: is it μg or mg? If misread, it would lead to a dose error out by a factor of 1,000. The recommended solution is never to use μ, whether in handwriting or in digital displays, which may be copied and written down. Instead, *always* write mcg. Certainly low-resolution digital displays must never be used, as they have the same legibility problems as handwriting.

then an intended μg may be misread as a mg, which means a milligram — a thousand times larger. Equally, of course, a handwritten m can be mistaken for a μ, thus causing a number to be misread as a thousand times smaller.

🜚 ISMP is clear you should write mcg if you mean microgram: instead of writing μg, you should always write mcg. Equally, all systems should use mcg to be consistent, and not tempt anyone into ever using μg, for instance when they remember or write down what a screen has shown them. Sadly there are plenty of examples of death from μ/milli confusions and other handwriting misreading errors.[54]

🜚 ISMP has similar safety rules for other abbreviations, such as never using IU for international units. It is too easy to misread IU as 1 U or even as 10 if the U is written badly. Imagine writing — or the computer displaying — 2IU in a prescription; it would be easy to misread this as 21U, which means 21 units. IU can also be misread as IV, which is an abbreviation for intravenous. Instead, always write IU out in full as "unit." It takes a little extra time to write it in full, sure, but if doing this ever saves an error it will more than recoup the time! Also, of course, all digital systems should write it out in full too.

🜚 These rules are very easy to implement if you are a programmer: using mcg, putting spaces after numbers, writing out IU as unit, and so on — in a computer program this only needs doing once, and then every time the system is used, everyone benefits from the improved safety, with the busy clinicians doing no extra work.

The Abbott pump does not conform to ISMP's standard advice; it uses the Greek letter μ. It may seem to be sophisticated that the display can cope with Greek letters, but it would be better to prioritize patient safety. The

Figure 5.6. The Abbott "up" button (enlarged from figure 5.4) confusingly also serves as a decimal point.

developers had years to get the design right and safe,[e] and presumably they were experienced, and they should have known what they were doing.

Another quirky feature is the Abbott infusion pump's keyboard. Look at the up-arrow button one row up from the bottom of the keyboard (redrawn larger in figure 5.6). Putting the decimal point and up-arrow together saves a bit of space and saves the cost of another button — but it's at the risk of inducing use errors, as the user may press the button expecting it to do one thing and find it does the other.

The Abbott pump has lots of other odd features I think are unwise. Many of its buggy features are common to almost every bit of digital healthcare, particularly its poor handling of **interactive numerals**.[55] Rather than me going over a list of its design problems, a more direct approach is to see the effect the problems have on nurses.

The Canadian ISMP did a **root cause analysis** (RCA) of the Denise Melanson incident. Just as it sounds, an RCA seeks to find out the original cause of an incident. Unfortunately, it is rather hard to decide how to stop looking for causes, and it seems to me to be suspicious that RCA tries to find "the" cause — see box 7.1. We'll return to this problem in the next chapter.[f]

The ISMP took five nurses from an oncology clinic in Ontario who were familiar with the Abbott pump to go through the scenario that had led up to the drug overdose. This exercise took them just two hours. This is what the ISMP discovered:

- All of the nurses were confused by setup or selection of the mL per hour drug dose rate.

- All pressed the "Start" button incorrectly.

- Three nurses needed hints to use it.

- Three were confused by the decimal point button, which doubles as an up-arrow.

- Three of the nurses entered incorrect data, and didn't notice.

---

[e] See Chapter 24: Sharp-end of the wedge, page 325 →
[f] See Chapter 6: Swiss Cheese Model, page 61 →

⚫ Two nurses were confused by the user interface *but made no negative comments about the design.* The ISMP report says,

> This lack of insight into design issues is very common given that the healthcare world is filled with these issues and healthcare personnel are rewarded for working around them with little complaint.

⚫ One nurse entered 28.8 mL per hour and didn't notice the incorrect rate. This is the same erroneous rate that was entered in Denise Melanson's fatal treatment.

The nurses obviously need retraining if this is the equipment that they must use. But, you might ask, why didn't Abbott hire some nurses (ideally selected randomly from a range of hospitals), spend a few hours, and find out these problems *and fix them* before they started selling the infusion pumps? Lives could have been saved. Why didn't they participate in the investigation?

Why doesn't everyone do this sort of User Centered Design (UCD[g]) experiment routinely for every product — both during its design to improve it, and after it's on the market, to assess how safe it is? Why wait until somebody dies? Indeed, why isn't it a legal or regulatory requirement that digital systems pass rigorous safety tests before they are put on the market?

Why didn't the hospital do a quick and simple experiment like this while they were deciding which infusion pumps to buy? Maybe they would not have bought this infusion pump.

ISMP says (with my emphasis):

> The provincial cancer board where the event happened **took an exceptional step** and made the RCA [root cause analysis] report available on the Internet to promote learning across the country.[56]

Why was it an "exceptional step" to make the investigation public, even though, as ISMP says, the "Application of Lessons Learned Will Save Lives" in the title of their news report on the incident? Why are insights into drug bag label design, drug calculation processes, and digital infusion pump design routinely hidden? Why are recommendations for improving safe practice normally kept out of sight? It's as if, most of the time, healthcare institutionally doesn't want to improve.

———————————————■———————————————

If only somebody was curious and did experiments like the ISMP's investigation *before an incident,* and reported the results publicly, manufacturers would soon make better systems, and everybody would soon know how to

---

[g] See Chapter 22: User Centered Design, page 301 →

choose safer systems: a double benefit. Lives would be saved. I suppose, though, that while most people don't think digital healthcare, including digital infusion pumps, digital pharmacy systems, and so on, are risky, there will seem to be little point in doing the work. While it remains an "exceptional step" to make investigations public, the world will remain ignorant of the risks, and nothing will happen.

If we did a "root cause analysis" of this chapter, the underlying thing that made it possible was the generosity of Denise Melanson's family in allowing the investigation of her death to go public, supported by the Cross Cancer Institute and ISMP Canada in making the investigation and its lessons learned freely available.

If we make more incident investigations public, especially ones undertaken so thoroughly, *everyone* will be able to benefit. Furthermore, it'd be helpful if manufacturers also participated — as they do in the airline industry[h] — as only they are able to improve their systems. It would help everyone if they did.

---

[h] See Chapter 26: Planes are safer, page 347 →

Swiss Cheese famously has holes, which can represent the holes and oversights that lead to harm. The **Swiss Cheese Model** has become a powerful way to help think more clearly about errors and harm.

6

Swiss Cheese

James Reason has a fantastic way of reminding us that when bad things happen, *everything* has gone wrong. It is *never* just one person's or one thing's fault.

Reason's idea is the **Swiss Cheese Model**. Swiss Cheese is famous for its holes. Now imagine a block of Swiss Cheese cut up into thin slices. In the Swiss Cheese Model, each slice represents a defense against failure, but each slice is an imperfect defense because of its holes.

The Swiss Cheese Model, with its slices of cheese, is easy and memorable to visualize (figure 6.1).

The slices of cheese in the model shown (figure 6.1), called "Doctor," "Pharmacy," "Nurse 1," "Infusion pump," and so on, are names for the slices of cheese taken from the story of Denise Melanson, already covered in the last chapter.[a]

It is worth noting that some slices of cheese are more strategic than others. If the **standard operating procedures** (SOPs) are improved or if the pharmacy computer is improved, many things will improve to everyone's benefit. If instead an investigation focuses on the people at the sharp-end (here, it might be tempting to think that Nurse 2 "should have stopped it"), then nothing will be improved for future generations.

Some people take the Swiss Cheese Model as a literal, rigorous model, but that is being too literalist. For example, the diagram I've drawn, if taken literally, seems to suggest that the pharmacy allows something erroneous, such as an error in the drug or the prescription, through to the nurses who possibly allow something, through to the infusion pump allowing something. But the nurse has also got a lot more going on. They have their training, their experience, their knowledge of the patient from the patient records system, they may well have distractions, they've had a long shift, and lots more. The Swiss Cheese diagram doesn't show any of that complexity.

---

[a] See Chapter 5: Denise Melanson's fatal overdose, page 49 ←

Fix It: See and solve the problems of digital healthcare. Harold Thimbleby, Oxford University Press. © Harold Thimbleby 2021.
DOI: 10.1093/oso/9780198861270.003.0006

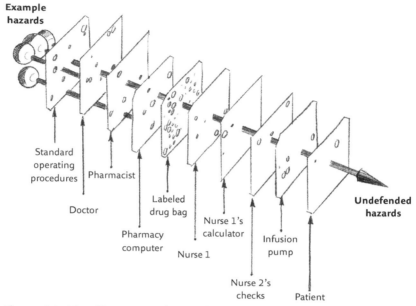

Figure 6.1. Most illustrations of Swiss Cheese Models don't go into details or show enough slices, but here's a worked example based on the previous chapter's case of Denise Melanson's fatal overdose. Each slice of cheese schematically defends against some errors, but no slice is perfect. If any holes in the slices coincidentally line up, then harm can and will eventually happen. Clearly, there is no one cause for the harm; *every* defense failed. (The drug bag label could be repeated as part of Nurse 2's defenses, but, logically, having the same slice in two places makes no difference to the outcome.)

The real value of the Swiss Cheese Model is how it starts conversations and stimulates thinking. In particular, it makes very clear that no failure, no patient harm, is ever the fault of any one thing or any one person. Several defenses have failed.[57]

For the various holes in the defenses to combine into a disaster, all the holes have to "line up." There has to be a problem in the first place (illustrated by the big ball on the left), and *every* defense has to fail. It isn't just the nurse or doctor closest to the patient. Fortunately, most of the time, one or other defense — another slice of cheese — blocks the problems and prevents them from escalating.

An interesting point is that adding more slices of cheese won't help much if their holes are in the same place as existing slices of cheese. For instance, more nurses adding checks probably makes little difference, because all people tend to make the same sorts of error under the same circumstances (as we'll discuss in the Human Factors chapter[b]). Indeed, research on double checking is ambivalent.[58] Perhaps one nurse acting alone would be more cautious? Perhaps the second nurse's check is not very thorough? It seems obvious to me that a computer being part of the checks would be better — computers don't work like people, so would tend to pick up errors humans don't notice; checking algorithms can be improved with data about experience; digital systems can be integrated with other systems so that some errors don't occur at all; and so on. Yet this is just me thinking it's obvious. There are lots of obvious things that aren't so, and almost certainly more research would uncover even better ways of making healthcare safer. More research is needed.

The idea is that accidents happen all the time, but occasionally every protection goes wrong and a catastrophe happens. Normally, at least one defense — another person, a digital device, even something as simple as a checklist — spots the problem, avoids it, or blocks it from escalating.

In reality, there are far more slices of cheese than I showed in my diagram, but the point of the diagram is to prompt discussion, not to be a rigorous and final statement of the causes of an incident. For example: how can we have more slices of cheese? How can we have smaller holes? How can we have fewer holes? How can we ensure holes don't line up?

In the Swiss Cheese diagram (figure 6.1), a doctor and a pharmacist are shown as each intercepting one error, and no patient harm occurred from those errors. I've also shown the patient as part of the defense system. Encouraging the patient to be part of their treatment, including questioning it, can reduce errors. The analysis of the Denise Melanson case doesn't mention Denise taking any part in her infusion or the calculations;[46] she had had treatment before. If she had been actively involved, perhaps she would have been surprised at being given a dose 24 times higher than last time, and queried it.

If you Google "pharmacy error" you are bound to find numerous lawyers telling you about how they can help get compensation. Here's my retelling of one tragic story of a child's death in hospital, taken from Medical Malpractice Lawyers, **www.medicalmalpracticelawyers.com**.[59]

In this story, lots of holes in many slices of cheese sadly lined up together. None of them on their own would have caused the death, but all the errors together were overwhelming. In the end, the hospital settled a medical malpractice lawsuit, costing it $8.25 million.

Using a digital system, a pharmacy technician entered incorrect data, which resulted in an overdose of sodium chloride, which caused Genesis Burkett's death. A hospital spokesman said,

---

[b] See Chapter 20: Human Factors, page 259 →

Box 6.1. Programming with better cheese

As this book shows, digital systems are often slices of Swiss Cheese with big holes in them. Computer programs are often very relaxed about errors.

Computers can be programmed in hundreds of languages (we'll meet some in this book).[60] JavaScript is popular, but is incredibly sloppy (as we'll see). In contrast, SPARK Ada is *much* safer. We'll talk about it later, but here are some key reasons to prefer SPARK Ada ...

Often people write programs and just hope they work. If they make typos, as they do, the programs will have bugs. In SPARK Ada programs have a lot of rigorous mathematics in them, and the programs must be *proved* correct before they are used. The proof process eliminates holes, and certainly finds numerous typos; it makes a tough form of cheese.

When you don't really trust somebody to do something, you get lawyers to write a contract, and all parties sign it to promise to do things properly. Likewise, SPARK Ada (like a few high integrity programming languages) has **contracts** built into it. People who want SPARK Ada programs to do things literally have contracts with their programs — and the programs have contracts with each other. These contracts are mathematical, and much more rigorous than contracts written by human lawyers! In fact, it's possible to tell automatically whether a program can fulfill its contracts. Contracts eliminate holes in the cheese.

With SPARK Ada many holes (bugs) can never exist in the first place. There are enormous advantages. The Millennium Bug[a] would have been impossible (unless everyone, for some reason, *wanted* the bug). Interoperability problems[b] can be avoided at the design stage rather than only be noticed too late, after the systems are in use in healthcare, causing chaos.

In short, SPARK Ada (and a few other modern programming languages) is much safer and can avoid a lot of harms and wasted time in healthcare.

---

[a] See Chapter 4: Millennium Bug (Y2K problem), page 33 ←
[b] See Chapter 19: Interoperability, page 245 →

> It was determined that a data entry error was made in the formulation of the IV [intravenous] solution. The dosage of sodium for an IV bag from an order had been incorrectly entered into the machine that mixes IV solutions.

The investigation says the death may have been avoided had automated alerts in the pharmacy compounding machine been turned on. The court case also argued the hospital staff then covered up the sticker on the IV bag, which correctly described the amount of sodium, with a sticker that displayed the doctor's original prescribed amount.

Identification of the mistake was delayed when a lab technician reading blood test results believed that abnormally high sodium levels were inaccurate test results.

> **Box 6.2.** Design errors cause use errors
>
> We think technology is extremely reliable, so when things go wrong it *must* be the user's fault. This lie bedevils investigations, and stops improvement — if it's the user's fault, then the system needn't change, and then things can carry on as before. The Swiss Cheese Model shows that when anything has gone wrong, *everything* has gone wrong. But Swiss Cheese is silent on where we should apportion blame (if at all).
>
> After World War II, the US Airforce wanted to find out why its Boeing B-17 Flying Fortress bomber pilots kept making mistakes. The prevailing assumption was **pilot error** — during the war there were lots of pilots rushed into flying to meet demand, so many of them must have been incompetent. But when Paul Fitts and Alphonse Chapanis interviewed pilots and examined the thousands of reports about plane crashes, they noticed there were patterns: the crashes were related to the aircraft and didn't have the variation you'd expect from "incompetent" pilots.[61] Instead of pilot error, what they saw was different: **designer error**. The planes were so badly designed they were too hard for even good pilots to fly safely.
>
> Today we can easily collect huge amounts of data from digital systems, and find out whether incidents are caused by doctors and nurses, or whether they are caused by the digital systems themselves.
>
> A large study, *easily* done digitally, covering 2,575,411 prescriptions for three critical drugs, found that GPs (doctors) breached NHS guidance in 12.3% of them.[62] But when the data was analyzed, the variations in errors were explained by the different digital systems the GPs were using. There were consistently more errors in one GP system, EMIS. Indeed, EMIS breaches NHS safety guidance: errors for prescribing the drug diltiazem were four times higher with it than with another system, SystmOne. Clearly this is a design error.
>
> Now we know — having collected the data — we can do two things. We can improve EMIS and other systems, and we can stop knee-jerk blaming healthcare staff for problems caused by bugs and poor design.

The lab technician's checks were slices of cheese; but, like Swiss Cheese, the technician's checks had some holes.

The slices of cheese are there — automated alerts, stickers, input validation, blood tests — but they had significant holes. Why didn't the digital system block the error, or ask for the erroneous data to be double-checked?

After the investigation, the hospital thought of new ways to block holes in some of its slices of cheese. The hospital implemented changes, including activating alerts in the pharmacy drug-mixing machines as well as improving checks before medications leave the pharmacy.

I wonder whether the learning here — making digital systems detect more errors, and not disabling their ability to help block errors turning into harm — has been passed on to other hospitals. Has the learning been passed on to device manufacturers — why not make it harder, if not impossible, to turn off safety features? The overdose has been reported as being 60 times too high, which was fatal. If the hospital needed to implement changes, it must have recognized that other errors were also being made (you don't need to change processes to stop a unique error), so why wasn't there a reporting system to pick up smaller, indicative, errors before a fatal error occurred?

How many near misses, where things would have gone wrong but for one slice of cheese stopping it? If a slice of cheese, thankfully, stopped a catastrophe, most people would think there was nothing to report. If the hospital had had more monitoring in place or a requirement to report "near misses," it might have discovered much sooner that its pharmacy machines had their error checking turned off. Then we should ask: why are we focusing on *that* hospital — surely some other hospitals are learning how to be safer, and why isn't the knowledge passed on?

I wonder why turned-off safety features don't automatically report problems that are passing right through their holes? If the hospital (or manufacturer over the internet) had been monitoring errors slipping through holes, surely somebody would have fixed the holes before the hospital ran out of cheese? If the manufacturer improved their pharmacy system, *every* hospital would benefit, and every patient, and every technician, and every nurse, and ... I don't know, but I doubt the manufacturer thought to improve their system because if they did they would have effectively admitted contributory liability, and they would have to have had contributed to the $8.25 million payout.

The only way to make something positive out of a tragedy is to make sure everyone learns the right lessons and puts them into practice. One tragedy of the story is that it focuses on one hospital, and neither emphasizes that learning should be spread around, nor emphasizes that learning elsewhere might have avoided the tragedy if only it had been spread around. Another tragedy is that the court case and compensation, however justified, make everyone else wary of being open about problems — note how many guesses I had to make in describing the case above. On the one hand, if the hospital or the manufacturers publicly disclosed more, they might be sued for more; yet on the other hand, surely, we want a safer healthcare system, and that will rely on learning as much as possible and not keeping anything hidden. I hope the manufacturers tried to learn as much as possible, for if they improve their systems with more cheese, then everybody benefits easily.

———————————————

When investigations are undertaken, the Swiss Cheese Model can do some real magic.

The Swiss Cheese model's slices of cheese do something very clever. They turn the *absence* of something, which allowed some harm to occur, into a *concrete*, very easily grasped, metaphor — that is, a slice of cheese and some holes.

It's helpful, then, to start any investigation by listing all the *things*, *systems*, *procedures*, and *people* that were relevant to the incident. Thinking about the obvious failures isn't enough, as it's too easy to miss some failures because they "don't exist." But slices of cheese do. The concrete stuff in an incident is much easier to list than the intangible, unseen — and perhaps still unknown — failures.

Everything corresponds to a slice of cheese, as they could and perhaps should have helped stop the incident happening. However, some of these things must have had holes that were relevant, which the investigation might otherwise have overlooked.

In particular, all the digital stuff is very relevant to any incident, but as digital is usually hidden from sight many investigations overlook it. Digital is in infusion pumps, drug dispensing machines, MRI scanners, implants, ventilators, even beds ... and it affects everything — hopefully blocking errors, but all too often letting the error trajectory just take its course unhindered. It's the job of an incident investigation to find out more. In turn, where were the slices of cheese to stop the manufacturers or developers making design errors in the digital systems themselves? Where were the slices of cheese that were in the training and Standard Operating Procedures (SOPs), so that everybody knew how the systems actually worked and knew what to do?

The Swiss Cheese Model has another advantage: the investigators will find it easy to explain to everyone involved, so they too can constructively help with the investigation.

--------------------◼--------------------

What the Swiss Cheese Model makes clear is that when the holes all line up, some catastrophe will eventually happen, and *every* defense will have failed. Just because the person at the sharp-end, the "last" slice of cheese, is a nurse who pressed the button or a car driver who didn't press the brake or a lab technician who didn't believe a test result does not mean they are the only person that missed stopping the error. Most often, "the system" — the design of the system — failed them.

Part I ◇ Diagnosis ◇ Riskier than you think

When patients are harmed, staff often get blamed — especially when nobody realizes how digital systems can go wrong and create the problems.

7

Victims and second victims

Teenager Lisa Norris was being treated for brain cancer at The Beatson West of Scotland Cancer Centre, in Glasgow. She was being treated with radiotherapy.[63] Tragically, she died after a radiation overdose.

Radiation therapy has to be precisely controlled. Too little radiation, and the cancer is not killed; too much radiation and other parts of the body will be affected, and more tissues than the cancer will likely be damaged. Working out how much radiation to give is a tricky calculation, especially as the radiation doses are spread over weeks to try to minimize damaging other parts of the body. In addition, the beam of radiation has to be shaped to shine on just the cancerous tissues and as little of the surrounding tissues as possible. The shape and intensity of the beam, combined with aiming it into the body from different angles, makes the radiation dose calculation very complicated.

Computers can help enormously with complex calculations.

Unfortunately, each time Lisa was treated, she was given a radiation dose that was 65% too high. Her body went red, broke out in sores, and her internal organs were affected. Understandably, her treatment was stopped, but her cancer continued to spread. Arguably, it isn't clear whether she died from the cancer spreading or from the error that meant that the cancer was not properly treated in the first place.

The official story is the radiotherapists were blamed for the error, and that Lisa died of cancer. However, as we'll see, if we want to improve, we cannot blame either cancer or the radiotherapists. We need to acknowledge that digital healthcare is risky, and that it needs improving.

There is a place to argue about the cause and the proportion of blame, if any, for each incident, but, like a car crash,[a] we should sort out these issues (and whether the crash is criminal ...) as a separate process from learning about what happened, and finding out how to stop it or anything like it happening again.

---

[a] See Chapter 11: Isaac Thimbleby's car crash, page 137 →

Fix It: See and solve the problems of digital healthcare. Harold Thimbleby,
Oxford University Press. © Harold Thimbleby 2021.
DOI: 10.1093/oso/9780198861270.003.0007

Lisa's treatment was complex, and I don't want to oversimplify and make things more clear-cut than they are. But there *was* a computer problem and it contributed to the mess.

Put briefly, the computer system was supposed to help calculate the radiation dose. The software was upgraded and changed the way it calculated radiation doses; in particular, it now performed a "normalization." Unfortunately, the radiotherapists were, for some reason, unaware of this change and continued to calculate doses the old way. So *both* the radiotherapists *and* the computer performed the normalization. As the official report summarizes it:

> Changing to the new Varis 7 system introduced a specific feature that, if selected by the treatment planner, changed the nature of the data in the Eclipse Treatment Plan Report relative to that in similar reports prior to the May 2005 upgrade. This feature was selected but the critical error was that the treatment planner who transcribed the resulting data from the Treatment Plan Report to the paper form (the planning form) was unaware of this difference and therefore failed to take the action necessary to accommodate the changed data.

The official analysis of the incident blames the radiotherapist (treatment planner), as they should have known better. (But how could they know better if nobody told them?) Secondly, and much more worryingly, at least to me, is the official report's statement:

> It is important to note that the error described above was procedural and was not associated in any way with faults or deficiencies in the Varis 7 computer system.
>
> [...]
>
> Particular reference is made to Varis 7, Eclipse, and to RTChart (registered trade marks). In this regard, it should be noted that at no point in the investigation was it deemed necessary to discuss the incident with the suppliers of this equipment since there was no suggestion that these products contributed to the error.

So far as I can see, the incompatibility between the Varis system and what the radiotherapists were doing was the cause of the calculation error. Why does the official report argue that the error was the radiotherapist's fault, when — equally — the change to the software was the other side of the problem? Indeed, the manufacturers knew about the improvements to the Varis system that led to the upgrade, so why didn't they make sure the operators knew the consequences? The official analysis makes no mention of this, as, from its point of view, the blame centers on the local operating procedures and on the local people thought responsible.

The Beatson Oncology Centre investigation was undertaken by the inspector appointed by the Scottish Ministers, and its finding was essentially to blame the staff, and solve the problem by retraining them. It thus absolved itself — the Beatson Centre — and the manufacturers of any problems. A report on the report is worth quoting:[64]

> The decision to ignore machines and their interactions with humans is typical of novice inquiries into accidents that involve human operators. The resulting narrowness is characteristic of stakeholder investigations and the Scottish Executive is an important stakeholder. The findings of the report are little more than the usual "blame-and-train" response that is a staple of medical accident investigations ... The report lodges failure in a few individuals while keeping the expensive and complicated machinery and procedures out of view.

The original investigation, and its blame game, focused on the sharp-end (where treatment happened),[b] explicitly ignoring the system failures — for instance, as I quoted above, it ignored any design or management issues to do with the digital system. It missed the opportunity to help improve the Varis system to make every radiation center using it safer. The investigation should have explored the digital healthcare failure, not scapegoat the radiotherapists.

———————■———————

Lisa Sparrow was a nurse caught up in an incident that left a patient dead. Here's how the *Daily Mail* newspaper headlined it:[65]

> Mother-of-four dies after blundering nurse administers TEN times drug overdose

The patient, Arsula Samson, had been prescribed potassium chloride for her low potassium levels. Here, the patient died after a ten-times overdose of the prescribed level.[c]

The *Daily Mail* story carries on:

> Instead of pressing the 10ml per hour button, the nurse admitted tapping in 100ml per hour on the drug infusion pump.

Did the nurse "blunder," or was it a design blunder?

---

[b] See Chapter 24: Sharp-end of the wedge, page 325 →
[c] See Chapter 12: Never events and always conditions, page 149 →

The pump may have had a numeric keypad, and the nurse could have used it to enter any dose, like entering a number on a calculator — in this case, the nurse may have pressed 0 once too often, and got the intended 10 mL entered as 100 mL. Throughout this book, we're seeing just how error-prone digital things are and how they encourage unnecessary errors.

The nurse, Lisa Sparrow, may have correctly entered 10 milliliters per hour, but the pump then incorrectly delivered 100 milliliters per hour *and* recorded that dose of 100 mL per hour on its log — again, we'll see just how easily this can happen *because of bad design* later in this book.[d]

When the nurse was confronted with the "infallible" log that she had delivered 100 milliliters per hour, she would have known it was pointless arguing and she may as well plead guilty — our legal system penalizes people who plead not guilty but who are later found guilty. If this explanation is right, the pump has set the nurse up.

Apparently,

> No error was found with the infusion pump and investigators ruled the death was due to 'individual, human error.'

But then,

> A Trust action plan after the death saw new infusion pumps and software that reduce the risk of error brought into all wards, medical staff retrained and warned over the dangers of potassium chloride and advice on the importance of a second nurse witnessing medication being given.

That admits the hospital recognizes that the bad design of the infusion pump as well as poor staff training contributed to the death. It doesn't admit it in so many words, but replacing infusion pumps is costly — they can cost thousands of pounds each. This is money that would not have been spent without good reason. It seems, then, that it wasn't simply a "blundering nurse" so much as a nurse caught up in a blundering system that did not train staff adequately and which had inadequate equipment.

Why didn't the infusion pump itself make it much harder to give the patient an overdose of potassium chloride, a drug that's well known to be dangerous?

Perhaps this was not the first time Arsula Samson had been treated with this infusion pump. If so, why did the infusion pump allow the nurse to give a dose ten times higher than the last time without warning? Why didn't the infusion pump use speech to say "100" so that the nurse (and the patient) could hear the actual dose — this would have helped stop an error if the nurse had slipped and simply pressed the wrong button in error.

---

[d] See Chapter 14: B-Braun infusion pump, page 187 →

There are lots of ways the infusion pump might be improved. Since infusion pumps have been made for many years, one wonders why they aren't getting any safer. They could, as we'll see later.[e]

Unfortunately, describing the inadequate equipment and training rapidly becomes a complex story. It is much easier to ignore it and focus exclusively on the "blundering nurse." We understand "blundering nurse." We'd feel betrayed by one, so it makes a good headline story. But it makes a misleading story, and misdirects attention away from the whole, complex system that failed. If we fix the system, every nurse and every patient benefits; if we scapegoat and witch-hunt a "blundering nurse," we'll feel very satisfied, but we'll miss the opportunity to improve. We've even got rid of the one person who was probably most motivated about improving.

Scapegoating results in an interesting effect called **impossible error**. If somebody is blamed and sent off as the "bad apple" into the wilderness, the classic fate of the scapegoat, then the ward or hospital has nobody left in it who has ever made the error. If you now go into the ward and ask, people will say, "Nobody here does that; it's impossible for that error to happen here."

In a wood workshop, everybody has two hands. No woodworker ever cuts off their hands on the table saw: it's an **impossible error**. Actually, of course, sometimes, woodworkers *do* lose their fingers or hands, but then they stop being woodworkers. So the error disappears from sight and soon it seems impossible. There is never anybody working in a workshop who has cut their hands off. Cutting your hand off seems to be impossible!

What impossible errors do is to create a cover story to help stop thinking: the error "doesn't happen here" (phew!) and clearly can't happen here now the woodworkers-with-no-hands no longer work here, so we don't need to do anything at all to make the saws safer.

Whether the woodworkers made a mistake or not, it's clear that the system as a whole *also* failed to stop the incident. For instance, maybe the saws did not have working guards to protect the woodworkers' hands? The system is therefore almost certainly part of the problem. The flawed systems still need fixing.

> ⓘ Impossible errors are the flip side of success bias.[f] Success bias is that we see success everywhere because failures disappear. Impossible errors happen because disappearing failures mean that the errors that caused the failures also disappear. Thus if we want to learn how to be successful (to have fewer errors and less harm), we have to dig deep to uncover the full stories of the errors.

---

[e] See Chapter 29: Safety ratings will improve healthcare, page 401 →
[f] See Chapter 3: Success bias, page 29 ←

Olivia Saldaña González and Alveo González worked at the National Cancer Institute of Panama. They were radiotherapists who treated patients with radiation, mainly to treat cancers. Both went to prison, on 12 counts of murder.[66]

If the patient is the first victim, the staff who get burdened with the horror are the **second victims**.[67] There is some debate about calling the clinicians the *second* victim, when it seems that the relatives and friends are being demoted by this ranking, but there is something deep about using the word **victim**.

We think we are good (I think most of us do) and if we thought that bad things could happen to good people, then it would follow that bad things could happen to us. That's not a nice thought. So it's far more comfortable to believe bad things happen to bad people — phew, so we are safe. Hence there is this strong urge to blame staff who get caught up in problems; they must be bad if bad things happened to them.

Now add to that complex mix that most people think that computers are good (why would we buy bad computers?), and we have a very powerful recipe for blaming staff.

The key problem in Olivia and Alveo's case is that they used radiation treatment planning software, manufactured by Multidata Systems.[68]

I'll describe what happened.

Here, in picture 1 below, is the shape of the basic square beam going straight through the machine. If this was used, the patient would be irradiated with a square beam, but a square is very unlikely to be the shape of their cancer that needs treatment. Certainly, you do not want to irradiate healthy tissue around a cancer, so the radiation beam must be restricted, tightened down from the basic square to become the best shape to treat the cancer. In short, picture 1, a simple square, isn't likely to be the right shape to treat any real cancer.

1.

Cancers come in all sorts of shapes and sizes, so movable blocks of metal, usually lead or a special metal called Lipowitz's alloy (made out of lead, cadmium, and bismuth), are moved into the square to adjust the shape of the beam.

Box 7.1. The Blame Game

When things go wrong, we like to blame somebody, preferably somebody else.

The **Blame Game** thrives on four fallacies:

► The professional staff fallacy. If only people were professional or tried harder, nothing would go wrong. Therefore, if something has gone wrong, somebody was not professional. They have failed.

► The punishment fallacy. If bad people are punished, they will behave better in the future, and then make fewer errors. Therefore we should punish wrong-doers. Even better, if we sack them, then no more errors will happen because they don't work here anymore.

► The perfect system fallacy. The management, the hospital **standard operating procedures** (SOPs) and the computer systems are all perfect. So if anything ever goes wrong, it must be something else, like the clinician in the room.

► The stopping fallacy. An investigation, often called a **root cause analysis** (RCA), has to stop somewhere. So once we find somebody to blame, we stop investigating. This is a fallacy, as the "root cause" always has further underlying causes: it's a symptom, not a cause. There are always *lots* of reasons why things go wrong — see my longer discussion of Swiss Cheese.[a]

Playing the Blame Game makes everyone much less likely to report or investigate errors, so nobody learns how to avoid errors. Worse, when errors do get reported, they seem to be worse, because most of the time it seems — because nobody is reporting them — that errors are not happening. If you are the first person to report an error this year, that seems much worse than if errors are regularly being reported. Of course, many errors do not lead to patient harm, so these are great opportunities to learn that are being wasted.

[a] See Chapter 6: Swiss Cheese Model, page 61 ←

By way of example, picture 2 shows a slightly more realistic shape, with four blocks cutting into the corners:

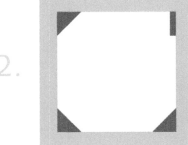

2.

In this example, the four differently shaped metal blocks in the corners of the square make the beam a sort-of octagonal shape. I know this isn't a very realistic shape, but it shows clearly how it works in principle.

The beam is now smaller than the original square shape was, and the blocks will also cause some reflections and losses when the cobalt 60 gamma radiation hits them. The blocks of metal change the radiation dose to the patient in a very complicated way. Allowing for the shapes and sizes of the various metal blocks that are needed so the patient gets the right radiation dose to treat their cancer means the radiotherapist has to do a complicated calculation.

Doing complicated calculations is a perfect job for computers, right?

The Multidata system allows the operator to draw the required blocks on a computer screen, a bit like in picture 3, below. I've drawn the four blocks, one in each corner of the square, and arrows that the user would follow to define each block's shape and position. The patient will now be irradiated by gamma rays in the shape that passes through the smaller hole.

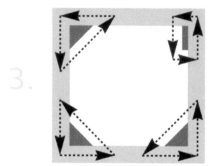

The Multidata system then calculates the right dose, given the new size and shape for the treatment.

Sometimes, however, the beam needs to be a more complicated shape, perhaps as shown in picture 4, below. Remember that the treatment beam is the white shape not interrupted by the gray metal blocks pushed in from the edges.

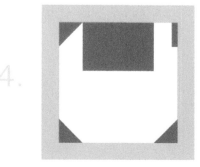

As it happens, this treatment shape in picture 4 needs to be created using at least five metal blocks — using a triangular block in three corners, a rectangular block in the top right corner, and a fifth rectangular block dropped in from the top. In reality, the blocks would be more interesting shapes, but for our explanation the actual shapes of the blocks doesn't really matter.

Unfortunately, the Multidata system handles at most four blocks, so this beam shape cannot be drawn on the computer.

However, the radiotherapists discovered that the system would be happy doing the calculation when the blocks were drawn *as a single piece*.

Anyone familiar with drawing shapes on a computer can see how to end up with the right shape. For instance it could be drawn like I've shown in picture 5, next. Just follow the arrows, and you end up drawing the five blocks as one shape.

5.

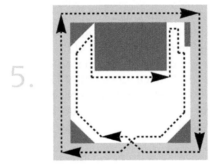

The final shape looks perfectly alright and, indeed, it is accepted by the Multidata system.

Unfortunately, although the *picture* is right, Multidata's *calculation* goes wrong. The patient's radiation dose will be *double* what it should be.

The manufacturers say the radiotherapists should have checked its results, but then I am not sure why you would bother using a computer if it is so unreliable it needs checking every time it is used — and if you have to do the check, the computer is creating more work, not saving work. The picture it lets you draw looks fine, and the computer accepts it without complaining. If the Multidata can't do a correct calculation because the user has drawn blocks in a novel way, it should tell the user it can't accept the drawings.

Certainly, radiotherapists should check what they are doing is correct, perhaps getting a colleague to double check their work. But I think Multidata are using this normal precaution to deflect from their responsibility for their part in the calculation. One wonders whether the Multidata program checks its own calculations? If it does, its checks were not adequate to spot this bug.

I'd say the software was buggy. The software happily allowed the radiotherapists to use it to do the calculation, but *it* made mistakes. Apparently, if the inside and outside lines are drawn in opposite directions, the Multidata

Part I ◇ Diagnosis ◇ Riskier than you think

calculation is almost correct — which makes the bugs even more bizarre and much harder for users to spot. Why should the radiation depend on which way a user draws blocks? It's a bug.

Like many computer programs we've seen in digital health, there were no internal checks that worked. The radiation overdose went unnoticed by the computer. Only after people started to worry about the deaths was the problem tracked down. Unfortunately, investigators decided that "the problem" was that the radiotherapists were incompetent. Not that the computer, the training, equipment maintenance, or regulatory oversight — or perhaps some combination of all these things — was to blame.

The investigators' hands were twisted by the manufacturer's instructions which say, along with their original capitals ...

> it is the responsibility of the user to validate any RESULTS obtained with the system and CAREFULLY check if data, algorithms and settings are meaningful, correct or applicable, PRIOR to using the results as a part of the decision making process to develop, define or document a course or treatment. In particular, a USER SHOULD VERIFY THE RESULTS OBTAINED THROUGH INDEPENDENT MEANS AND EVALUATE ANY DISCREPANCIES CAREFULLY until the USER'S PROFESSIONAL CRITERIA HAS BEEN SATISFIED.

Yet the software gave no warning on the computer when blocks were drawn in a manner different from the one described in the instructions. This is an elementary oversight in the software.

I'd suggest that when instructions say "USER SHOULD VERIFY THE RESULTS OBTAINED THROUGH INDEPENDENT MEANS," the manufacturers are admitting they are worried they may not have done a very thorough job. Like, why doesn't the software itself use some independent means? What's the benefit of a computer if it isn't helping you do your job more reliably? At the very least, the software should prompt the user to do any necessary checks, if, as the instructions make clear, those steps are an important part of the process the computer is supposed to be supporting.

———————————◼———————————

We've known for a long time that unprofessional programming is dangerous. The Therac-25 is a classic story of at least six radiotherapy overdose deaths in the late 1980s, using a computer-controlled radiotherapy system a bit like the Multidata system. The Therac-25 incident happened *two decades* before the Multidata deaths, and it makes it look like Multidata learned nothing from the Therac-25 story.

The Therac-25 problems were described at the time as the worst accidents in the history of radiotherapy. At least one patient ran out of the therapy room screaming. They later died.

The manufacturers, Atomic Energy of Canada Limited (AECL) did not believe the complaints from hospitals.

Later investigations showed that AECL had not had their programming checked by anyone else. They thought it all worked just fine. The trouble with being incompetent is that, generally, you don't know it. Programmers *must* work in teams, preferably including external and independent experts.

The Therac-25 story is taught to Computer Science students, so there is no excuse for industrial programmers not to know about it.[69] It will also give patients food for thought — more so, in that the problems keep happening.

Thirty years later, after the Therac-25 catastrophe, Nancy Leveson published a retrospective article about it.[70] Her article has lots of excellent advice for people who want to think about risky digital systems (and healthcare systems in particular). As she makes very clear, digital healthcare is *still* risky stuff. She makes the powerful point that the FDA (the US regulator) spends more time worrying about reporting incidents than on about preventing them in the first place. She also criticizes standards, because they may give manufacturers the impression that their obligations are fulfilled if they merely follow the standards. I think that's more a problem with the inadequate standards and regulations, but seeing as they are unlikely to be fixed any time soon, we need to think up some more effective alternatives to use as well.

I'll suggest many solutions later, but here's a suggestion for now: universities could step up and offer safety-critical software qualifications. Students who graduated from these courses would command better salaries, and companies that employed them would have reduced liabilities. It would be a win-win, and wouldn't need to wait for the slow wheels of regulators to catch up with the state of the art. Then purchasers — generally the hospitals — would ask how many qualified programmers the manufacturers used to oversee product development; this number would be then be compared with the procurement criteria.

Another approach would be to make the quality of healthcare systems visible to the people who purchase and use it, which would help hospitals and others buy safer systems — I'll come back to this very effective idea later.[g]

---

[g] See Chapter 29: Safety ratings will improve healthcare, page 401 →

We accept that medical interventions like drugs and X-rays have side effects. It makes a lot of sense to think of digital healthcare as having side effects too, and therefore it should be evaluated and regulated as carefully.

8

Side effects and scandals

X-rays were discovered by Wilhelm Röntgen in 1895. The first X-ray clearly showed the bones on his wife's, Anna Bertha's, hand as well as the wedding ring she was wearing (figure 8.1).

X-rays were so *obviously* useful that the world's first radiology department was set up the very next year, in 1896 at Glasgow's Royal Infirmary. X-rays were very useful for examining broken bones, and almost immediately they were invaluable for locating bullets in soldiers' bodies in the Second Boer War (1899–1902) and then in World War I (1914–1918). By the 1920s, X-rays were being used in shoe shops to help fit shoes.

Thomas Edison quickly got into the promising new X-ray technology, but his assistant Clarence Dally did the hard slog of regular experiments, as shown in a contemporary newspaper picture (figure 8.2).

Clarence Dally died from cancer caused by X-rays in 1904, just nine years after they had been discovered by Röntgen. Very gradually, the medical establishment learned that the apparently obvious benefits of X-rays had to be balanced against their not-so-obvious invisible dangers.

Today, X-rays are used *very* carefully to minimize their unwanted side effects, and to balance those side effects against the clinical benefits of doing each X-ray. Today, one would certainly not countenance a medically untrained shoe-shop assistant exposing children's feet to X-rays just to check if shoes fitted.

———————————————————

Thalidomide was a triumph of marketing in the 1950s. Thalidomide was marketed as a "wonder drug," a sedative with no side effects and no possibility of overdosing. It was good for anxiety, insomnia, gastritis, and tension, and soon it was used against nausea and to alleviate morning sickness. It was a lucrative drug sold over the counter with no need for a prescription.

Then the horrible side effects of thalidomide damaging the unborn baby were discovered.[71] By all accounts, its original manufacturer, the German

Fix It: See and solve the problems of digital healthcare. Harold Thimbleby, Oxford University Press. © Harold Thimbleby 2021.
DOI: 10.1093/oso/9780198861270.003.0008

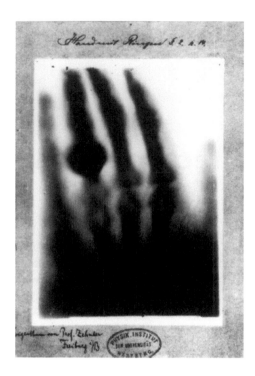

Figure 8.1. You can see Anna Bertha Röntgen's wedding ring in one of the first X-rays taken.

company Chemie Grünenthal was negligent with their research, and they dismissed many clear warnings of thalidomide's unraveling problems. It was a disaster for pregnant women, their children, and for families. Worldwide, it is estimated that about 24,000 children were born with thalidomide problems (perhaps another 123,000 were still-born or miscarried).[72]

There is something worse than those stark numbers: they're estimates, because *we just don't know*. The first problems were not recognized as thalidomide side effects, and then nobody was concerned enough or able at the time to count or do any systematic research to find out. There was no birth defects register.

The Thalidomide Society says the numbers do not include babies born alive but who were victims of State infanticide. Every country that was using thalidomide did things differently — thalidomide even has different names around the world: Asmaval, Distaval, Forte, Tensival, Valgis, and Valgraine. In Spain it was called Softenon, and Spain only recognized thalidomide as a problem 50 years after it was first used: 286 surviving victims finally managed to take Grünenthal to court in 2013, but Grünenthal successfully argued that there was no proof the deformities were caused by their drug.[73]

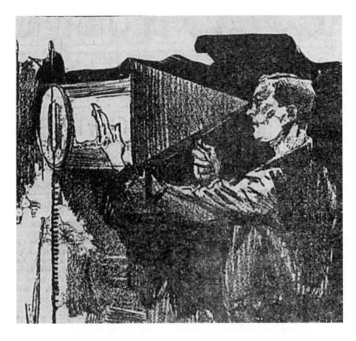

Figure 8.2. A newspaper sketch of Clarence Dally, Edison's assistant, routinely taking an X-ray of his hand, just five years after X-rays were invented. Clarence died of cancer in 1904.

Frances Kelsey was a reviewer for the US Food and Drug Administration (FDA) and she courageously refused to authorize thalidomide for the American market because she had concerns about its safety. Her concerns proved to be justified, and she became a heroine.[74] Thalidomide's horrific side effects thankfully stimulated a radical overhaul of drug regulation, so that drugs cannot now be released onto the market without thorough checks of their safety.

We now take drug side effects for granted, and know that finding the facts out about the side effects is hard work — it may take years for problems to become apparent well after a drug is in use. We have invented a new word for this: **pharmacovigilance**, which covers the entire life of a drug, from initial tests and authorizations, to long-term monitoring; the word is used so much it's often abbreviated as PV.

The World Health Organization defines **pharmacovigilance** as "the science and activities relating to the detection, assessment, understanding, and prevention of adverse effects or any other drug-related problem." However, side effects are not limited to drugs or to medical interventions like X-rays. Side effects affect everything in healthcare — nothing is perfect, and every treatment represents a trade-off.

Box 8.1. BRAN: Benefits – Risks – Alternatives – do Nothing

When the doctor recommends a treatment for you, it is very easy for both of you to focus on the cure. Unfortunately, things don't always work out positively — there may be side effects, it may be costly, whatever.

BRAN is an acronym designed to help both of you think more clearly. What are the **b**enefits of the suggested treatment? What are the **r**isks? What are the **a**lternatives? What would happen if you did **n**othing? BRAN puts some fiber into your thinking.

Our culture emphasizes the easy benefits of digital, and Cat Thinking means we are pre-disposed to be positive toward exciting digital ideas. I want a new iPhone, and I focus on my wanting and all the wonderful things it'll do, and I feel sure it'll help my work in hospital. But we should also ask, as well as the benefits that we tend to focus on:

- What are the risks? It will probably cost a lot of money. It will become obsolete. It may not work with other stuff, so will have knock-on effects. People will need training. There may be new types of error. It may get hacked.

- What are the alternatives? Paper is pretty reliable. Can we collect the information we want from some other source? Have you really understood the problem properly? Is there a better solution?

- What if we do nothing? If nothing else, if we wait, digital will become faster and cheaper. Somebody else may work out how to solve this problem, and we can then adopt some digital that works well. And anyway, your old digital system may last a while longer. (A nice bit of word play is: instead of solving your problem can you dissolve it?)

Some people add an **S**, as in **BRANS**. Get a **s**econd opinion!

I propose the word **digivigilance** (DVig?), analogous to pharmacovigilance for the science of digitally related effects. We need a new word to keep the risks of digital healthcare at the forefront of our thinking; we need to up our game — we need to get science and activities focused on detection, assessment, understanding, and prevention of the adverse effects of digital healthcare.

Gosport War Memorial Hospital is a small community hospital, which had just 52 beds in 2019.[75] Over the period 1989 to 2000, Dr Jane Barton worked as a clinical assistant and oversaw the deaths of at least 456 patients, many of whom had overdoses of opiate painkillers.

The Gosport War Memorial Hospital tragedy is of massive proportions, and many were caught up in the scandal.[76] The official report — taking four years and costing £14 million — makes it clear that there were system fail-

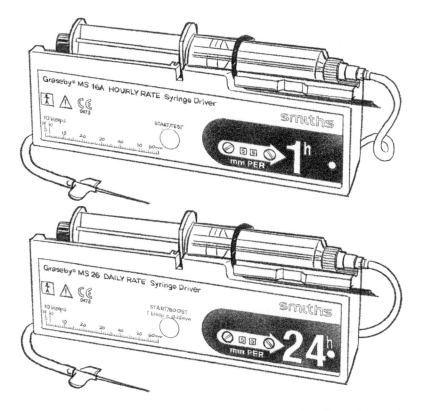

Figure 8.3. Two very similar Graseby syringe drivers: one is calibrated in the drug dose per hour ("hourly rate" model MS 16A, top) and the other in the drug dose per day ("daily rate" model MS 26, bottom).

ings. One wonders how much blame can be put on individuals at the sharp-end when the failings are institutionalized and go all the way up to management.[77] The substitution rule comes to mind.[a]

One nurse at Gosport, Anne Grigg-Booth, committed suicide when she was accused of murdering three of her patients.[78] She had been told to use Graseby MS 26 and Graseby MS 16A syringe drivers to deliver opiates to patients. We'll focus our discussion on the design of these things.

The two Graseby syringe drivers are very similar in appearance (figure 8.3). They are small, literally handy, and can be carried around by the patient, so they are very convenient to use. They are used for giving drugs intravenously (into a vein) continuously over a period of time.

These Graseby syringe drivers must be one of the world's simplest digital healthcare devices. There's just one button. On the MS 16A all it does is

---

[a] See Chapter 4: Just Culture, page 44 ←

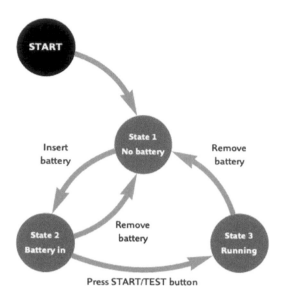

Figure 8.4. The Graseby MS 16A syringe driver is a very simple device, easily visualized as a finite state machine (abbreviated as FSM). A FSM has **states**, what it is doing, and **actions**, which change the current state to the next state. That's basically it. The MS 16A needs three states (though you can add more, depending on the detail you want, say to account for whether the syringe is installed or not, or whether the driver is locked inside its box). The advantages of FSMs include that they are *very* easy to program, they can do anything (if they are big enough), and they are easy to analyze to ensure they are implemented correctly.[79] It's surprising that FSMs aren't used a lot more in digital health.

switch the driver on; on the MS 26 it can also provide a bolus while it is held down to deliver a few extra milliliters of fluid (a bolus is used to initially fill up the tube from the syringe to the patient). It's surprising that two such similar-looking syringe drivers behave differently, potentially causing confusion. In addition, there are also two screws, which you need a screwdriver to turn to adjust the rate. Needing a screwdriver is quirky, but ensures that the rate is difficult to change accidentally.

You put the battery in, and the syringe driver will switch on straight away — you can't switch them off without removing the battery. Graseby make a transparent plastic box to put them in that can be locked shut so the patient (or a visitor) can't press the buttons or turn screws and overdose the drugs. It is easy to visualize how the syringe drivers work using a **finite state machine** (FSM) — figure 8.4 shows the MS 16A version.

Simplicity itself. What could possibly go wrong?

Unfortunately, several things.

> **Box 8.2.** Calculating drug dosage on a Graseby syringe driver
>
> Because the MS 16A and MS 26 syringe drivers are calibrated in millimeters, but patient drug doses are in milliliters, both syringe drivers require the user to do a calculation to convert milliliters into millimeters.
>
> Here's how. Suppose a syringe is filled with 8 mL of drug, which is to be given to the patient over a period of 12 hours, a rate of 0.67 mL per hour. Filling the syringe, the plunger will have traveled around 48 mm. The nurse will need to measure that distance. Then, calculating 48 mm divided by 12 hours, the duration of the treatment, will find a travel rate of 4 mm per 1 hour.
>
> The nurse will then use a screwdriver to set the MS 16A's left-hand screw to 0 and the right-hand screw to 4. The nurse should check the panel shows 04, the number calculated from the prescription.
>
> The nurse, or preferably an independent colleague, must also check that the syringe driver is the MS 16A and not the MS 26. If the MS 26 is used, the patient's dose will be 24 times faster, at a rate of 16 mL per hour, a potentially serious overdose.

The MS 16A Graseby syringe driver is calibrated in millimeters per *hour* and the other, the MS 26, is calibrated in millimeters per *day*. So if you use the wrong syringe driver, the patient could get an opiate dose 24 times too fast, which could easily be fatal, or a dose 24 times too slow, which wouldn't be very effective as a painkiller for the patient.

Another serious problem with the Graseby syringe driver designs is that they work in millimeters (distance in mm), but patients are treated with drugs that are prescribed by volume, usually in milliliters (mL), usually over a period of time.

You can see what a mess this is. I had to write millimeters and milliliters, using contrasting styles of underlining, because the normal way of writing — plain millimeters and milliliters, without any distinctive underlining — makes it far too easy to miss the potentially fatal difference.

The Grasebys, being calibrated in millimeters per hour or per day, measure how fast the syringe plunger moves, but the nurse or patient doesn't care how fast a plunger moves. They need to know how fast they get the drugs. Patients need a certain volume of drug per hour (or per day), and that's measured in milliliters per hour, not in millimeters per hour (or day). The fact that it's so hard to write clearly about the design just shows what a poor design it is.

If a syringe driver is calibrated in millimeters, as the Grasebys are, that means its correct use to get so-many milliliters depends on the exact type of the syringe it's being using with. Wider syringes will deliver more milliliters per millimeter than thinner syringes, and hence they will overdose a patient.

If a different type or make of syringe is used, it might well turn out to be the wrong diameter. The Graseby will deliver higher or lower doses, as it

> **Box 8.3.** Design trade-offs
>
> Any company, like Graseby, need to make cost-effective products, and they have to make design trade-offs between very safe but very expensive devices and devices that are less safe but are cheaper to make, and therefore can sell more at a lower price point. The Gosport hospital is complicit in this: they need to buy lots of syringe drivers, and they have to balance the cost of treatment with the likely outcomes for enough patients.
>
> At the time when the products were first purchased, probably nobody was aware of the potential problems: the tragedies had not yet happened. So, clearly, we cannot over-simplify and blame manufacturers for making unsafe products, nor blame hospitals for not being more careful.
>
> Different medical device regulations would shift the balance in the trade-offs, and different procurement — prioritizing safety — would have helped. The most serious criticism, though, is how slow healthcare and healthcare regulation are to learn and how slowly they improve. Inspired by Cat Thinking, the trap is: because we think digital is wonderful, why bother to collect good data? You don't need data if you already know the answer is it's good.
>
> The hospital was not recording relevant data, and the syringe drivers being used couldn't record any data anyway. This, of course, made everything cheaper, but in the long-run ignoring learning was probably the most serious oversight in the original trade-offs made by both the manufacturers and the hospitals that bought the products.
>
> We'll see trade-offs discussed throughout this book.[a,b,c]
>
> ---
>
> [a] See Chapter 9: Trade-offs in ease of use and safety, page 112 →
> [b] See Chapter 29: Trade-offs with numbers, page 409 →
> [c] See Chapter 29: Trade-offs with abbreviations, page 412 →

cannot check or make any allowance whatsoever for the actual diameter of the syringe installed in it. Surprisingly, there is no warning on the Graseby syringe drivers to use any particular size or make of syringe.

Twenty years *after* the Gosport problems came to light, the UK's National Patient Safety Agency was still needing to warn everyone:[80]

> The use of millimetres rather than millilitres (ml)[81] as a basis for medication calculation is unique to ambulatory syringe drivers. This is not intuitive for many users and not easy to check. Errors include the wrong rate of infusion caused by inaccurate measurement of fluid length or miscalculation or incorrect rate setting of the device. Errors can also be made through confusion between models calibrated for mm per hour or mm per 24 hours. Syringes in some of these devices can become dislodged in use. Some have inadequate alarms and no internal memory (which makes establishing the reason for any over or under-infusion difficult). Because

> ambulatory syringe drivers are often used to deliver opioids and other palliative care medication, over-infusion can cause death through respiratory depression while under-infusion can cause pain and distress.

Hospital harms need to be carefully monitored, and that monitoring *must* be a national exercise. If we had the data from a lot of hospitals and could compare them, some of them would have been using Grasebys and some would not have been. The data would have quickly raised concerns that the Grasebys could be a factor in the raised death rate. The Graseby syringe drivers do not record anything, so they wouldn't have been much help here.

To be charitable to the manufacturer Graseby, it is of course possible that clinicians made errors or maybe deliberately killed everyone (and different clinicians will likely have behaved differently) so the Grasesby equipment was merely an unwitting bystander to a tragedy. However, as the Swiss Cheese Model makes clear,[b] the Graseby *was* a slice of cheese whoever or whatever else contributed to the tragedy. And it had big holes.

Although it took 25 years from the start of the Gosport tragedy, the NHS did eventually rule that the Graseby syringe drivers were unsafe and should be banned, following earlier New Zealand and Australia bans.[82] And what did we do? We donated the banned syringe drivers to other countries, including Bangladesh, India, South Africa, and Nepal.[83] We ought to distinguish between surplus and banned equipment when donating.

Rather than donating the obsolete devices to other countries, we might have tried returning them to the manufacturers to recycle them. The user manual for the Graseby syringe drivers has a web link for compliance to the European WEEE (Waste Electrical and Electronic Equipment) directive: www.smiths-medical.com/recycle, but the page says "Sorry – the page you are looking for cannot be found!" Searching for WEEE, recycle, and other similar terms gets "No record found." So it isn't that easy to recycle them — though if only few people try to recycle, it'll carry on being hard to recycle, because the manufacturers won't bother to help when there's little demand.

It's interesting to compare the status of these medical devices with popular consumer devices. Apple, for instance, has a helpful scheme that works like this:

Apple GiveBack

> Turn the device you have into the one you want. Trade in your eligible device for an Apple Store Gift Card. If it's not eligible for credit, we'll recycle it for free. No matter the model or condition, we can turn it into something good for you and good for the planet.[84]

---

[b] See Chapter 6: Swiss Cheese Model, page 61 ←

> **Box 8.4.** Side effects and the Principle of Dual Effect
>
> Drugs often have side effects: curing one health problem often skirts around causing or exacerbating some other problem, the **side effect**. Aspirin, for instance, helps reduce the risk of stroke, but also unavoidably increases the risk of bleeding, a particular problem for people with stomach ulcers. A more dramatic dilemma is giving painkillers that, as a side effect, accelerate death. Clearly, giving a painkiller to cause death is wrong; giving a painkiller to reduce pain is good; but giving so much that death is inevitable walks into an ethical minefield.
>
> It's tempting to think of side effects as being an impersonal property of drugs, but anyone prescribing a drug makes an ethical decision: do its benefits for the patient (at this dose, under these circumstances) out-weigh its risks? The **Principle of Dual Effect** asserts that giving a drug with the intention of curing, while recognizing the risk but not intending it, is ethically acceptable. The Principle, though, has further criteria: the good effects must out-weigh the bad, and there must be diligence to minimize the potential harms (plus a few other details I won't consider here).[85]
>
> With digital healthcare, the Principle of Dual Effect looms large — or it should do. A developer writes a program intended to help staff or patients, but any program may have bugs, which could be counter-productive. The Principle of Dual Effect says that it is ethical to develop digital healthcare *provided that* the risks — primarily of bugs, cybersecurity problems, design faults and their effects — are properly managed. Developing software without considering the trade-offs is unethical. Developing life-critical software without exercising due diligence in exploring and managing the risks of bugs and other unintended side effects is unethical.

Meanwhile, the Grasebys are *still* for general sale in the UK. Here's a typical advert that I copied from eBay in 2019:

> GRASEBY MS-16A HOURLY RATE 1HR SYRINGE DRIVER & CASE. It is the most cost-effective syringe pump for this procedure using inexpensive syringes and subcutaneous infusion sets. Easy to use — load syringe, set rate and push start.[86]

The Gosport tragedy took years to even get to a national inquiry. One wonders, then, what might we be missing today if, for so long, we could miss such massive, growing catastrophes? How could we get better data on patient harm and error, and take monitoring more seriously? We must learn from Gosport that there is more to what is going on in error than blaming doctors and nurses.

Today, with the internet and more sophisticated digital medical devices, it's very easy to get data, along with the device identities and where they are used. If anybody wanted to get the data, that is.

Before Ralph Nader's landmark book, *Unsafe at Any Speed* published in 1965,[c] car manufacturers pretty much ignored accidents and safety: they "weren't the manufacturers' fault." Thankfully the culture has changed:

Old culture $\left\{ \begin{array}{l} \text{Car drivers have accidents} \\ \text{It's not the manufacturers' fault} \end{array} \right.$

New culture $\left\{ \begin{array}{l} \text{Car drivers have accidents} \\ \text{Manufacturers must make safer cars} \end{array} \right.$

In words, it seems a subtle difference; in culture, it's a radical change. We have all benefitted because car manufacturers have made cars safer. In contrast, at least so far as I can see, Graseby as well as the NHS for years ignored the *known* problems with their syringe drivers. This "conspiracy of silence" would have reinforced the hospital's view that they were safe.

Since the thalidomide scandal, we have tightened up drug regulations, tightening up both the approval processes and the monitoring processes after drugs are in use (called **post-market surveillance**). Never again do we want a drug that has such appalling effects as thalidomide did. Therefore our regulations today require drugs to be very carefully tested and certified, and there is a long, complex process that all manufacturers and their employees must follow. Employees even have a duty if they learn of problems with a drug they are not directly involved with.

The Graseby syringe drivers deliver drugs to patients, and can accidentally deliver fatal doses. Surely they should have been tested as carefully as the drugs they deliver? A drug is not safe if it is handled by a device that can deliver 24 times what it should and kill a patient. There is really no reason to assume an infusion pump or syringe driver is safe without rigorous testing to *prove* that they are safe. Devices and digital systems need to be tested as rigorously and as thoroughly as drugs are tested (though obviously they would be tested in rigorous digital ways rather than in pharmaceutical ways).

Rigorous testing must be done in realistic situations. The Graseby drivers used alone and with only the right type of syringe would probably be relatively safe, but used on a real ward with both 1-hour and 24-hour variants, with different syringes, with different drugs, with busy nurses, and no doubt lively patients and visitors, things can clearly get tricky. In real life, you'd have problems like the batteries going flat, drivers being dropped or knocked, or the syringe being dislodged.

Laboratory tests help, but they are not good enough, other than as preliminary checks. It's a bit as if laboratory tests check one or two slices of cheese but, by their nature, they cannot explore how all of the slices interact with each other.[d] Indeed, this issue is widely recognized with a special

---

[c] See Chapter 11: *Unsafe at Any Speed*, page 140 →
[d] See Chapter 6: Swiss Cheese Model, page 61 ←

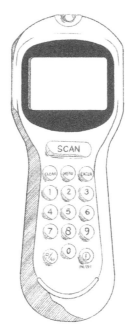

Figure 8.5. The Abbott XceedPro blood glucometer fits nicely into your hand.

word: **ecological studies** (or ecological experiments) are studies done "in the wild" to see how stuff *really* works. So when you buy things, don't be fobbed off with claims that it is safe or "easy to use" (a common, vacuous claim) — ask *exactly* what ecological experiments did you do, and what did you find?

We need an inquiry into the digital healthcare law and regulations as a whole, to cover medical devices and medical apps and software inside systems like MRI scanners, and how to make the laws and regulations fit for purpose in the twenty-first century with the added complexity of digital.

———————————————————

The next story came to court in 2015. The investigations started at the Princess of Wales Hospital in Wales, and focused on alleged misuse of blood glucometers, which are devices used to measure and record the blood glucose levels of patients. They are familiar to diabetics.

Nurses were taking blood glucose readings because their patients were diabetic. They were using Abbott XceedPro blood glucometers (figure 8.5) and writing down the test results on paper notes.

Seventy-three nurses allegedly omitted to record patient data properly, or made false or incorrect recordings of patient blood glucose levels. For diabetic patients this could have had serious consequences.

The paper records made by the nurses working on the wards and the computer records of what they were doing were different.

The Abbott XceedPro blood glucometers, which the nurses used, automatically upload tests to a computer system. There were no computer records of some tests the nurses had written on paper, so it appeared that the nurses had written down tests they hadn't done. It was therefore alleged that the nurses must have made up fake results, and written them down on the paper notes but without actually performing any tests on the patients, perhaps because they were lazy.

Since some of the patients lacked mental capacity, some of the nurses were charged with "wilful neglect" contrary to the Mental Capacity Act.[87] The allegations were that the nurses had made fraudulent patient records, and 16 nurses, who had apparently made more than five errors, were suspended and referred to the Nursing & Midwifery Council (NMC). Of these suspended nurses, five were charged with criminal offenses. Once the police criminal investigation started, the hospital halted its internal investigation.

Some nurses pleaded guilty, so it seemed straightforward. The case progressed to court.

An Abbott representative was the first person in the court to be cross-examined. Their opening comment was that the XceedPro glucometer was CE-marked, meaning that the device was certified for use across Europe, and therefore any problems would have to be the fault of the nurses using it.

I was an expert witness in the case, and I was present throughout the trial.[88] My first suggestion was that you might have one bad nurse, but to have 73 was implausible. Perhaps there had been a computer failure that affected all of their records? Perhaps some technician with access to the computer databases inadvertently deleted data? Perhaps someone had a grudge, maybe against the nurses, and messed up the data deliberately? Swiss Cheese[e] suggests several things *must* have gone wrong — so what were they?

The prosecution ignored all of these possibilities, and just thought the ward had a bad culture and that all the nurses were "in it together."

I analyzed the computer records, which had been managed in an Abbott database called PrecisionWeb. The data was very strange; a lot appeared to be missing — but because the database was so poorly implemented,[89] it was impossible to be certain what was missing or how data might have been corrupted, if it had. Although I had lots of ideas, I could not be certain *why* the data was so strange.

When a nurse takes a blood glucose reading, they first have to tell the glucometer who they are, which they do by scanning their staff ID card. They then have to scan the patient's barcode. Now the glucometer knows who is using it, and it knows whose blood results are going to be recorded.

---

[e] See Chapter 6: Swiss Cheese Model, page 61 ←

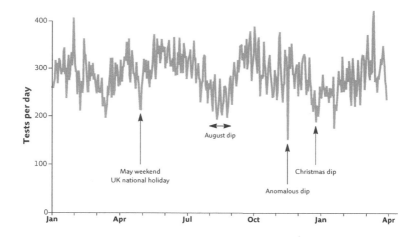

Figure 8.6. Blood glucose tests per day taken just over a year by 938 nurses working in 60 wards and clinics. The data is very "noisy," meaning that there is a lot
of variation from day to day. The anomalous, big dip on 17 November *might* be
random noise, some nurses may have been away, or it could suggest a problem with
the data that day, such as an unusually large number of rejected tests (figure 8.7).
Since correct blood glucose measurements are a patient safety issue, this sort of
data should be routinely scrutinized for anomalies like this.

Sometimes, nurses don't scan the patient barcode for some reason (perhaps because it's inaccessible or it's wet), and as a shortcut they scan their
own staff code again. The glucometer accepts this, but of course it now
doesn't know who the patient is. The glucometer displays the test results on
its screen, and the nurse can write them down in the paper patient records.
However, the glucose reading, instead of being recorded in the database, is
automatically rejected and stored separately from the normal digital patient
records. The idea is that later the nurse (or somebody else) will sort out
whose test data it is.

I drew a graph from the data taken from over a whole year (figure 8.6).
The numbers of test readings tally very closely with the numbers of patients
on the ward — you can prove this statistically, but it's pretty easy to see
there's a dip on Christmas Day (25 December), when you'd expect there
to be fewer patients on the ward, and there's a broad dip in August when
wards are less busy with people taking summer holidays. You'd expect that,
and when there are more tests, you'd expect there'd also be proportionately
more rejected tests too. But most — but not all — of the graph (figure 8.7)
of reject readings seems to be completely unrelated to the successful tests. I
haven't shown the analysis here, but it seemed that something very strange
was happening that wasn't anything to do with the patients.

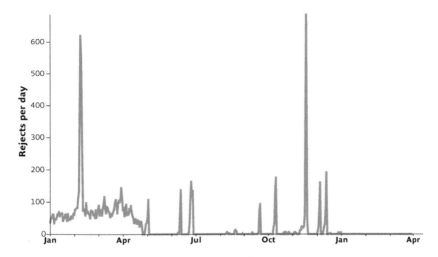

Figure 8.7. The number of rejected tests per day, from the hospital data we later found had been "tidied up." Some days have hundreds of rejected tests, and there are implausibly long runs of absolutely no rejects. Perhaps data has been deleted?

I couldn't see any useful pattern in this, and I couldn't see any general, consistent connection between the two graphs. For instance, there are long runs of zero rejects but a few days when there are huge numbers of rejected tests. No rejects *at all* for long periods of time seems very improbable to me. It made me get suspicious about the quality of the data. I plotted lots of graphs and did statistical analysis; I saw the same problems all over the data. It made me think of cyberattacks.

The data I had included the number of nurses taking tests, the ward temperature, the devices' battery voltages ... you name it. It had got the names of nurses and everything they'd done, but no nurses stood out as notably "bad" nurses with consistently high reject rates. None of the data correlated with the rejections. In other words, it looked to me like something was going on, or had gone on, that was not connected to anything (such as the nurses, wards, or numbers of patients) that had been recorded. Was it a bug, was it malicious intervention, was it a strange configuration problem perhaps being affected by some other issue somewhere in the hospital? In the thousands of pages of evidence, there was an admission that a server often crashed, but "often" wasn't often enough to explain the missing data, and crashes would probably have affected everything equally.

After three weeks in court, an Abbott support specialist was called to testify. While being cross-examined, he happened to mention he'd visited the hospital. I got a barrister to ask when, and what he'd been doing.

He had "tidied up" the data.

> **Box 8.5.** Design awards ignore safety
>
> The XceedPro was awarded the Japanese Good Design Award in 2010.[90]
>
> I admit the XceedPro is a certainly nice-looking device, but there's surely more to design than what the device looks like? Especially devices used in hospitals to care for patients? Things have to be designed well *and* have to work safely in the complex hospital environment. The XceedPro failed the nurses who used it because the system was not programmed by Abbott to detect errors in its database.
>
> | **The Good Design Award** | |
> | --- | --- |
> | HUMANITY | the creativity that guides the making of things |
> | HONESTY | the ability to clearly see the nature of modern society |
> | INNOVATION | the vision to open up the future |
> | ESTHETICS | the imagination to evoke a rich life and culture |
> | ETHICS | the thoughtfulness to shape society and the environment |
>
> The Good Design Award criteria are very positive and worthwhile, but they aren't complete. They are certainly of limited value in healthcare. The Abbott XceedPro's case shows that the criteria ignore the critical design issues in digital technologies. They say nothing about whether things work dependably in healthcare. I think "safety" and "reliability" need adding to design awards as explicit criteria.

At this point, the whole case started to unravel.

The Abbott support specialist had been called in by the hospital because the police were going to seize the data, and I guess the hospital wanted the data to be nice and ready for the police. Unfortunately the engineer sorted out the data *and deleted lots of it.* He took no notes of what he had done (he hadn't been told there was a criminal investigation going on).[91]

The judge then ruled the computer evidence had no value to the case and he excluded it, so the case collapsed. Two nurses who had been behind bars in court for three weeks were freed.

The case took three weeks to unravel in court. There were some further interesting points:

- The prosecution referred to published peer-reviewed papers on the quality of the XceedPro glucometers, claiming they were accurate and effective devices. I pointed out when I was being cross-examined that these papers evaluated how accurate the XceedPros were at measuring blood glucose levels; although it made them sound good, how accurate they were wasn't an issue for the case. The case centered on the reliability of the *whole* XceedPro system — whether and how glucometer readings, however accurate they were, actually end up in the database. The court was not interested in the measurement values; it was interested in whether measurements actually took place.

In contrast to the many papers on measurement accuracy, there were no papers assessing the system reliability that I could find — which, when you think about it, is a serious oversight of the research work being done in the area. What use is a glucometer or glucometer database if it is not reliable? It might measure reliably, but if the results aren't recorded reliably, what use are its measurements? Why wasn't reliability being tested? Why don't the medical device regulations *require* tests to prove it is working reliably "end to end"? Recording blood glucose levels, however accurate they are when they are taken, will lead to confusion if the computer systems then don't correctly record some of the test results. (And that is what had happened.)

① The prosecution argued that, as nobody had reported problems with XceedPros to the US or to the UK reporting systems,[92] then there could be no problems with the device. Of course, this argument assumes that people are aware of risky digital healthcare *and* also report faulty devices. In fact, the research literature — had the prosecution looked — has papers discussing similar problems in other hospitals. The Baystate Health System found they had 61 patient identifier errors per month, matching one of the problems at the Princess of Wales Hospital.[93] So there *are* recognized problems with the XceedPro encountered at other hospitals *but* these problems are not being reported to regulators. As usual, the prosecution didn't look for (or didn't admit to finding) evidence not supporting its case.

① Even if you do notice problems, they are hard to explain (because such problems tend to be technical) and therefore they are very tedious to report.[94] Many bugs are hard to reproduce to get the details for a useful report, and unfortunately many clinicians don't know how to report technical problems. Much better would be for backoffice technicians to be routinely checking data for anomalies; they have the time and skills to report technical problems. Many anomalies become obvious when the data is visualized — figure 8.7 being a simple example.

① There is a lot of excitement about healthcare going paperless,[95] but if the Princess of Wales Hospital had gone paperless there would have been no contradictory evidence at all, and none of the problems would ever have been exposed. If we are going paperless, digital needs to be a *lot* more reliable — and where is the research on that?

Part I ◇ Diagnosis ◇ Riskier than you think

And "digital being more reliable" means not just digital technologies alone, but also the management of them, staff awareness of cybersecurity issues, and vulnerabilities. Digital is tightly integrated with the delivery and management of healthcare, and reliability is a whole-system issue; it is a mistake to think of it as a "just get the best technology" problem.

There's a lot more interesting stuff to this story at the Princess of Wales Hospital.[87] For instance, the police seized the wrong glucometers for their prosecution evidence. They went into the ward and seized the glucometers that happened to be there on the day they visited, not realizing that glucometers wander around the hospital, as they are borrowed from other wards, repaired, and replaced. Seizing all the glucometers from one ward probably did more harm than everything the nurses had been accused of — indeed, it had been admitted in court that no patient had been harmed by the alleged "fraudulent" recordings.

I did find lots of problems that the court never needed to explore; the case collapsed as soon as one serious problem was found with the prosecution evidence, and once the case had collapsed, none of the other problems were of interest to the court.

I was fascinated that the prosecution (that is, the police) emphasized that they had used forensic methods to handle the data. They had encrypted the Abbott data *after* they had copied the data from the hospital. In fact, they had to do this manually. They had only used "forensic software" to store it *after* it had been exported from the database onto a USB stick and transported to the police offices. Yet the data they were analyzing was originally from CSV files edited in the hospital — these are text files, often made from spreadsheets, made up of comma separated values (hence CSV).

A well-known problem with CSV files is that they can easily be edited, corrupted or tampered with, whether accidentally or deliberately, leaving absolutely no trace at all: nobody will be any the wiser. The police might have used forensic methods *after* they'd collected the data, but forensic methods were worthless as the evidence wasn't forensic to start with, nor did the Abbott system itself work to forensic standards anyway. It was obvious to me that the police had no way of knowing what the data meant; their discussion of their forensic methods just emphasized how digitally illiterate they were.

The Abbott PrecisionWeb database operator's manual — which provided the main prosecution evidence — itself says:

> This product is not for diagnostic use; all patient diagnostics should be based on results reported by the point of care instrument.[96]

It's understandable that glucometers require monitoring and management, for instance to detect dud batteries, so PrecisionWeb could be useful without being relied on for diagnostic use. But why did Abbott design a system for monitoring blood glucose meters in a hospital that was, as it admitted in its manual, fundamentally unreliable? Why weren't there, at least, end-to-end checks that data successfully gets from the glucometers to the database? These are simple bugs that could — and should — have been automatically detected and avoided. PrecisionWeb could have been designed for clinical use, but it wasn't. Finally, why did the police and prosecution rely for their evidence on data that the manufacturers said was not even good enough for clinical use, questions of which were what the whole case was about?

Why didn't the hospital IT management notice that huge amounts of data had been deleted? Deleting data is practically a cybersecurity attack — but it wasn't noticed. Worse, a malicious attack by a nasty hacker could easily *change* data, not just delete stuff. If your blood type was changed in a hack, or your drugs were changed, it could be lethal, not just a "disciplinary problem."

———————————■———————————

The Princess of Wales Hospital blood glucometer case, with 73 nurses disciplined, some taken to court and some pleading guilty, has striking parallels with a UK Post Office case, where hundreds of employees across the UK were prosecuted after computer records showed discrepancies in Post Office accounts. The Post Office story is salutary because financial accounting is far, far simpler than digital healthcare records, yet it can still go horribly wrong — and still be denied.

In 2003, Lee Castleton became a subpostmaster — that is, he bought a franchise to run a post office as his own business. He invested his life savings in setting up his new business; and on their part, the Post Office provided the computer system, called Horizon, that he'd use to run the business.

Soon, the Post Office found Lee had a shortfall in his financial accounts of £25,858.95. They took him to court.

Lee's horrendous story is told in full by Paul Marshall, a barrister who has been helping him.[97] Lee was not only found to be liable to the Post Office, but the court also awarded the Post Office's legal costs against him, so he was burdened by a further £321,000 to pay to the Post Office. It remains extraordinary that the Post Office was willing to spend £321,000 to pursue an alleged debt of just £25,858.95.

Lee was one of over 900 subpostmaters that the Post Office brought civil claims or criminal prosecutions against; the majority of the subpostmasters were found liable (in civil courts) or convicted (in criminal courts). Many accused subpostmasters were shunned by their communities — in the UK, Post Offices are often centers of the community, especially in villages. Many went to prison; many went bankrupt; and some committed suicide.

Between 2000 and 2014, the Post Office was prosecuting its subpostmasters at the rate of about one a week. The subpostmasters were in no position to be able to prove that the Post Office's Horizon system they were using had bugs, and therefore that the errors and alleged shortfalls in their financial accounts were due not their fault, but to those bugs. The defendants were hamstrung partly by the Post Office's arrogance, but also by the UK legal framework that takes it for granted that computer evidence is reliable.[98] It's extraordinarily hard to argue in your defense, especially if nobody discloses the details about computer unreliability, known bugs and errors, and their effects on your day-to-day work.

In 2019, the Court of Appeal quashed an unprecedented number of convictions of the subpostmasters. There will be more to come. The scandal hit the news again in 2021, when judges called it "an affront to the conscience of the court." It's exposed one the largest miscarriages of justice in the UK ever, possibly the largest miscarriage of justice ever. Lee Castleton ultimately received in his hands less than £20,000 compensation — most of which will have been used to pay his costs. I hope that this inadequate compensation for all the consequences of a serious miscarriage of justice will be increased as the case continues.

As Paul Marshall wrote,

> It is now known that well-over 900 subpostmasters were prosecuted. The vast majority were convicted. Those convictions were secured by unreliable evidence of an unreliable computer system that judges, juries, and lawyers failed to properly understand — and the failure by the Post Office to give proper disclosure. [...] I would add that the thesis of *Electronic Evidence*,[99] namely, that electronic evidence is poorly understood by judges and lawyers has been all too plainly validated.[97]

Even the many subpostmasters who pleaded guilty to criminal charges have now been completely exonerated.[100]

- ⓘ It's possible to think, at least for the first few cases brought by the Post Office, that the legal teams believed they were in the right. But as the cases mounted, this charitable interpretation becomes implausible. There's now clear evidence that the Post Office and the manufacturers of Horizon knew about the bugs for many years. Indeed, Horizon's manufacturer, Fujitsu,[101] was able to remotely edit Post Office accounts without the local subpostmasters knowing anything. Naïvety (if, initially, that's what it was) drifted into institutional corruption.

- ⓘ Some of the defendants pleaded guilty, for instance to fraud, as they tried to manage their overwhelming debts as reported by the buggy Horizon. The vast majority of those who appealed had their convictions completely quashed, even though in many instances they'd pleaded guilty: the prosecution was unfair, and in addition an affront to justice. In effect, this was a finding that they should never have been prosecuted — it was a total exoneration. The Court of Appeal signalled that the conduct of the Post Office as prosecuting authority was such as to undermine the integrity of the criminal justice system and public confidence in it. Such a finding against a prosecuting authority is unheard of. If we are charitable to the Post Office, perhaps this blindness to computer bugs started with Cat Thinking:[f] if computers are wonderful, then any problems must be caused by the users. The first conviction didn't need much thought, but it seemed to confirm the criminal

In UK law, pleading guilty saves the court a lot of work, and someone pleading guilty almost always gets a lighter sentence. The defendants had no effective evidence to support their case that they were innocent (because the Post Office failed to disclose that material), so the prosecutions would very likely succeed with the weight of computer evidence seemingly on their side. In these circumstances, it would've seemed a good trade to concede guilt, typically to a lesser charge such as false accounting instead of theft. Indeed, the legal system supported the prosecutions with the structural assumption that computer evidence is reliable.[98]

The Post Office situation was comparable to the Princess of Wales Hospital being unaware that Abbott, the XceedPro glucometer manufacturer, had changed patient data.

- The nurses who pleaded guilty in the Princess of Wales Hospital case would've been presented with lots of data and discrepancies going back years previously — could any nurse accurately remember what they had done so long ago, and could they prove it better than a computer? Of course not. The computer evidence would've seemed unassailable at the time of prosecution.

- Again, the legal system supported the Princess of Wales Hospital's prosecutions with the structural assumption that computer evidence is reliable.[98]

The Princess of Wales Hospital and the Post Office are both respected organizations; they are both effectively State institutions. Yet they clearly didn't have adequate processes in place to check whether their computer systems were working reliably — though, really, that's the manufacturers' responsibility. The simplicity of blaming individuals for computer problems clouded their judgment, as well as their humanity. Both lost sight of, and failed to take account of, basic concepts of just culture. The NHS has an

---

[f] See Chapter 3: Cat Thinking, page 25 ←

official policy for Just Culture, and it's surprising this wasn't raised in the disciplinary process before the issues reached the courts.[g]

It's baffling that Abbott, Fujitsu, and other manufacturers don't routinely build in safeguards to detect computer problems. Furthermore, such safeguards have to be easy to use — a hospital should not need to call in the manufacturer's expert to sort out a database of routine patient records.[102]

In both the Princess of Wales Hospital and Post Office cases, there was a huge asymmetry between the people affected and the organizations owning the computers, who held all the information and refused to properly disclose the information and knowledge they had, even as they brought the cases to court.

People assume that digital systems are reliable. Cat Thinking is built into our culture. Indeed, as the Post Office has already paid millions in compensation and it is having financial difficulties itself, the costs of Cat Thinking, and the harms they can do, are unlimited.

I wonder, then, how many other misdiagnosed computer bugs continue to cause problems that are mistakenly blamed on staff? How many systems have *unnoticed* bugs that harm patients or staff? Meanwhile, customers — such as hospitals — buying computer systems should demand safeguards, such as: "If data is moved from A to B, or any other operation is performed that is not intended to change data (including doing nothing), we contractually *require* that the system check that the data is unchanged. [...] We also require that the system keep accurate logs that are of sufficient quality to be used in evidence, should the need arise."

The claim that something must be true is called an **assertion**. For example, to say that data at A and at B will be the same is an assertion. Unsurprisingly, assertions are standard good programming practice. The fact that many programs don't bother to make adequate safety assertions (or, too often, don't even make any) is why front line workers get blamed rather than buggy digital systems — because nobody knows the digital systems have bugs and have failed to work correctly. The Princess of Wales Hospital and the Post Office stories illustrate this, and we will see many more cases throughout this book.

———————————◼———————————

It's very important that hospitals (and other healthcare practices, like dentists and GPs) continually check patient data and ensure it is not tampered with. The Princess of Wales Hospital clearly wasn't monitoring its data closely enough. I don't think there's anything unusual about the Princess of Wales Hospital; this problem could've happened anywhere. What was special about the Princess of Wales Hospital, though, was that the police came in and seized data and started collecting evidence to support a criminal case. I wonder what would happen at any other hospital if the police came in and

---

[g] See Chapter 4: Just Culture, page 44 ←

seized patient and staff data? What would they discover? How much of what they uncover would be true, and how much would be as misleading as the Princess of Wales Hospital data?

This is not idle speculation: cybersecurity and hacking are serious problems.[h] To give an idea of the scale of the problem, a recent survey of just medical images found 400 million images and other patient details had been hacked and made freely accessible.[103] Serious problems were identified in 52 countries around the world. This huge treasure trove of patient data was uncovered with no effort, but when you take account of how highly motivated criminals are to access patient data for financial and personal data, for blackmail, for repurposing for fraudulent billing, or for just the thrill of hacking, the realistic potential for disaster from poor cybersecurity is astronomical.[104]

If we believe digital healthcare is infallible, as many do, we'll end up taking doctors and nurses to court, as in this Princess of Wales Hospital story.

It's a great shame that the Abbott XceedPro *by design* does not ensure that data it records is reliably and securely recorded on the Abbott database ("handshaking" is one standard method that was missing). In my first report to the court, I had pointed out this uncertainty that was built into the design of the Abbott systems. Without auditing based on a reliable system, you can't really be sure of anything. In the Princess of Wales Hospital case, this really mattered. Without auditing (let alone reliable auditing) the hospital had no idea things were going wrong with their computer databases. The nurses became scapegoats for digital shortcomings.

This chapter opened with the horrifying problems of the misuse of X-rays and thalidomide, and the devastating impact these innovations had on people. Those historic stories provide a background to the Gosport War Memorial Hospital, the Princess of Wales Hospital, and the Post Office Horizon cases.

In every story, individuals were at a huge disadvantage in disputes with large organizations that held more information, and which controlled what information was used. It's charitable to think that these organizations "didn't know" but this begs serious questions about the quality of the systems they were using: if they didn't know the systems were buggy or encouraged use errors, why didn't they know?

Patients and staff harmed have no way of knowing whether digital failures are a contributing factor, and, if so — without a lot of inside knowledge — it's impossible to find the evidence and the informed expertise to interpret it. If they fight in court, they are at a huge disadvantage. In the UK, even the law is set against them: computers are assumed to be infallible unless you can prove otherwise.[98] And how can ordinary people do that?

---

[h] See Chapter 17: Cybersecurity, page 211 →

It's instructive, now, to think about Swiss Cheese again.[i] So, in hindsight, which slices might have been better at stopping problems? What new slices could there be to stop problems happening elsewheree?

The Princess of Wales Hospital court case typified all of the problems. The case assumed the nurses' slices of cheese had the big holes; in fact, the nurses were alleged to be criminal. This misconception was so deep it drove the investigation and prosecution for several years. The ultimate collapse of the court case hinged on discovering that an Abbott employee had exploited different holes — holes in the digital systems. Those holes were there because neither the hospital nor the police understood how the digital systems worked, nor what precautions should be taken to properly manage patient data. Ultimately, those holes were there because the Abbott implementation had bugs that allowed unauthorized deletion of data to go completely unnoticed.

Possibilities include: the nurses could have been better trained; Abbott could have programmed the system more reliably; the hospital could have procured a more reliable system for their needs; the regulations could have been tighter to avoid unreliable digital systems being used in hospitals.

All of these groups might enjoy reading this book, of course, but where should we best focus attention?

There are several priority areas where the holes could have been avoided:

① Manufacturers should develop systems to be more reliable and to be able to demonstrate they are reliable. In turn, those of us teaching Computer Science need to be more effective so that manufacturers can get better programmers to make these more reliable systems.

① Given that cybersecurity is a huge problem (which I discuss later[j]), we all need better ways of avoiding, and, when they happen, detecting and recovering from, cyberattacks. Improving defenses against cyberattacks would have avoided the Princess of Wales problem: simply, the actions of the Abbott employee would have been detected as soon they happened. They could then have been repaired before any serious damage was done. Improving cybersecurity should be done *now*; it's an urgent problem.

① The regulators should tighten medical device and other IT regulations and regulatory processes so that systems in healthcare improve. The regulatory problems need fixing now, because improving them will, inevitably, take years to take effect in the world (which, again, I'll discuss later[k]).

---

[i] See Chapter 6: Swiss Cheese Model, page 61 ←
[j] See Chapter 17: Cybersecurity, page 211 →
[k] See Chapter 16: Regulation needs fixing, page 201 →

🦋 In seeking blame for the problems, the big holes were the failures to think clearly. Nobody thought that if tens of nurses or hundreds of employees are all being investigated for the same problems *very likely* there's a common factor. Maybe the computer systems they all use are unreliable? Unless you can show that all these people colluded to do the same wrong things, the presence of bugs is a far more reasonable explanation that should have been carefully checked first. It's important to note that this hole is, at least in principle, the easiest one to tackle.

🦋 The digitally-illiterate culture goes all the way to the top. In the UK, Common Law has a presumption that what it quaintly calls a "mechanical device" (which includes a digital device) has been properly set or calibrated. This is carried over into the Criminal Justice Act 2003,[99] so — if you end up in court as a defendant — the presumption in law is that the digital healthcare device is correct and its log is correct. If you don't want to be convicted, you will need a knowledgeable and persuasive expert witness who can survive the cross-examination's attack on their credibility to persuade the court against them. To make progress, we have to recognize that digital healthcare is risky, and hence the Criminal Justice Act, and the "justice" flowing from it, is flawed if it's applied to cases involving digital healthcare.

🦋 I'd add that if manufacturers cannot *prove* their systems are reliable at the time in question, then investigatory, disciplinary, and legal processes must assume that the systems are *not* reliable. Try reframing any failure like this: "The alleged failure has been blamed on a nurse [or other person], but it could've been concocted by the system; can anyone provide evidence — at least to the same standard you'd demand of a nurse — that the computer couldn't have done it?" Surely, if the computer, or infusion pump ..., is in the room (or networked into the room) for every murder, as it usually is, then it must be a prime suspect until proven otherwise?

🦋 AI and ML systems are becoming more sophisticated than humans. There is no reason for AI systems to be thought more reliable than any other sort of digital system. They should not be treated more leniently than any other sort of digital healthcare, and certainly not more leniently than humans would be doing the same job.

Meanwhile, bad things happen, and sadly bad things will always happen from time to time. Some may be missed, some may be covered up, but in the best case we'll want to learn from them so things improve. What's the best way to do that? Use **multi-disciplinary teams**; deliberately seek different views and different areas of expertise.

Part I ◇ Diagnosis ◇ Riskier than you think

Part I ◇ Diagnosis ◇ Riskier than you think

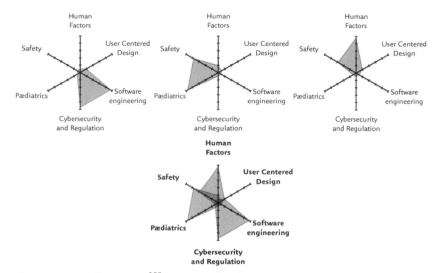

Figure 8.8. Skill mapping[105] a team to develop a system. For illustrative purposes, six skill areas have been identified as critical to success. Three individual team members' skill sets are mapped out on the top row — the values along each axis represent the competency of each person in the specified skills. The lower skill map shows the team's combined skill set. Given the requirement for these particular skills, it's clear from the skillmap that this small team needs to recruit more expertise in User Centered Design.

In all the cases I cover in this book, involving appropriate experts sooner would undoubtedly have helped head off problems. The problem is that we (on our own, without the right experts) don't know what we don't know. To get around this chicken-and-egg problem teams should be made multi-disciplinary and diverse; we should do this even before we know what disciplines may be needed. That's easily solved by starting with as many eyes involved as possible to review the problem, and only then specializing to the critical areas. Digital, for the time being, is an area where problems are too often out of sight, so in my view we should prioritize involving digital expertise in investigations and learning processes.

Here's an important note to end this chapter on: many "multi-disciplinary teams" are fiction. A software engineer, a cybersecurity expert and a medic with some safety experience *sounds* multi-disciplinary, but it may miss critical areas of expertise, such as User Centered Design (figure 8.8). The skill maps[105] shown in figure 8.8 were based on six skills picked to illustrate the idea: in a real project, you would work out which skills are needed, what is needed for each phase of the work, and what competencies each team member has — also including diversity, deliberately seeking different types and backgrounds of people for the team. Skill maps let teams think and talk about multi-disciplinarity, rather than just assume it happens automatically. You have to take multi-disciplinarity seriously, and not just pay it lip-service. Note that in my example, I included Human Factors. I meant not just Human Factors for the problem the team is working on, as Human Factors also applies to how the team itself is working — for instance, how can the team best work, so the different disciplinary contributions are properly heard?

Part I ◇ Diagnosis ◇ Riskier than you think

We don't know how many
people are dying or being
harmed from errors in
healthcare, let alone those
caused by digital errors.
What are the facts, and what
can we do about it?

9

The scale of the problem

As the famous statistician and founder of modern nursing, Florence Nightingale, said,

> The very first requirement in a hospital [is] that it should do the sick no harm.[106]

Nightingale worked in the hospitals at Scutari (now called Üsküdar, in Turkey) during the Crimean War in the 1840s. She soon become famous for her shocking analysis of the hospitals caught up in the conflict: she showed that poor hospital conditions were killing more soldiers than the fighting itself.

Today, we are killing more people because we do not understand error. We don't understand how bad computers contribute to error, and we don't take full advantage of how professionally programmed computers could protect us from error and its consequences. We don't even take full advantage of computers to collect data so we can reliably analyze what's going on and work out how to improve.

My father, Peter Thimbleby, died from a preventable error in hospital. I know this because the doctor told me just after I'd seen my Dad's body in the morgue. I'd got to the hospital too late to see Dad alive for the last time. The doctor told me an infusion had been left to free-flow, so that Dad had got too much fluid, which filled his lungs, so he drowned (pulmonary edema).

I talked to the doctor about reporting the incident, but he did not want to report it. I had to explain I was not blaming him, but a report would mean the hospital might learn something useful. Maybe there aren't enough nurses? Maybe the infusion pump had bugs? Maybe ... I don't know what, but please report it. How will we ever learn anything if you don't report it?

When the doctor reported the error officially, he selected standard text from the formal Datix computer reporting system,

Fix It: See and solve the problems of digital healthcare. Harold Thimbleby,
Oxford University Press. © Harold Thimbleby 2021.
DOI: 10.1093/oso/9780198861270.003.0009

> Avoidable short-term, non-permanent harm or impairment of
> health — full recovery in up to 1 month.

Yet Dad was already dead when this was entered into the Datix reporting
system. The "description of the incident" details on the Datix reporto goes
on to say,

> The patient got better but later that day he went into acute
> LVF [Left Ventricular Failure] again and died. The underlying
> diagnosis is likely to be ACS [Acute Coronary Syndrome] and
> that his death was unavoidable [...]

In fact, the unnoticed free-flowing over-infusion of fluid caused pulmonary edema (lungs filling up with fluid, making breathing difficult or impossible), which caused the LVF heart failure — not the other way round.
The written Datix report contradicts what the doctor himself told me.

The Datix report makes out that nobody was responsible: the patient was
ill and died, as they do. Nobody wanted to know why the error happened
that caused the heart failure, because, as officially reported, no error had
occurred. The doctor went on in his report:

> Family informed in [sic] details (they are happy not to take
> this matter further)

That's not true either. I'd been very clear at the time the doctor spoke to
me that I wanted the incident investigated to see what might be learned. In
fact, the misleading errors in the report led us to take the matter further.

When nobody is aware an error has been made, nobody is going to know
there are problems that can be fixed. In Dad's case, nobody is going to realize
that improving drips and making them safer would save lives. More importantly, if all issues are reported, the national data can be used very effectively
— without the national data, nobody knows whether my Dad's death was a
one-off story or representative of a trend. Unfortunately, what my Dad's
story shows is that national data is unreliable.

According to the Duty of Candour, there should have been a written
record, but none was made. To make such a record would have been an
admission that a "notifiable event" had happened. Clearly, trying to create a rigorous legal framework around errors creates barriers to honesty and
learning; if the doctor can instead make it appear it isn't sufficiently serious, then nothing need happen, and the doctor is off the hook. Learning
from not-serious-enough-to-be-reported errors would make a huge impact
simply because of their large numbers.

Manufacturers, not just doctors, try very hard not to be in a position of
being accountable, let alone being blamed. They dare not , because that
would be an admission they might be liable. As a result, digital healthcare

isn't improving. It may be getting more exciting but it isn't getting safer. This abrogation has been picked up and "legalized" in digital technology's so-called warranties; so far as the warranty is concerned, the developers aren't accountable either.[a]

The World Health Organization (WHO) maintains a huge and comprehensive classification system to manage data, called the International Classification of Diseases (ICD)[107] to categorize any disease and to help collect useful statistics. The WHO has no useful classification for medical errors, let alone digitally related errors.

The WHO ICD classification is used worldwide, including on death certificates. Death certificates register the causes of death, but don't collect statistics on errors because "error" isn't a disease. Yet, curiously, there *are* codes for things that have obviously got through the committees, like being struck by blunt object with undetermined intent (code PH00) and unintentional land transport traffic event injuring an occupant of an animal-drawn vehicle (code PA0F), so WHO could have handled errors if they wanted to.

Among other inevitable oversights, there is no classification for any error that does *not* cause harm, so it is not easy to learn from **near misses**, nor from problems specific to digital systems that don't directly lead to a harm. They can't be categorized in the WHO system. I'll discuss how useful it would be to record and learn from near misses and other "non-events" later, when I discuss the concept of Safety Two.[b]

It gets worse. The ICD documents themselves admit that many coding errors arise when ICD codes are used. The IDC coding is concise, but on the other hand it has no redundancy to help detect or correct errors. For instance, the ICD code NE2Z means "burns, unspecified," but a simple one letter error writing DE2Z instead means "diseases of the digestive system, unspecified." Box 9.1 pulls together some lessons about usability and safety, putting this digression into WHO coding into a larger context.

There are several versions of ICD and the latest ICD is copyright and expensive — usually country healthcare systems pay to use it — so it is hard to access the correct codes to develop digital systems to correctly use whichever the current code is. Instead, earlier versions that have been released into the public domain may be used instead, causing further discrepancies, and other errors in coding. Many countries, such as the US, have developed variants of the ICD. For instance, the US extended it for the exceptional needs of recording COVID-19.[108] Obviously, WHO will sort out COVID coding in their ICD system, but it seems strange to me that coding isn't managed centrally, digitally, internationally, and in real time — COVID isn't unprecedented as a new disease in needing rapid classification. It's the sort of thing the internet could do easily.

There are blindspots all the way down. The final statistic, the death cer-

---

[a] See Chapter 15: Who's accountable?, page 193 →
[b] See Chapter 12: Safety One & Safety Two, page 145 →

> **Box 9.1.** Risks of making computers "easier to use"
>
> People who work all day on computers are at risk of repetitive strain injuries (RSI — nerve damage, often taking the form of painful carpal tunnel syndrome). Understandably, everyone gets frustrated with having to do too many mouse clicks or keystrokes. Making the user interface easier to use is surely important, and would release time to do more important things? Unfortunately, making something easier to use *also* means making it easier to make errors that can't be blocked. All errors eat up *more* time to correct, likely far more than any time actually saved — worse, errors can destroy lives, and possibly can end up being fought, taking months in court. Is "ease of use" always worth it?
>
> The World Health Organization's ICD codes, discussed in the text, make a simple example of ease of use/error trade-offs.
>
> There aren't many ways to make a mistake typing "osteoarthritis of hip" which would make it unrecognizable, but it gets tedious to type so much, especially if it's your job to do ICD coding day in, day out. An expert might well know the right code, FA00, and prefer to type only the four keys.
>
> Yet a single keystroke error typing FA00 can make 40 very different codes, including JA00 for abortion, NA00 for superficial injury of head, or FA30 for acquired deformities of fingers or toes. There are tricks that can be used to help — knowing the clinician's speciality can help automatically cut down on the valid choices, but these often need to be overridden. For example, if an oncologist is helping out in an emergency COVID-19 episode, their usual pre-COVID-19 oncology codes are not going to be helpful. Even so, while typing "osteoarthritis of hip" may be tedious, it's safe and hard to make any meaning-changing mistakes that won't be detected.
>
> The same ease of use/error trade-offs happen with mouse clicks. If fewer mouse clicks are required to select a code, the user could also hit a nearby wrong code more easily.

tificate, doesn't record errors as a potential cause of death. A death certificate has the actual cause of death (like pulmonary edema), the clinical cause of that (like left ventricular failure), and other conditions like diabetes or pneumonia that were present but not a direct cause of death. So the data is misleading; there are virtually no proper records anywhere. We know some examples where official national databases are deliberately circumvented and not used to record problems.[109] Florence Nightingale said as far back as in the 1860s: "accurate hospital statistics are much more rare than is generally imagined."[106] Little has changed since then.

In other words, nobody has reliable statistics for errors, harms, or fatalities caused by errors. So there's no choice but to estimate the figures.

While adverse events are under-reported and errors are under-reported, digital and other system problems that may underlie those problems are even less likely to be reported.

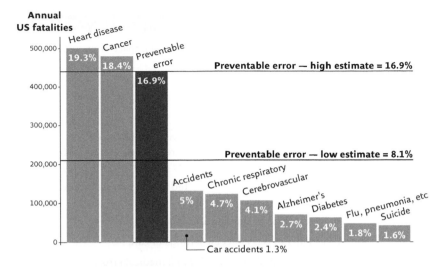

Figure 9.1. The top ten causes of death, from US data.[110] I've shown percentages on each bar, so the figures can be easily applied to similar Western healthcare systems. Note that there is a long tail of 23.1% of deaths from all the other various causes not shown in the bar chart.

Some estimates of death from error in hospitals puts it, astonishingly, on a footing with cancer and cardiovascular disease deaths.[110] When I combined these estimates with death certificate causes of death, I got the bar chart in figure 9.1. This shows preventable error, the highlighted bar, as the third largest killer: preventable error in secondary (hospital) healthcare may be around 17%. The data I used to get these estimates predates the horrific huge numbers of deaths from the COVID-19 pandemic (which are a mixture of political errors, lack of resources, and, inevitably, some preventable patient harms), but the figures should give a reliable impression of what happens in normal advanced healthcare situations. We'll talk more about COVID-19 and its relation to *digital* healthcare, specifically, later.[c]

In the chart, the two horizontal lines (marked 8.1% and 16.9%, respectively) cover the range of estimates. There is a *lot* of uncertainty. The lower estimate is close to Lucian Leape's estimates from way back in 1994.[111]

Leape points out that doctors might be performing at 99% proficiency, but this is very much lower than would be accepted in other industries. At an airport like Heathrow in London, having a 99% success rate would mean messing up over 2,000 passengers a day — and Heathrow isn't even the busiest airport in the world. Heathrow performs at a much higher level of safety than hospitals achieve. A 99% success rate, which is acceptable in

---

[c] See Chapter 31: The pivotal pandemic?, page 437 →

Part I ◇ Diagnosis ◇ Riskier than you think

> **Box 9.2.** WHO's global facts on patient harm
>
> The World Health Organization's facts on the global impact of preventable harms on patients:[112]
>
> ▶ Patient harm is the 14th leading cause of global disease burden, comparable to tuberculosis and malaria
>
> ▶ 1 in 10 patients are harmed
>
> ▶ Medical cost associated with error affects millions and costs countries between 6–29 billions[5] of dollars annually [it's really much worse since healthcare offloads many costs to social services and community care]
>
> ▶ 15% of healthcare spending in Europe is wasted dealing with all aspects of adverse events
>
> ▶ Investment in safety can lead to significant savings
>
> ▶ Inaccurate or delayed diagnoses affect all settings of care
>
> ▶ Administrative errors account for up to half of all medical errors
>
> ▶ In the US, focused safety improvements saved Medicare $28 billion[5] between 2010 and 2015.

hospitals, would be a national scandal in any safety-critical industry like air travel.[113]

The little segment at the bottom of the "accidents" bar (figure 9.1) shows car accidents. Car accidents contribute 1.3% of all deaths. Although this is US data, we all take car accidents seriously, and cars are getting safer and safer. Why don't we take the much higher numbers of healthcare accidents seriously? Why don't we do something about them? Even if you disagree with the estimates of preventable deaths, it's clearly something we should be very concerned about.[114]

———————————◼———————————

We shouldn't ignore preventable death, but we should also be concerned about preventable *harm*, like removing the wrong kidney. Harm has huge impact for the patient and carers for the rest of their lives. The numbers for preventable serious harms are about 20 times higher than those for preventable deaths.[115] We need to do something about it, and if we go about it the right way, the figures for *both* preventable death and for preventable harm will come down dramatically, lives will be saved, and people will be healthier — and staff will be happier.

From a purely financial point of view, preventable harm is much more expensive than preventable death. The healthcare system, or its insurer, has to provide extra treatment for recovery — hoping it's possible — and, as needed, care and support over the lifetime of the harmed patient, rather than just a financial transaction. Perhaps there will be costs to modify the family house and to provide daily care? What about education and care costs? If we took serious harm seriously, then preventable death would also be reduced.

———————————■———————————

The horrific Gosport tragedy in a UK hospital,[d] which involved hundreds of preventable deaths, could have been identified before so many patients died, had anyone been collecting the right data and looking at it. I am sure some data is collected, but as the syringe drivers are "dumb" and they don't record anything at all, accurate, objective data was *not* being collected. As an added benefit, the same data — if only it was routinely collected — would identify hospitals with unusually low preventable error rates, and we could go along to them and find out what good practices they were using or see if their digital systems had nice features that made them safer. As it is, we have no idea.

We know many people, fearing blame, do not record errors. If you go into hospital with cancer, you will most likely "die of cancer" instead of the hospital admitting that (if so) you caught a preventable infection or that some other preventable error killed you which should have been avoided. They'll say you were very ill, and what do you know? Yes you caught an infection, but you still died of cancer.

———————————■———————————

In 2019 four doctors reported some errors they had made with X-rays, thanks to problems they were having with their IT systems. They worked in Rhode Island Hospital in Providence, a city in Rhode Island (the smallest state in the US). The consequence of reporting problems: they received subpoenas.[116] Subpoenas force people with the threat of legal penalties to disclose evidence, so they are one step, in this case, before formally accusing people of crimes. The subpoenas said "medical misconduct," yet the doctors' reports were meant to draw attention to the problems they had with the hospital's computer systems.

Blaming the doctors kills the messenger. If this is the culture, why ever risk reporting any computer problems?

Chitra Acharya — who has a PhD in Computer Science, so she has an eye for detail — had the misfortune and opportunity to be with her son in two pediatric intensive care units for over a year.[117] For this one poorly patient, she recorded 120 errors a month (that's about four a day) on average. Some days were worse.

The incidents varied in severity; there were 11 **never events**, which are defined as serious incidents (such as wrong site surgery) that are wholly preventable. August had the highest rate of incidents and the highest rate of incidents weighted by severity; perhaps something could be tracked down to understand this and then fix it? In the UK — where Chitra was — junior doctors "rotate" in August, so they will have had no experience with any

---

[d] See Chapter 8: Gosport War Memorial Hospital tragedy, page 84 ←

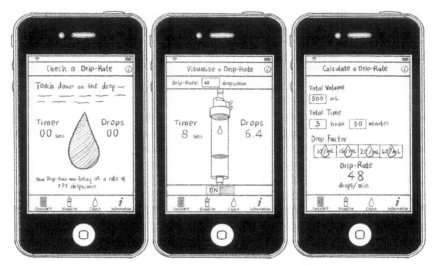

Figure 9.2. An app for setting up drip infusions.

systems they have not encountered before. If this is the explanation, it is a
serious criticism of the variation in design of medical systems and the lack
of interoperability between them.[e]

When James Macdonald had radiotherapy to the left side of his neck to
treat a cancerous tumor, unfortunately, the tumor was in fact on the right
hand side of his neck.

James died, and the official cause of death was cancer, which, yes, did
kill him. But had it not been for the left/right mix-up, the cancer would have
been treated and may not have killed him. The error directly resulted in his
untimely death but was unreported on the death certificate.[118]

My father died from an over-infusion from a gravity drip. Drips are literally drips: a bag of fluid drips into a tube that goes into the patient. A nurse is
supposed to check the drips are going at the right rate, so the patient gets the
right amount of fluid at the right rate. If this step is missed out — perhaps
because the nurse has to rush to another patient — there is a risk that the
whole bag of drugs empties quickly, as happened with Dad.

Timing drips is a bit complicated and very easy to get wrong, especially
on busy and distracting wards, so my student Mark Davies[119] designed and
built an app that helps (figure 9.2). We used User Centered Design to ensure
the app best met nurses' needs.[f]

The app animates drips so you can see them drip on the screen, and it
becomes a lot easier to get the drip rate exactly right. And the app does not

allow you to walk away without finishing. As you can see from the old iPhone in the picture, this app has been around for a while, and it could have been used to help, as another slice of Swiss Cheese,[g] when my Dad was admitted.

It's worth saying there isn't a conspiracy. There's a lack of interest and a lack of awareness, which feed each other, and result in a culture everyone is in and nobody notices. Certainly nobody is surprised or shocked by patient harms any more, and few places have any process to learn from error. Nobody has a preventable error registry. In law, death certificates do not record errors. Statistics are based on things we can count; since we don't have good definitions of "preventable death" and we aren't counting error, let alone error caused or exacerbated by or not stopped by digital systems, then we have bad statistics. With bad statistics, we can carry on in a state of not knowing what to do. Worse, it's frequently denied that proposals (which might cost money) to improve safety have no evidence in their favor — there's simply a vacuum instead of evidence.

We should ask why healthcare *system* accidents aren't getting inquiries, and nobody is worried about the reasons why digital healthcare systems and devices may be helping cause them. That's not entirely true; individual cases do sometimes get inquiries. The Beatson Oncology Centre got an inquiry,[h] the Mid Staffs Hospital got an inquiry,[39] and the Gosport War Memorial Hospital got an inquiry;[i] these inquiries were all focused on staff and culture. There have been (so far as I know) no inquiries on the whole systems, and next-to-no attention paid to the digital systems involved.

It might be because our culture just accepts the legal disclaimers (it is ridiculous to call them warranties) and accepts the thinking that goes along with them.

I described my father's preventable death above.[j] Tragic stories quickly get very complicated, and therefore difficult to communicate. I complained about the incident, and it just got more complex and intricate, and slowed to a crawl. You experience what's called **delay and deny**. The system, or the bit of it handling complaints, seems intent on ensuring as little change as possible. Complaints are handled as local problems, on a case-by-case basis. We need ways to transform complaints into learning.[120]

Prue Thimbleby, my wife, leads a digital patient storytelling program for the NHS. I worked with her to make a Digital Story. A **Digital Story**[k] (spelled with capitals) is a short, first person voice recording edited together with images to make a video clip. It isn't easy to make a short story about a complex complaint, but doing it carefully with a storytelling facilitator is an enormously helpful and therapeutic process. There are usually so many

---

[g] See Chapter 6: Swiss Cheese Model, page 61 ←
[h] See Chapter 7: Beatson Oncology Centre, page 69 ←
[i] See Chapter 8: Gosport War Memorial Hospital tragedy, page 84 ←
[j] See Chapter 9: Peter Thimbleby's preventable death, page 109 ←
[k] See Chapter 30: How to make Digital Stories, page 422 →

things that go wrong, sifting it down to what *really* matters to communicate as a coherent, punchy story helps you separate the niggles from the serious things. After you've made the story you feel heard — and you also have a clear message to share.

I sent my finished Digital Story[121] to the Chief Executive. I said it's only a few minutes long, and I'm sure you've got time to watch it. He wrote back to me and said,

> At the staff briefing session with clinical leaders and managers
> [...] I played your video about the death of your father and
> failures of our organization and systems. The reaction from
> colleagues was immediate and strong — there was an
> emotional reaction and an expression of shame from many
> colleagues. We had an open and honest discussion. We will
> be using this video in many fora across the organization.

I was also asked to do some workshops. The hospital had listened, and I felt listened to! Short, carefully focused stories can transform healthcare. For me, this was all a very positive resolution of the incident, a common result from using Digital Stories for patient complaints.

We've got lots more to say about Digital Stories later.[1]

---

[1] See Chapter 30: How to make Digital Stories, page 422 →

Part I ◇ Diagnosis ◇ Riskier than you think

Medical apps are very popular, but they are as prone to bugs as any other digital system. This chapter gives some typical examples and begins to suggest solutions. Like all digital healthcare, apps could be designed to block bugs and avoid the harms that follow.

10

Medical apps
and bug blocking

The medical app market has exploded with hundreds of thousands of medical apps. As a computer scientist, I can see problems with many of them — with such rapid, explosive innovation, quality control has become a serious issue. There are situations where apps give incorrect results and may be unsafe. These problems are caused by bugs in their designs. The bugs should have been avoided by better programming or by better testing and more careful user studies. There are also bugs that probably have little clinical impact, but are just frustrating.

Medical apps are the future, and where better to start than with a multi-award winning app that has been in the news for its clever design? I decided to have a look at Mersey Burns. It's used for assessing burns patients to see how much fluid to give them, depending on how badly they are burned.

Mersey Burns runs on iPhone and Android as well as on ordinary web browsers.[122] Anyone can download and try it, and it's a very nice visual app that is easy to explain in a book. I don't want to make a fuss about Mersey Burns in particular; so, at the end of this chapter, I'll look at a completely different app, and show that poor programming is a widespread problem.

I chose Mersey Burns as the first case study for this chapter because it was the first app in the UK to get a CE marking, and it has won several prizes and awards, so it is widely recognized as cutting-edge and innovative.

CE marks are supposed to be a basic quality mark to show that a product is appropriate for its intended use within the European Union (EU). So if a children's toy has a CE marking it means it isn't covered in toxic paint and doesn't have small bits that will fall off it, so it's safe for a child to play with. Of course, the CE marking requires different standards for different things. In principle, a CE-marked medical device should be fit for purpose.

Fix It: See and solve the problems of digital healthcare. Harold Thimbleby,
Oxford University Press. © Harold Thimbleby 2021.
DOI: 10.1093/oso/9780198861270.003.0010

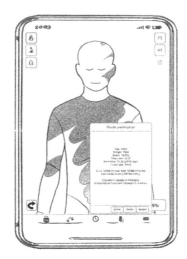

Figure 10.1. A drawing of Mersey Burns, version 1.6.4. The drawing shows how burns can be "painted" (in a distinctive red) on the patient's outline body with your finger. Here, the screen shows Mersey Burns showing the fluid dose the app recommends for this case.

I'll explain CE markings in more detail later[a] — we'll see it's a problem and guarantees nothing useful for digital healthcare.

A typical review of Mersey Burns on the app store says,

> **Excellent**
> This app is brilliant! As an EMT [emergency medical technician] I went to a gas cylinder explosion yesterday, this app was so helpful in working the total percentage of burns, was so easy to use and it worked it all out for me!

Figure 10.1 shows a drawing based on a screenshot of it.[123]

By the time you read, this I hope Mersey Burns will have fixed the bugs, which I'll describe over the next few pages. Fixing the bugs will be worthwhile, but really the bugs should be taken as *signals* that their development process missed them — the bugs should not have happened (and should not have been left around for the several years since the app was launched). Although the bugs are fixable, what really needs fixing is the process that lets them slip through. The app doesn't provide any direct way of sending the developers feedback, so they are unlikely to learn of bugs from experience in the field, so they will also miss bugs found by others after they've finished development.

---

[a] See Chapter 16: CE marking, page 201 →

> **Box 10.1.** Always say "use error" not "user error"
>
> Errors happen, and it's tempting to talk about user error.
> Please don't.
> The correct term is **use error**.
> Use error means an error occurred while a system was being used, which is what happened. If you use the incorrect term user error, by your language you are immediately assuming *the user* made the error. Maybe they did, and maybe they didn't. If the user didn't, and in fact even if they were part of the problem, then you are going to miss other causes of the problem.
> "The user did not respond to the alarm properly." Sounds like a user error, right? No; it's really a use error.
> Use the term use error, and it's now much easier to explore the other causes. Perhaps — and actually much more likely than "user error" — the alarm was vague, the alarm message was indecipherable, or the message was obscured, it was just a beeping sound that could have meant anything, and — very often — it was lost in an overload of a million other alarms and essential activities. All of these problems are system errors, indeed system *design* errors, not user errors.

The development process for Mersey Burns is comparable to the development processes used throughout digital healthcare, which is why it's important to describe some of the app's bugs here. They aren't complicated.

Although Mersey Burns has bugs, it's important to see them in perspective. A doctor treating a burns victim without the help of an app might wrongly estimate the burned body surface area, they may not know the right calculation, and they may get their calculation wrong. Using a good app should fix these problems. On the other hand, doctors rarely get things wildly wrong, but if an app is buggy (or is hard to use), everybody who uses it is a potential victim to being caught out by one or other of its flaws when it's used. One should do thorough studies to find out which is safest in practice. Indeed, Mersey Burns did user studies and User Centered Design (UCD),[124] which ensures apps (or, in general, any digital systems) are easier, safer, and more reliable to use — we'll give some more examples from Mersey Burns later in this book.[b,c] Good UCD helps reduce the impact of any bugs that the development process misses.

So, how is Mersey Burns used?

Imagine a burns victim turns up in the Emergency Department.

In the old days, you'd have to do a rather complicated assessment and calculation. Where are they burned, and how badly? How long is it since the burn happened? Each part of the body is different — for instance, burns on the neck are worse than burns on feet. How old is the patient? What do they

---

[b] See Chapter 21: Mersey Burns user guards, page 293 →
[c] See Chapter 29: Mersey Burns roller number entry, page 410 →

weigh? Are the burns partial thickness or full thickness? If they are badly burned, the patient may be dehydrated and will risk kidney problems, so you'll infuse them with some fluids. But how much, and for how long? All of these details then go into a calculation, and you end up with a prescription for giving the patient a resuscitation fluid. This is where Mersey Burns shines.

You draw the burns on the screen. Compared to the traditional method, this is very easy. You then tap an icon near the lower right of the screen, and a "Fluids prescription" box pops up and tells you what to do (figure 10.1).

Strangely, Mersey Burns doesn't require you to specify the age or weight of your patient before you get a fluids prescription — it'll use the age and weight from your *previous* patient. In the picture (figure 10.1), the age and weight are some patient's details from the last time it was used. This is a bug; the app should confirm the age and weight of the patient. One hopes the doctor notices and corrects the patient details — fortunately, Mersey Burns lets you do that without having to re-enter the burn details as well.

Let's carry on entering data for the same patient (figure 10.1), as they probably have burns on their back too.

Tap the ↻ arrow button and the body drawing flips over. Now you can draw the burns on the back. If the user draws the burns, then the app recalculates the percentage of burned body area, as you'd expect. Alternatively, the user can enter the percentage directly as a number, which will generally be quicker than drawing the details of the burns. Anyway, experienced clinicians will know the percentage of many common burns. Let's say we want 10% burns, and we enter it.

We now click on the prescription button. The patient still needs fluids, but the app is saying none should be given. What's happened is that entering a number has cleared all the drawing we did on the front. Because we'd turned the body over, we can't see that's what's happened.

The bug works like this. Whenever a numerical percentage is entered into the app, all drawn burns are cleared. Conversely, when you draw any entered numerical percentage is cleared. I imagine the designers thought you would not want to both draw burns and enter a percentage, so you can do one or the other, but not both. Unfortunately, if you have turned the body over, you can't see that your hand-drawn burns get cleared. The way the app is designed, it's a silent error if the user both does a drawing and gives a percentage. The app takes whatever is done last — the drawing or the percentage — as the definitive thing, and silently deletes the other. The bug "makes sense," but it is a silent bug — it could catch a user out and cause patient harm and nobody would be any the wiser.

One can argue whether the user "should not" make this error, perhaps because it seems to make little clinical sense, but given that errors can always be made, the app should block the error or point out the problem so the user can correct it and work out how to do what they intended. Apps should report, block, and manage all possible errors.

In general, if an error is possible, eventually somebody will make that error. Designers of systems should therefore always ask themselves if an error is dangerous (could it ever lead to delays or to patient harm?) and, if so, how should their designs warn users or, better, how should they block errors so the consequences are trivial. In other words, we do not say "the user should not make that error," but, rather, "how can we make the design safer in case use errors happen?" Furthermore, to ask these design questions, designers need a systematic way of finding *all* such possible errors — we'll explore how this can be done throughout Part II of this book, coming next after this chapter.

When such errors occur, it's no help saying the user made the error because that's how it's designed. This was the problem with the National Cancer Institute of Panama incident[d] which led to the imprisonment of radiotherapists who allegedly killed patients. Mistakes were made *but ended up with serious patient harm* because of a bug.

Back to Mersey Burns ... if a user is trying to do both drawing and percentage (in either order), then there are conceptual problems in the program that need to be avoided. Here are some design alternatives that avoid the bug:

- A redesigned app could give the user a choice to resolve the problem — see the sketch mock-up in figure 10.2.

- The percentage display tells the user something useful, but perhaps it need not allow any interactive input: it could just be a number confirming that the patient has such-and-such percentage burns. It the user cannot enter a new percentage, the drawn burns will never be deleted by mistake.

- Once drawing starts, the percentage could disappear, or once a percentage number starts to be entered, drawing burns by painting them is blocked.

Without doing experiments with users *actually* doing real work with the app, it isn't obvious which the best approach is. Indeed, it's likely with observing and talking to users — who would be professional clinicians — that they will propose more good design ideas, which in turn need more experiments to evaluate. One of the key attractions of Mersey Burns is it allows people to draw burns and it works out the percentage, so ideas to redesign will require UCD[e] evidence to make good design decisions — any redesign may introduce more problems than it solves. Indeed, I think that introducing the percentage number entry was originally suggested during UCD, but, evidently, the new feature added because people wanted it wasn't thoroughly tested.

---

[d] See Chapter 7: National Cancer Institute of Panama problems, page 73 ←
[e] See Chapter 22: User Centered Design, page 301 →

> You have drawn some burns, and you are also trying to enter a number
> for the percentage of burn area.
>
> Do you want to keep the drawing (and lose the percentage),
> **or** do you want to keep the percentage (and lose the drawing)?
>
> [Keep the drawing]   [Keep the percentage]

Figure 10.2. A mock-up of how Mersey Burns might be modified, to handle an
error that is currently not noticed by Mersey Burns and therefore could cause problems. The choice above could be given to the user so they can sort out the ambiguity — what did they want?

Let's interrupt the Mersey Burns bug story with an actual drug overdose story ...

In July 2013 doctor Jenny Lucca thought she had ordered a drug dose of
160 milligrams, but her computer took this to be 160 milligrams *per kilo-
gram*. As a result, her 16-year-old, 39 kilo patient, Pablo Garcia, got a dose
ordered that was 39 times too high.[125]

A dose 39 times too high? You'd expect the computer to give a warning
and check if such a large dose is what's really wanted.

The computer Jenny was using certainly warned about overdoses, but it
also warned about even small 0.1 mg overdoses, which rarely matter. So everyone has learned to ignore its alarms — there are thousands of them a day,
and most mean nothing critical.[126] Staff get what's called **alarm fatigue**,
and start ignoring alarms and even taking action to silence alarms, which can
have knock-on effects. Patient harms and deaths have happened because of
alarm fatigue.[127] Even patients have been known to silence irritating alarms.

We've talked about the Swiss Cheese Model already.[f] Here one of the
defenses, one of the slices of cheese, doesn't just have a big hole — the whole
slice of cheese has intentionally been *removed*.

The University of California San Francisco (UCSF) Medical Center's Be-
nioff Children's Hospital, where Jenny worked, had a new $7 million phar-
macy robot, which had been bought to eliminate error.

The robot obeyed its instructions flawlessly: it packaged exactly what had
been prescribed. It eliminated any errors human pharmacists might make,
but at the same time it also eliminated the human oversight the pharmacists
previously would have provided.

---

[f] See Chapter 6: Swiss Cheese Model, page 61 ←

Like many digital systems, the robot had only been designed to do what it was told.

Back on the ward, Brooke Levitt, Pablo's nurse, took the pills packaged by the robot. She scanned their barcodes, all 38½ of them, which the computer duly dispensed to match the prescription. This system has been installed to be perfect and eliminate error, after all.

About six hours later, Pablo's arms and legs started jerking. He stopped breathing.

The point is: a bug allowed an error to happen unhindered, and the app or the pharmacy robot didn't notice — and the preventable error turned into an incident. It's a bit like a car crash happening and the seat belts or the air bags failing and not reducing driver and passenger harm, so that a bump escalates into injury.

The *idea* to catch errors would improve any medical system. Errors happen. If the computer can spot errors and warn the user, or block the errors, or even correct the errors, then the errors won't cascade into patient harm. The computer should be part of the team that makes healthcare safer, not a disinterested bystander that lets anything happen without comment. The computer, robot, app or medical device should be another slice of cheese in the Swiss Cheese Model.

I personally would make digital system manufacturers liable for ignoring bugs. I'd also have a rule that if a system alarms more than (say) 5 times an hour, then the manufacturer is *automatically liable* (legally called a strict liability) — a busy nurse *cannot* be expected to respond to each of 5 alarms, and the manufacturer knows that before they start.

The actual number of alarms (5, for example) should be chosen after doing some experiments,[g] and would probably need to be different for intensive care, general wards, home use, and so on. Even better might be a legal limit on the number of alarms per hour on the ward divided by the number of nurses on the shift. However it's done, manufacturers would then start to make their devices work together to stay within the law, and this would improve interoperability.[h]

Alarms, as they are currently done, are one way of the manufacturers saying they are not accountable for what goes wrong. Alarms are often used as an excuse to move blame onto the nurses or doctors. Of course, *sometimes*, but not very often, alarms are caused by doctors or nurses doing the wrong thing, not very often, or by patients rolling over and pulling lines out, but the point I'm trying to make is that the assumption should not be that it's always the clinicians' fault for not responding to an alarm. Sometimes the alarm problems are induced by the poor designs of the systems clinicians have to use. Instead of first blaming clinicians, then, we need to change the incentives to improve the designs.

---

[g] See Chapter 22: User Centered Design, page 301 →
[h] See Chapter 19: Interoperability, page 245 →

The question is, why do these bugs happen? For Mersey Burns, the answer is that the designers over-simplified the app. When they developed it and tested it, as I am sure they did, they knew what they had designed. They tested whether it worked. And it did. If they demonstrated the app, it would have seemed to work perfectly.

But they did not test it as it would be used. Sooner or later, real users use systems in unexpected ways. People using an app (or anything else) don't have to behave as you expect. A digital healthcare system *must* be able to handle errors and unusual behavior, because they will all eventually happen in pressurized healthcare.

———————————■———————————

Now returning to the Mersey Burns app story.

Chris Seaton, the Mersey Burns programmer, has written candidly about his experience developing Mersey Burns. His writing has its fair share of insightful comments. Here's one:

> Developing a safety-critical app for multiple platforms is an absolute nightmare. I never want to develop this kind of front-end software ever again. Just the mundane problems of iOS [Apple's iPhone/iPad operating system] key management and working with all the different SDKs [software development kits] drained my enthusiasm. Maintaining a project on top of constantly changing platforms is also demoralizing. People would email me and say it didn't run on some Android phone variant I'd never heard of. All the ecosystems are a mess.[128]

Yes, the programming problems don't stop in the app, but go all the way down to the various operating systems and vast software libraries (for instance, for graphics and internet connectivity) that were never intended for digital health applications.[i]

In fact, Chris Seaton took a great deal of care to ensure that the calculations that Mersey Burns does are correct. The calculations are based on the Parkland formula. Every time the app is used, the program runs 5,000 separate tests to check the app is calculating the prescription formula correctly. These 5,000 tests were themselves generated by another program (hopefully *that* program was checked independently).

Ultimately, all medical app calculations have to be referred back to the original medical research literature, and here's a serious problem for every digital healthcare system and their developers: *the medical literature is not interested in programming or in digital risk.*

Unfortunately, most of the medical information on the Parkland formula, the basis of Mersey Burns, is behind pay walls (which means that you have

---

[i] See Chapter 27: Heartbleed bug, page 369 →

to pay to read it), but Wikipedia has an accessible article.[129] In brief, the formula for the volume of fluid to be prescribed, V in milliliters (mL), is given as $V = 4 \times m \times A \times 100$, with the patient weight m in kilograms, and A being the percentage body area of the burn (hence the 100 in the equation).

That formula might seem simple enough, but where Mersey Burns helps is how magically it works out the percentage burn area from just knowing where you are burned: for example, if your head is burned, that's 9%, but if you're a young child it's more like 18%. Your arms are about 18% (9% each). The percentages change with your weight and age, as, for instance, obese people have relatively smaller heads, and younger people have proportionately larger legs ... and so on. An app that keeps track of all those details helps a lot, especially when the user is under pressure — as they will be with most burns victims being in pain and needing quick assessment.

A formula like $V = 4 \times m \times A \times 100$ doesn't say how to program it. Clinical details don't say how to get numbers into a computer reliably. They don't say how to associate the right numbers with the right patient, nor do they say critical things like a valid percentage burn area must be a number between 0 and 100. The weight has to make sense too: although the formula happily works with negative numbers, patient weights have to be positive. In the US, weights may be entered in Imperial (pounds) as well as metric (kilograms), so an app will have to provide units and conversions if it is to be used internationally. In France and Italy, the decimal point can be a comma rather than a dot. And so on.

Of course, *we* may take all these details for granted. The clinical literature doesn't even mention them. They all seem trivial. Unfortunately, computers don't think like humans. Computers don't know any of these critical details unless they are *very* carefully programmed, so these and other such details are, in practice, likely to go wrong. Any errors or oversights in the program will exacerbate any errors the user makes. If anything goes wrong, harm can happen, and if harm can happen, eventually it will happen.

In other words, while doing 5,000 tests on the correctness of the Parkland formula being used in the Mersey Burns app is essential, it is not sufficient. A good app has to have many more safeguards, particularly for managing use errors.

Despite the very extensive medical literature on burns, there is nothing (that I could find) on calculating the dose reliably *by computer* covering the sorts of design issues listed above.[130]

The Mersey Burns app has other problems I won't discuss here — such as problems with the time of the burns[131] — but these are harder to explain and to understand. The bugs I've shown you here are easy to see, and easy to learn about to avoid, but bugs you *can't* see are more dangerous.

After complaining a bit about Mersey Burns, I need to emphasize that it has been given accolades, and represents the current state of the art. Many

Part I ◇ Diagnosis ◇ Riskier than you think

other healthcare systems and medical apps have worse problems than Mersey Burns!

———————————■———————————

The POTTER app's claim to fame is that it's based on Machine Learning (ML), and it claims to be highly accurate. It also has a peer-reviewed paper about it in the journal *Annals of Surgery*.[132] From the journal's website, it's evident that this is a popular paper, which has been read and tweeted pretty widely (compared to other articles of a similar age). So it's a good app to explore further.

POTTER is a medical app for assessing emergency surgery risk. POTTER is available as an app that runs on both Android and iPhone, so it's easy to check out.

Potter was developed by a team of four people from Massachusetts Institute of Technology (MIT), Massachusetts General Hospital, and the Harvard Medical School, with two PhDs and two MDs between them. Its Machine Learning approach is based on data from 382,960 emergency surgery patients, so it all sounds very impressive. It should be noted that the *Annals of Surgery* will have had peer reviewers approve the paper for it to get published — indeed, the paper itself is followed by some enthusiastic discussion from four doctors from around the world.

Here are two screenshots from POTTER combined into a composite (figure 10.3), which I took from it on 16 January 2019, the day I downloaded it. Unfortunately, the app has no version information at all, so I can't say which version of the app I was using to make these screenshots. Hopefully when you check, it will have been improved. The app has no warranty or CE mark, so it cannot be used in the EU. It provides no warnings, meaningful use or contact information, either, if you need support.

Clearly, the app does little, if any, data validation. There is no warning that none of the data I entered made sense, or even that the numbers I entered, if taken seriously, would indicate seriously ill patients.

You may think my data — answering "1000" for everything — is nonsense. It is! But it's clear proof that *the app does not notice errors*, even gross errors. What more likely errors, probably more subtle errors, will it also fail to notice?

The POTTER app ignored my data errors and suggested that the patient mortality risk is 9.16% of mortality in the next 30 days. The app gives the impression that this erroneous data matches 192 out of 2,096 patients. For fun, if you enter –1000 (yes, I mean you enter a negative number) instead of 1000 for all the numeric answers, it still ignores the nonsense, but it gives 1.09% as the estimate, which is nearly ten times safer! Yet the app is claimed to give surgeons "objective data" on "meaningful survival" so patients at significant risk can forgo surgery.

Obviously, in normal practice, nobody would ever intentionally enter a negative number for a patient's age. There are a huge number keyboards

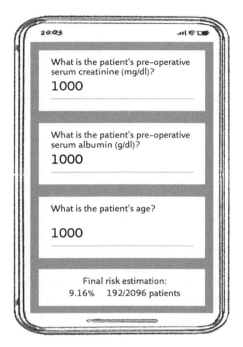

Figure 10.3. Composite drawing of screenshots from the POTTER ML app (version 1.1) for estimating emergency surgery risk. The app ignores gross errors in the data given to it, like entering 1000 for every numeric answer, as shown here. The app still provides an unqualified "final risk estimation" that is nonsense. Reasonable ranges for this data are shown in figure 10.4.

on mobile devices, but the minus key is next to digits on many standard keyboards. One day a negative number *will* be entered accidentally. It's astonishing that an app ignores use errors in its input. Ignoring errors with obviously nonsense numbers makes it plain that the error checking in the app is inadequate.

POTTER uses grams per deciliter, which is the preferred unit of measurement in the US. However, the preferred units to use vary around the world. For example, normal serum albumin levels are 35–50 grams per liter, as opposed to 3.5–5.0 grams per deciliter, which are the units the app uses. This makes the numbers ten times higher than this app expects, and it doesn't notice such errors. Creatinine levels may be in different units (such as μmol/L), which means that a clinician entering numbers in this app is very likely to make massive errors. A medical app like POTTER should check data is entered safely. Clearly, POTTER cannot be used safely internationally outside the US, although the app store makes it available to use anywhere in the world.

Part I ◇ Diagnosis ◇ Riskier than you think

Patient data	Healthy range	What I tested
Age	0–120 yr	1000
Albumin concentration	3.5–5.0 g/dL	1000
Creatinine concentration	0.6–1.3 mg/dL	1000

Figure 10.4. Safe data ranges, compared to the out-of-range extreme test data I entered into the POTTER app, getting the results shown in figure 10.3.

Incidentally, you can't tell from my composite screenshot (figure 10.3) that when the actual POTTER app provides the answer it doesn't summarize the patient data that led it to its conclusion. There is no second chance to notice that the patient's age has been entered incorrectly ...

It is understandable that an experimental prototype app ignores errors, but the paper claims the app is "easy to use." Normally, one would need to do experiments with users to find out if an app is easy to use; the paper provides no evidence of any user experiments whatsoever. Standard easy to use features like "undo" are missing; indeed, pressing the app button resets the entire session (apart from the first answer!), so losing almost all work you've done if you try to correct any of it. An "easy to use" app should not be so easy to use to do the wrong things — especially in a safety-critical area like healthcare.

It's surprising that the paper about POTTER says that it's "highly accurate" and that it "outperforms, in accuracy and user-friendliness, all the current existing risk prediction tools." No evidence is provided for these claims, and the bugs discussed above raise doubts about its quality. In addition, you can't say something is "user friendly," as the paper does, without providing evidence — there are standard ways to assess usability, and none are mentioned. You'd expect something in the appropriate technical language like, "90% of users completed 85% of tasks and reported on a Likert scale that ... [and give the details ...]"

I think it looks like excitement over ML (Machine Learning) has clouded the developers' and the journal's and peer reviewers' collective judgment. One important lesson, then, from POTTER is that just because something is ML or AI or an app doesn't, as such, mean it's ready for clinical use; it just ticks Cat Thinking boxes.[j] It would have been legitimate for the paper to explain the interesting application of ML, which it is, but the paper presents it as an easy to use clinical product. A clinical product must do much more, including error handling, else it cannot be used safely.

I emailed the authors of the paper a copy of this book and pointed out my criticisms above.

Here's their response:

---

[j] See Chapter 3: Cat Thinking, page 25 ←

> [The POTTER app's] ML is designed to function around break points of "less" or "more." So if the algorithm reads, age>65; then you entering 1000 still kicks in towards that wing of the tree.

So *any* age larger than 65 is taken as "older than 65," even if it is an impossibly large age, like 600, as might happen if the user, meaning 60.0, accidentally omitted a decimal point — for instance, a child's age of 10.00 could be accepted as 1,000, and hence treated as if they were over 65 without warning that the age is exceptionally large. (There can be reasons why huge patient ages may be critical, so apps should generally provide overrides.[133])

The POTTER authors continued ...

> It goes without saying that goal of POTTER is to help surgeons and physicians counsel patients, and not to be a pandora's box of trials of "can we beat the machine?" Having said that, we are aware of this shortcoming, and trying to design technological solutions to the users who still want to "mess" with it and enter non-realistic values.
>
> You are correct in that POTTER now uses the units used in the US and not several areas in Europe. We are actively working on finding the way to accommodate any unit in the answer with automated behind the scene conversions to make it easy for non-US users.

There's seems to be a confusion here. As the author of this book, I deliberately "messed" with POTTER to see how it responded to use errors. To see if the app validates numbers, such as ages, the simplest thing is to enter an impossibly large number and see if the error checking kicks in. In POTTER it doesn't. But of course real clinical users won't "mess" like me; instead, they will make different errors by mistake, and any app must respond appropriately to errors. Although the POTTER developers rather dismiss it as "messing," it is, in fact, a professional technique for testing programs and for finding bugs, properly called **fuzzing**.[k] If you miss the obvious errors, you're likely to have missed other errors.

I am glad the POTTER developers are aware of problems and are actively trying to design technological solutions for these simple problems; however, two years later (at the time of writing), there have been no new versions and the app's bugs have not yet been fixed.

———————————————————

I'm by no means the only person finding bugs in medical apps. The authors of a paper[134] found bugs in apps: a small survey of 10 apps they did

---

[k] See Chapter 28: Testing and fuzzing, page 389 →

Part I ◇ Diagnosis ◇ Riskier than you think

Box 10.2. Using wild data as a workaround

I enter extreme data like 1000 to help test how apps like POTTER handle use errors with patient ages, but sometimes users enter outlandish data deliberately as part of their work.

Ben Shneiderman was asked to look at the age statistics of an emergency department. Rather than looking at ordinary statistics like the average, he drew pictures of the data, drawing graphs to visualize it. It was immediately obvious to the eye that there was an extreme outlier in the age distribution. Some patients were recorded as being 999 years old![135]

What was actually happening was in the emergency department, patients turned up and nobody knew how old they were, so they were entered in the computer as 999 — the computer doesn't permit "don't know," so the doctors and nurses invented a workaround. If we don't know, we say 999.

That workaround works absolutely fine, until somebody wants to use the data, as the hospital was doing. Unfortunately, the analysis — without the workaround knowledge — is useless. Maybe my entering 1000 to check systems isn't so silly.

---

in 2018 found *three* different answers (36.8, 50, and 375) for the *same* oxygenation index (OI) calculation.

The paper says "it is therefore important to confirm how the website or application calculates the OI before relying on it," whereas I'd suggest, rather, that it'd be far better for the developers to get it right, not leave it to the clinician using it to sort out the problems when they're busy looking after a patient. They have much better things to be doing than debugging apps. The developers should be using professional development methods, including User Centered Design[1] — including doing representative experiments with real users doing real tasks. In particular, without the insights of UCD, developers will underestimate and ignore use error.

As well as bugs caused by poor programming, there's also the possibility of deliberate faults, the possibility of fraud. Some developers want to make money by attracting investors regardless of whether their apps really work. It's very easy — it's very tempting — to demonstrate unfinished products as if they are more polished than they really are. It's clear from discussions throughout this book that the regulators for digital health still have to catch up with the technology even when you assume the developers are doing their best. If, as sadly happens, some companies and developers are devious, then the current regulatory systems are completely inadequate. And it's not just the regulators: if bugs lead to anyone getting harmed, the legal profession is way behind too.[87] The company Theranos is a case in point: a high-profile Silicon Valley medical start-up, involving plenty of digital healthcare

---

[1] See Chapter 22: User Centered Design, page 301 →

promises, was into wholesale fraud.[136] The moral of the Theranos story is that fraud happens so easily, especially when so many people don't understand the technical issues, so they are too easy to fool. Sensible people get sucked into the hype.

Although medical apps have bugs, they are used by trained medical professionals who know what they are doing. They may notice the bugs and so will competently manage any problems that arise. In contrast, there are more "wellness" apps that are used by people who are not medically trained. "Wellness" and health apps cover a huge range of issues, from suicide prevention to hair styling, from social running to mind games to delay dementia. Many wellness apps fall into the public health arena, which also includes targeting pollution, poor education, poverty, obesity, smoking, excess drinking, and drug addiction — all major causes of premature ill health and excess death. Partly because manufacturers are able to reduce the liabilities of their business by down-playing the medical relevance of their products, wellness apps are not regulated.

Not surprisingly, wellness is a huge growth area. There are over 300,000 health apps, including tens of thousands related to mental health. Unfortunately, most have the usual range of bugs as well as dubious clinical effectiveness. For instance, a popular mindfulness app rated with five stars and having half a million downloads is no better than a placebo (non-effective) version of the app.[137]

———————————————■———————————————

It seems that enthusiasm for apps trumps rigorous assessment, evaluation, and safety. (Yet another case of Cat Thinking.[m]) Certainly, people have rushed into developing medical software, all of which may be fine for exploring the territory, but without rigorous programming — and rigorous regulation requires rigorous programming — they are not going to be safe for serious clinical use. I also predict that when things go wrong, the compensation and legal systems will have trouble sorting out where blame lies.

I hope you've enjoyed this chapter, but I know talking about bugs can be boring, especially talking about ones that aren't spectacular and can't be seen without getting into details. The problem is, as we tend to avoid talking about boring bugs, we tend to ignore them the rest of the time — and then staff get blamed for bugs we aren't noticing and aren't talking about.

[m] See Chapter 3: Cat Thinking, page 25 ←

Part I ◇ Diagnosis ◇ Riskier than you think

The car industry has made cars much safer since the 1960s. What can we learn from car safety and from why car safety improved to help improve the safety of digital healthcare?

11

Cars are safer

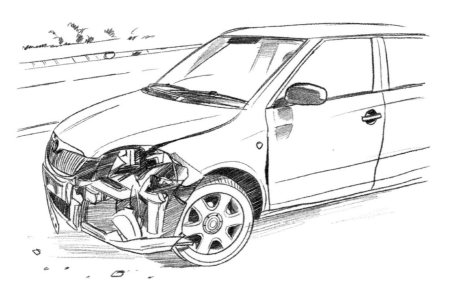

Figure 11.1. My car, after its crash in 2014.

The day before he got married in 2014, my son Isaac asked to borrow my car, a silver Škoda Fabia. Well, of course he could! ... about an hour later, the police telephoned me to say there had been an accident (figure 11.1).

Isaac had hit another car.

It's hard to talk about the crash without saying something like "Isaac had an accident" or "Isaac had hit another car." I doubt that the parents of the other driver talk about Isaac having a crash; if their daughter was called Jane, her parents are likely to talk about the crash *Jane* had. They'd say something like "Jane had hit another car."

Fix It: See and solve the problems of digital healthcare. Harold Thimbleby,
Oxford University Press. © Harold Thimbleby 2021.
DOI: 10.1093/oso/9780198861270.003.0011

It is very hard to talk about an accident without starting to lay the blame on the people we know. It's hard for me to say something like "Isaac was driving the car when an accident happened to him." It would just sound suspicious if I talked in such a convoluted way!

The police said there was a crash at that road junction every week. Put in other words: it doesn't matter who is driving, accidents happen regularly there. So, really, the road junction had the accident. Which in turn means that the local council, who designed and maintain the road junction, caused it. Somebody in the road junction planning department caused the crash.

When we say Isaac had the accident, it's so much clearer, but its simplicity stops us thinking about all the other possibilities. It's too tedious to say some unknown person or persons in the council or maybe somewhere else caused the crash. Simply saying that Isaac had the accident saves us a lot of troublesome thinking and pedantic wording.

So we avoid thinking and talking about the more complex reasons accidents happen, and we avoid a lengthy process of working out the true causes and liabilities. Sadly, the road junction is never going to get safer unless we work out how to make councils more accountable. Perhaps they should pay for every accident? If so, they would soon make dangerous junctions safer. Currently they have no incentives to do so. Since in the way we talk about road accidents we all blame the drivers, we end up using car insurance to pay for everything, and the "cure" is found in repairing the cars (and paying for personal injuries if they happen) rather than fixing the roads and their design.

Likewise, when things go wrong in hospitals, it is so much easier to blame the nurse, the "driver in the room." It is far simpler, and we do not need to start thinking about whether the design or programming of an infusion pump or some other gadget had anything to do with the incident. If we suspect an infusion pump is part of the problem — like the road junction was — we have set ourselves an important, but complex task. We need to understand the inner workings of the thing and where it may have gone wrong. In hospitals, we've the problem of tracking down everything that was in the room — most infusion pumps and other devices are rarely treated in a forensic way: the hospital will have moved the stuff around long before any investigation starts. Far easier to just say Isaac (or whoever the nurse was) "had" the accident. Then we can stop thinking. If we blame the nurse, we can sack them or even send them to prison, and thereby "solve" the problem.

Everyone believes we solved the problem; the bad nurse who let us all down has lost their job — this is a great story for the media. Nurse betrays our trust! Yet the truth is that the real causes have not been uncovered. The system has not changed. The accident can happen again.

There are more interesting things to say about the accident that happened when Isaac was driving. You can see the car has a crumple zone at the front, which has crumpled. The air bag also went off, and it saved him. This is

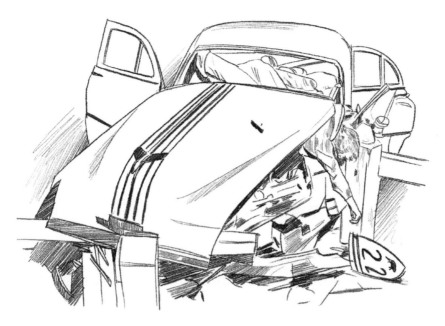

Figure 11.2. A fatal car crash in 1950.

Part II ◇ Treatment ◇ Finding solutions

what crumple zones and air bags are supposed to do: they absorb energy in crashes and save people from more serious injury.

There are also many safety features in modern cars that are harder to see or recognize as such, like the seat belts, the ABS brakes, the "crash box" or rigid frame to protect the passengers, and more. Car manufacturers today want drivers to survive car accidents, or, better, to *avoid* accidents. If your tires and brakes are good (and properly maintained), you can stop in a controlled way, and you may never have an accident, because your car stops before it hits anything or anyone. It's important to buy safe tires, just as it's important to know how to buy and use safe digital healthcare.[a]

Despite the speed of the impact, and the damage to their cars, Isaac and the driver in the other car walked away uninjured.

Safety technology works.

But car accidents weren't always like this.

If Isaac had driven a car fifty or so years ago, perhaps the police would have called me to the scene of a fatal accident. The drawing (figure 11.2) shows a car accident that happened in the 1950s, and which happened at about the same speed. It's comparable. And utterly catastrophic.

Originally, when they were first made, cars were unsafe. Just getting them to work was the main problem! Then the manufacturers said, "drivers

[a] See Chapter 29: Safety ratings will improve healthcare, page 401 →

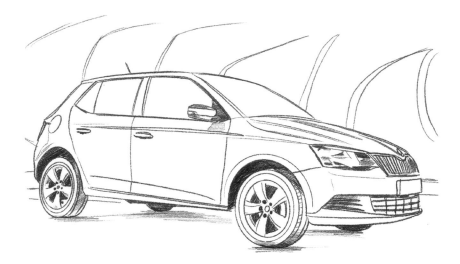

Figure 11.3. A Škoda car poses for promotional literature. Since Ralph Nader, extolling excellent safety ratings helps market a car. Unlike cars, digital healthcare doesn't have safety ratings so nobody can create informed market pressure to improve safety.

have accidents." So, just from the way they talked, it couldn't be the manufacturer's fault, as obviously the drivers had the accidents. Also, drivers of the day wanted fancy cars, and safety wasn't on their agenda either. Everybody, then, blamed the drivers for *their* accidents. How safe the *car* was wasn't part of anyone's thinking.

Then Ralph Nader wrote the shocking book, *Unsafe at Any Speed: The Designed-in Dangers of the American Automobile.*[138]

Ralph Nader's book changed everyone's attitudes to car safety.

Nader pointed out how cars had poor brakes, poor steering, and poor tires, and how manufacturers blamed the drivers. I recommend reading it, as, although he's talking about cars instead of medical systems and devices, he could have been talking about today's hospitals and the "unsafe at any speed" digital systems in them.

I think the most important change Ralph Nader brought about is that instead of saying "drivers have accidents, so it's not our fault," car manufacturers have now changed their emphasis to "drivers have accidents, *therefore we must make safer cars.*"

Now that car safety is recognized as important, car manufacturers compete over safety. Now that there is legislation that requires all manufacturers to build-in safety features, it's no longer uncompetitive to be a manufacturer that invests in safety. Indeed, the Škoda Fabia that Isaac was driving has top safety ratings.

Box 11.1. The problems of buying lemons and selling peaches

New cars come with a specification and a warranty, and customers know what they are buying and the manufacturer sorts out unexpected problems. Nader's achievement was to put safety on the customer's radar, and then this transparent safety market helps it improve — because customers want safe cars, and they may well pay premium prices for safer cars.

New cars are getting safer, but, currently, digital healthcare is much more like the second-hand car market. Customers rarely know enough about what they are buying. The sellers may be concealing problems. There is much more at risk in the second-hand car market because customers are so easy to exploit. Customers often end up with lemons.

On the other hand, if you have a good car that you want to sell — a peach — nobody will trust you, and you won't be able to get a good price for it.

This book shows clearly that many digital healthcare systems are lemons. They have unacknowledged bugs, and the system is set up so that the customers — the patients — are unaware of the risks, and they basically have no recompense. And, on the other hand, if you are a new digital start-up making a safe healthcare product, you'll find it very hard to cover your costs because you can't prove — within the current healthcare regulations — that you've got a peach product.

Maybe this all sounds obvious, but it isn't. George Akerlof's paper "The Market for 'Lemons': Quality uncertainty and the market mechanism" was so insightful it won the 2001 Nobel prize in economics.[139] The digital healthcare market is not yet willing to open itself up to transparent market forces. The resistance to transparency in digital healthcare comes from *all* sides: neither manufacturers nor healthcare organizations, like hospitals and regulators, are happy to go public. Unlike other industries, we take it for granted that patient confidentiality and commercial confidentiality trump the need for transparency, learning, and improvement. Sorting out the digital healthcare market might win another Nobel Prize.

Part II ◇ Treatment ◇ Finding solutions

NCAP, the New Car Assessment Program, is an organization that rates cars for safety.[b] Škoda want us to know they make safer cars (figure 11.3), and NCAP ratings provide a trusted way of assessing safety.

Because the Škoda car has a high NCAP rating, and people want safer cars, it sells well, and thus I ended up with one.

Just as it's easy to talk about *Isaac's* accident, speaking, and thinking as if it was his fault rather than go into a complex story about road design, we make up simple stories when things go wrong in hospitals: we quickly speak and think as if we were let down by the person at the sharp-end. We understand people. People make mistakes. End of story. Sometimes, of course, we *may* have been let down by someone, but our simplistic scapegoat think-

---

[b] See Chapter 32: NCAP mission statement, page 467 →

ing latches on so fast, it's hard to think clearly about the details that matter. (Scapegoat thinking is a very seductive case of attribute substitution, an error we talked about earlier.[c])

When road accidents happen, the police record the types of cars at the scene. If we combine this data with other things we know about cars, like their mileage, we can estimate the riskiness of each type of car.

With medical devices and digital systems we have no idea, because we aren't collecting the data. We don't even know what devices are in use. If we just kept track of what systems hospitals had and combined these with basic statistics on health, such as how long patients stay in each hospital, how many die, how many incidents are reported, we would immediately get some insights — and no doubt lots of interesting questions — into which systems were riskier and which were safer.

But, apparently, we're not interested.[140]

———————————————

Wouldn't it be good if medical devices were as safety conscious as cars? Wouldn't it be good if, when there is an incident in a hospital, manufacturers step in and say, "how can we make our systems safer"?

What do we need to do to change the culture so that hospital safety is improving — just like car safety has improved over the last 50 years, and continues to improve?

---

[c] See Chapter 3: Attribute substitution, page 28 ←

Focusing on the bad stuff is the traditional **Safety One** approach. Safety One is unconstructive. Instead, **Safety Two** means focusing on doing more good. Safety Two emphasizes doing more good things and therefore squeezes out the bad things.

12

Safety Two

We *obviously* want fewer bugs in digital healthcare. If we drew a pie chart of everything that we are doing, it might look like this:

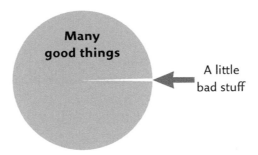

Almost everything we do is good, but a small fraction of what we do sometimes goes bad. This is true whether we are talking about programming, or whether we are talking about what goes on in patient care in hospitals (most patient care is amazing, but some of it falls short). Rather like programming, though, patient care that seems to work perfectly well can suddenly go wrong when something else changes — just like programs always have bugs, but the bugs only surface when the environment pushes the programs into handling something unexpected. The bugs are bad things, whether in programs or how we do patient care. Systems are not perfect. Very fortunately, most of the time we can get away with these lurking problems, but then one day it really matters and something bad happens.

Thinking and worrying about the bad stuff makes us focus on "the bad people," and that's actually counter-productive. The bad things are already past, but what we want is fewer bad things *in the future*. What's happened has happened, but if we can learn how to fix things, we'll be able to avoid *many* future bad things.

Fix It: See and solve the problems of digital healthcare. Harold Thimbleby,
Oxford University Press. © Harold Thimbleby 2021.
DOI: 10.1093/oso/9780198861270.003.0012

Box 12.1. What encourages success?

If you study the bad things that happen in hospitals, the adverse incidents, you are very likely to find workarounds, shortcuts, miscalculations, guidelines not followed, poor use of technology, and other failures. These are all obviously bad things, and they should not be happening. Each problem is caused by staff, so therefore there is a natural tendency for us to blame people and require them to improve.

Sidney Dekker asked what happens in the other incidents — the successful ones are in the majority, after all.[141] If you know what's going right, you can find out how to do better.

What did he find? *Exactly the same things happen.* Workarounds, shortcuts, miscalculations, guidelines not followed, unfriendly technology, and more failures.

So the seemingly "obvious problems" found in adverse incidents do not cause the problems! These things *always* happen. Something else must be making the difference. Dekker and his team dug harder into their data. They found some things were consistently present more frequently when things went well, including:

- Diversity of opinion and people raising dissent.
- Discussing risks.
- Not relying on past success as a guarantee of present success.
- People able to say "Stop." Other people may notice problems.
- Low barriers across seniority and departments.
- Not waiting for audits or inspections before starting to improve.
- Pride in good workmanship.

All these findings can be summarized in just one word, **civility**. There is direct research showing civility makes healthcare safer.[142] Civility is something that computers are generally very bad at.

The people caught up in bad situations, or caught up in situations that were *nearly* bad ones (often called **near misses**), have fantastic insights into how to help improve. They could become helpers rather than scapegoats.

Here's the thing. As the pie chart above makes clear, it's obvious that doing a higher proportion of good stuff is *the same* as doing a smaller proportion of bad stuff. When we know how to do more good stuff tomorrow, doing so will inevitably squeeze out some of the bad stuff that might have happened. If we don't learn from bad stuff, it'll just happen again. Indeed, as any Human Factors specialist will tell you: the first thing to do to fix a problem is to redesign the system to help stop the problem happening. The first thing to do is to learn.

As Ignaz Semmelweis found out:[a] if someone gets infected they may die, but it is far better to wash your hands and avoid passing on infection in the first place. Worrying about the mistake somebody made to get infected is **Safety One** thinking. Washing hands is **Safety Two** thinking — it avoids the problems Safety One obsesses about.

This isn't to say that inquiring into bad things is wrong, but *only* thinking about what went wrong and who to blame is wrong.

At the sharp-end of clinical practice, focusing on the bad things and "bad people" doing them (adverse incidents, patient harm ...) is called **Safety One**.[143] It is the traditional approach. Clearly we want to reduce error, so when it happens, we focus on it and its causes.

Typically in Safety One we blame the staff involved, but, interestingly, as we succeed in reducing problems, we are increasingly unaware of what is actually going wrong. We have less data about problems to analyze. Ironically, Safety One leads to what's called the **regulator's fallacy**: the more you regulate problems, the less data you get to help you improve. The incident data becomes noise. And who wants to admit harming a patient? If we maintain the fiction that nothing has gone wrong *yet* ("we don't have problems here!"), who wants to be the first person to report an incident? Nobody.

In contrast, the more you employ Safety Two thinking, the more good ideas you get, and the easier it is to be safer. (And that's without taking into account the infectiousness of celebrating successes.)

Safety Two focuses on the good things that are being done. The problems that are being solved. How we helped patients go home happy and healthy. As Safety Two succeeds, it gets *more and more* success stories. It gets more success data to go on, and creates a virtuous cycle.

Crucially, focusing on the good stuff instead of the problems changes our perspective. We can learn to do better. Doing better is systematic, whereas each bad error — as Swiss Cheese makes clear[b] — is mostly a chance combination of factors, usually from which we can learn little other than that we were just unlucky. Swiss Cheese makes clear that those hazardous factors are around all the time. The thing that's interesting is how we can best avoid them. Without Safety Two thinking, we may never work it out.

Would you learn how to make houses safer if you only studied houses that fell down? You could learn a bit, but you'd learn far more if you also studied successful houses that stayed up and why they stayed up. In particular, if you don't investigate anything until something falls down, then you only learn about the accidental particulars of the failure. To be able to build safe houses, you need to know what safe engineering practice is: what are the principles that ensure houses are stable and that keep houses *up*?

I heard of a sailor on an aircraft carrier who was given a decoration for picking up a wrench. If an aircraft had landed on the flight deck and hit the

---

[a] See Chapter 2: Ignaz Semmelweis, page 15 ←
[b] See Chapter 6: Swiss Cheese Model, page 61 ←

> **Box 12.2.** The orange-wire test
>
> Conventional accident and incident investigations try to find out what went wrong. This is Safety One thinking. It has its place, but rarely makes much difference to the rest of the world. With Safety Two thinking, incident investigations try to find out what went right, and also what can be put right for a safer future.
>
> Liam Donaldson's **orange-wire test** is an analogy made with aviation safety.[144] Imagine an airline engineer finds a faulty orange wire on a plane. Suppose the state of the wire suggests a systematic fault, which will affect all planes of the same type. In aviation, it's standard practice that all planes in the world will be prioritized for inspection and fixed as appropriate. In healthcare, currently, when there is an investigation, the investigation looks backwards to determine what caused the adverse event — and because the investigation is couched in local terms, nobody else is much interested in it. But like the orange-wire test, the incident analysis should also be proactive: what has it learned that can help improve healthcare worldwide? And how can healthcare worldwide respond to fixing the problems identified?
>
> Incident reporting systems need modifying with Safety Two in mind. Investigations must know what digital systems are relevant to an incident, and they should seek out the "orange wires" — the bugs, the system flaws still lurking to keep on causing problems. Immediately all manufacturers should be informed, as well as all healthcare organizations using those systems. (This is easy using the internet, of course — provided there is an incident reporting system that supports doing so.)
>
> When manufacturers and local IT managers respond and fix the problems, the orange-wire test has been passed.

wrench, the accident of dropping the wrench would have turned into the catastrophe of a fast jet hitting it and causing chaos. The sailor was given an award for stopping an accident turning into a catastrophe. The interesting thing is that nobody was interested in who dropped the wrench — it could even have been the very person who picked it up. Worrying about blame — who dropped the wrench? — is Safety One thinking. Instead, the award celebrated safety and helped improve safety through Safety Two thinking — yes, accidents happen, but the important thing is avoiding catastrophes by doing the right thing more often.

In my imagination, somebody would have debriefed the sailor, and found out what good ideas they had for improving things. Maybe sailors working on the flight deck will then be given better tool belts so they are less likely to drop wrenches? Who knows, but if Safety One had been used to blame the sailor, many ideas for improvement would never have been considered. The sailor would have been disciplined and sidelined. Improvement would not have happened.

The analogy with healthcare is closer than it might at first seem. Aircraft

> **Box 12.3.** Never events and always conditions
>
> There are some sorts of bad incidents that seem so horrible that we never want them to happen. If, further, we think they should have been prevented, then we start on the route of defining **never events**. Here're two standard never events: "Intravenous administration of mis-selected concentrated potassium chloride," and "Patient suicide." The idea is that when a never event happens, it is investigated and taken very seriously.
>
> Never events are Safety One thinking. One problem with never events is that there are lots of horrible things that can happen, and an official list of never events will never be long enough. Another problem is that if certain events should never happen, when they do happen it seems that somebody must be to blame. Conversely if there is an incident that is not a Never Event, it won't be taken so seriously — though the patient might be unable to tell the difference, especially if they died.
>
> In contrast, Safety Two encourages thinking about **always conditions**. What can we *always* do to make the best outcomes happen more often?
>
> Needlestick injuries happen when somebody jabs themselves with a sharp object, like a syringe needle. If the needle was contaminated, typically by blood, needlestick injuries can be very serious.
>
> One approach to needlestick injuries would be to say we must *never* have needlestick injuries — if so, we'll likely end up with rules that blame anyone who hurts themselves. Alternatively, we could *always* buy syringes like VanishPoint,[145] where the needle is automatically retracted after use. With VanishPoint, it's almost impossible to get a contaminated needlestick injury by accident.
>
> One of the key lessons to learn from needlestick injuries is that better-designed technology can reduce errors and harms. Especially with digital technologies.

maintenance crew are obsessed with Foreign Object Damage (FOD), such as dropping nuts and bolts into aircraft and losing tools. Tools are counted in and out and signed for so they don't get left behind or left on the flight deck, just like surgical instruments and swabs in an operating theater are double-checked so none are accidentally left in the patient.

Safety One is the dominant cultural assumption in healthcare, as well as in wider society, including the media. It is so easy to blame "blundering" doctors and nurses in a witch hunt — there are many examples in this book where poor digital systems caused problems that were blamed on the health-care staff. The "blame game" achieves nothing, but exacerbates the blame and then the self-blame of people caught up in the incidents. It then badly, sometimes catastrophically, affects mental health, and therefore undermines the effectiveness of all of healthcare.[85]

A memorable way to summarize Safety Two thinking is, "Start with what's strong, not with what's wrong."[146]

There's a lot more to digital health than being excited about digital computing. We need to learn how to think computationally to take full advantage of digital. **Computational Thinking** is the mature way to think about computing — and digital healthcare.

(Don't forget that the computer chip means that this is a more technical chapter.)

13

Computational Thinking

When Charles Babbage started to design the world's first digital computer in 1822,[147] he was so far ahead of his time that he had to build it out of brass gear wheels. He was very excited by the potential of his Difference Engine, as he called it, and as he built it he had so many new ideas he could not resist abandoning it to start building an even more powerful successor, the Difference Engine No 2. He never finished Difference Engine No 2 either, because by 1837 he had become obsessed with new ideas for an even more exciting computer, one that he called the Analytical Engine.

Apart from the fact that he failed to finish his Difference Engines and see them work, on the plus side his Analytical Engine would have been the world's first ever programmable computer.

He didn't finish his Analytical Engine either.

Babbage did, however, inspire Ada Lovelace, who has gone down in history as the world's first programmer. (The programming language Ada,[a] which we'll meet again, was named after her.) Ada, Countess of Lovelace, was way ahead of her time, and she is noteworthy for realizing that one day computers would be able to do far more than mere calculation — they could, for instance, compose music. She wrote this prescient piece in 1843:

> Supposing, for instance, that the fundamental relations of pitched sounds in the science of harmony and of musical composition were susceptible of such expression and adaptations, the engine might compose elaborate and scientific pieces of music of any degree of complexity or extent.[148]

Ada also anticipated mathematical modeling of the human body, in particular she thought about the nervous system, so in some ways she anticipated modern digital healthcare. Her notes[148] have been called the most

---

[a] See Chapter 27: SPARK Ada, page 375 →

Fix It: See and solve the problems of digital healthcare. Harold Thimbleby,
Oxford University Press. © Harold Thimbleby 2021.
DOI: 10.1093/oso/9780198861270.003.0013

important document in Computer Science before modern times, and, certainly they are full of fascinating analysis and insights.

The London Science Museum constructed a replica of Babbage's Difference Engine to the same engineering standards as were available to him in the 1800s. It performed its first calculation in 1991.[149] The Science Museum then built Babbage's printer, just as he'd designed it, and finally got it to work in 2000.

You can argue that Babbage, the archetypal British eccentric inventor, was nearly two centuries ahead of his time, or you can argue that his Difference Engine certainly set a very high bar for the longest delay to computer projects.

Over a century after Babbage, during World War II (1939–1945), Alan Turing helped design some amazing electro-mechanical devices to crack Germany's secret Enigma code.[b] Years ahead of his time, by 1950 Turing had also anticipated and worked out some of the key ideas about Artificial Intelligence.

But back in 1936, three years before the war, Turing had already published a very remarkable article about a simple but general purpose computer, which has now come to be called the **Turing Machine** in his honor. He wrote this before any computers had actually been built, but he showed that, in theory, once you build a sufficiently powerful computer it can do anything. *Anything at all that any computer can do.* This is a stunning insight.

Turing designed Turing Machines as very simple computers. He made them so simple so that he could explore the fundamental limits of computing. What Turing found was that once you've got a few bits of a computer working, it will be powerful enough to simulate *any* computer, and so it can do all the things that any computer can do.

It is easy to make a Turing Machine, as they are so simple. Anything powerful enough to behave like a Turing Machine is now called **Turing Complete**, because, as Turing showed, no computer can do anything more powerful than a Turing Machine can. As if to prove the point, Turing Machines have been built out of Lego and even out of wood (figure 13.1).[150]

Many things are powerful enough, but nothing is more powerful: nothing can do more sorts of computing than Turing's original machine. This discovery has an amazing implication: there is nothing that is more powerful than a Turing Machine, and every form of computing is equivalent to a Turing Machine. Your brain, for example, cannot do more powerful computing than a wooden Turing Machine! (Though it may well do it faster and more quietly.)

It happened that Alonzo Church had gone down a very similar line of thinking, and so in their joint honor, the **Church–Turing Thesis** is that *all*

---

[b] See Chapter 24: The Enigma Code Machine, page 329 →

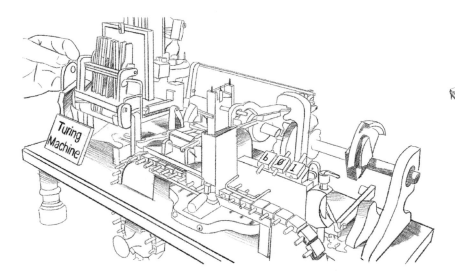

Figure 13.1. The amazing wooden computer built by Richard J. Ridel. Because this machine is a Turing Machine it can (eventually) do anything any computer can do, provided it doesn't run out of wood first. The point is, computers can be made out of anything and they can simulate anything.

forms of sufficiently powerful computing are equivalent. In fact, all sufficiently powerful computers are equivalent to Turing Machines and everything that being a Turing Machine implies, namely that they can simulate any other computer. As the wooden and Lego Turing Machines make clear, computers don't have to be very powerful before they can do *anything*, and they don't have to be made out of digital electronics. The ideas of Turing Completeness and the Church–Turing Thesis are BIG.

If your mobile phone can run apps, it is essentially Turing Complete. In principle, it can run *any* app and do practically anything, so long as you don't run out of memory (or battery). Indeed, being Turing Complete, it can even simulate any computer doing anything. It was a remarkable discovery of Turing's, and firmly established the profound power of computers over our lives. There are now numerous Turing Machine apps that you can run on your mobile.

The amazing visual effects you see in films like Star Trek are just one example of the power of Turing Completeness. Films can now create *any* imaginary world, and they can create the illusion of anything happening — whether that is visualizing ordinary machinery (like spacecraft) doing things, or visualizing computers on a spaceship doing anything computers can do, and so on recursively.

While Turing Completeness enables films to be compelling, as they can simulate anything (they can even do the animations for physically impossible fiction), equally, the power of Turing Completeness creates profound problems at the heart of digital:

> Computers can generate images and experiences that can simulate absolutely anything we can imagine. They can look and feel incredibly realistic, whether they are just a designer's ideas about screenshots or full-on interactive virtual reality. Anything in any film you've ever seen, like Star Trek, can be created and made into a persuasive world. We can imagine a Star Trek doctor and medical suite that does amazing things, and it can be made visible and appear as if it really worked. With computer game technologies you can interact with it as if it was real.

> However, what computers can actually do is logically restricted. In fact, the human limitations of programmers puts further practical restrictions on what is possible — some things are too big or too complex to get our minds around to program correctly. Our creative imagination is not sufficient to ensure things work reliably.

> Digital things that look good may not be good. They may be imaginary. Despite the apparent realism, we have no idea how imaginary they are. We have no idea how many bugs there are in reality. Unless we have an actual, rigorously worked out and confirmed plan, it won't work as we expect.

When I first started teaching programming (in the early 1970s, when everything was much simpler), a first exercise was to write a program to read two numbers and print their sum. In those days, just getting your program into a computer on a stack of punched cards and getting the answer back was quite a learning experience. If your program was accepted, the computer printed the answer on paper, which was then put in a pigeon hole for you to pick up the next day. Our students needed a simple exercise so they could first learn all the arcane procedures, and this was it.

One student handed in a program that said WRITE 15, and it was followed by 7 and 8. I'm simplifying a little bit: the correct answer was a bit more complicated, as it had to be written correctly in a proper programming language — FORTRAN in those days — but this gives the idea the student had.

Yes, the program did print the sum of those two numbers, 7 and 8, perfectly well, as of course $7 + 8 = 15$. But it did not actually read those numbers, nor did it add those numbers and print their sum. If the numbers 7 and 8 were changed to 17 and 25, the program would not print their sum, 42; instead, it would still print 15. The student was thinking that a program that looked like it worked would get marked as correct. His program read two numbers and printed their sum, but what was wanted was a program that could add *any* two numbers and print their sum. This story illustrates some profound problem. It's easy to make a program look like it works if you don't look too closely, but it may be incomplete, imaginary, have bugs, or even be faked to look better than it is. Another problem is that we all knew what the question meant, but you could say the student had legitimately found a buggy interpretation of what we asked them to do, and what he did wasn't what we meant. We asked for a program to add some numbers; his program could do that. What we had *meant* to ask was for a program that could add *any* two numbers. Even then we didn't mean *any* two numbers, as computers can't handle any numbers — we hadn't asked for any error checking! There are limits. So there is a whole mess in what the question actually meant, as well as a mess in what this student gave as an answer.

These quirky problems arise in a very simple example: a first student program. Imagine how complex the problems become in real questions like how to design a hospital computing system. There are fundamental gulfs between what we want digital systems to do, what we tell them to do, what we program them to do, what they really do, and what we realize we meant after things go wrong. And like the student exercise, many of the problems aren't at all obvious until you get something in front of you that is obviously wrong — but you didn't have the foresight to avoid it happening. Bridging all those gulfs is not just hard work — in fact, it's strictly impossible.

This example makes many important, profound points — in fact, too many points to follow up here.[151] For instance, testing a program is not enough to establish whether it's correct. This student's program does pass a test: it adds 7 and 8 and correctly gets 15. Unfortunately, this test is inadequate, as is obvious — but it's only obvious in hindsight, because we've understood the conceptual error in the student's program. Usually, we can't see the program, and therefore testing in general can *never* be sufficient — they may seem to work, but still have bugs we've missed. And real programs are *far* more complicated than this utterly trivial student example. Potentially, they pass every test you throw at them, yet they still have bugs lurking somewhere that you've missed.

Turing also showed that there are some things a Turing Machine cannot do, regardless of its power — these things are now called **non-computable**.

If something is non-computable, a computer cannot do it. More precisely, it cannot do it correctly — there must be bugs. So, before you start programming, you need to show your ideas are computable, that they will work in principle.[152] If you try to develop a program that does something that in principle is non-computable then your program *must* have bugs.

It's possible, unavoidable even, that many things humans do informally in healthcare are non-computable — if anybody wrote down precisely what a computer had to do to get these things done, it would in principle show up the inconsistencies. There'd be bugs as the computers make the inconsistencies visible — computers don't do *ad hoc* workarounds when things are strictly impossible to do by the letter. When computers crash or have interoperability problems, they are just making the bugs visible.

Turing showed that if something is computable, there are any number of ways you can do it. In contrast, if something is non-computable, it won't work correctly however you try to do it. A practical insight following from this rather technical idea is to try to avoid **implementation bias**: that is, avoid premature concern for *how* something is to be done, before working out *what* is to be done and whether it will work. For example, many people want healthcare to move away from paper and faxes to modern email. But email is just a faster way of doing what paper and faxes do: it's just a change in implementation and it doesn't change what the computation is. The question should be not can we do what paper does but faster, but *what* does paper do? What does paper compute (or what do people compute with paper)? Paper keeps clinicians up-to-date with patient information, for example. What would be a good way of doing that? Possibly, having a shared database. That would mean clinicians could share all information and you would not need email.

The point here is: paper can't provide a shared database. To improve paper, you want to find out what you were trying to compute, not just try to make paper more efficient. Making paper more efficient — computerizing it — doesn't address the fundamental problems that need solving.[95]

The point is, email does what paper does and certainly much faster and in many ways better. But paper is an implementation trying to solve a problem. We need to find out what the problem is, not think paper is the problem that needs solving. Computerizing what we are already doing — replacing paper with computers — is having implementation bias. We end up with computers highlighting the problems paper has, so much faster that we complain about the problems of computers, when really the problems are the previously unappreciated problems that paper has made an inadequate attempt at doing.

———————————————■———————————————

But back to the history of computing. It took another ten years after Turing's ideas for the world's first recognizably modern computer, the ENIAC, to be built. The ENIAC was built at the US University of Pennsylvania, and was working properly by 1946.[153]

Before John Mauchly and Presper Eckert had finished building the ENIAC, they had already started work on its successor, the EDVAC, which they proposed in 1944 for $100,000. They got it working seven years later, delivered at a cost five times higher.

All this ancient history of digital computing has set precedents we haven't shaken off. It's still considered normal to be continually updating and revising digital systems. Life-critical systems, in some areas like aircraft and space-flight software, however, are remarkably stable and reliable.

The furthest humans have ever traveled from Earth was in the very nearly

> **Box 13.1.** The British EDSAC computer
>
> The British competitor to ENIAC and EDVAC was EDSAC, the Electronic Delay Storage Automatic Calculator. EDSAC was the first computer to run a video game, and was the world's first proper digital computer with a completely stored program. EDSAC was constructed by Maurice Wilkes and ran its first programs in 1949. (I am a proud holder of the British Computer Society's Wilkes Medal.)
>
> Wilkes is famous for this 1949 quote about bugs:
>
>> It was on one of my journeys between the EDSAC room and the punching equipment that the realization came over me with full force that a good part of the remainder of my life was going to be spent in finding errors in my own programs.
>
> Emphasizing the fact that any sufficiently powerful computer (human brain or actual computer) can simulate any other, the EDSAC can now be simulated on Windows, Macintosh, and Linux computers.[154] The project that built the EDSAC simulator quotes this from 1949:
>
>> There are not enough "brains" to go around at the moment, but a dozen would probably be sufficient for the whole country ... The future? The "brain" may one day come down to our level and help with our income-tax and book-keeping calculations. But this is speculation and there is no sign of it so far.
>
> Computers were specialized and might do tedious numerical work for us, but networks, social media, and entertainment — let alone digital healthcare — weren't anticipated.

disastrous 1970 space flight of Apollo 13, dramatized in the film of the same name.[155] It flew around the moon using computers that were huge, filling rooms, but were far less powerful than your mobile phone. It's amazing how computers have become so powerful and become so small. My iPhone XR, which easily fits in my pocket, is an amazing example of how computing has totally transformed in just a few years (figure 13.2). I wonder what technology will soon be able to do, eclipsing my iPhone in the same way my iPhone eclipsed Apollo.

In the early days of computing, computers weren't so powerful, and we struggled to get computers to do the work we wanted them to do. They were so slow, and they hardly had enough memory to do anything useful. Getting something as simple as doing a payroll — printing out checks to pay your staff — was a lot of hard work. The computers were only just big enough to handle all the data. So our programs had to be correct, small, and efficient, else nothing would work.

	1951 **EDVAC**	2019 **iPhone XR**
Cost	$500,000 (over $5M in 2019 money)	$900
Weight	7,800 kg	0.2 kg
Power consumption	56 kW	0.00173 kW
Floor space	45.5 sq m	0.00063 sq m (upright)
Bits of memory	44,000	2,048,000,000,000
Speed in operations per second	340	5,000,000,000,000
Active components in processor	6,000 valves	6.9 billion transistors
Error-free runs	8 hours	Months
Number of human operators	34	1
Other features	Oscilloscope for output	Wi-Fi, camera, microphone, accelerometer, GPS, phone, streaming video, and more

Figure 13.2. One lifetime of digital progress. Digital technology is not only unbelievably more powerful, but it's personal: almost everybody has far more powerful computing literally at their finger tips than could have been imagined only a few years ago. What's coming next?

We didn't realize it at the time, but we were developing the science of thinking clearly about how to tell a stupid thing, the computer, how to solve a problem quickly. Soon, that process got to be called **algorithmics**,[156] and finding the best, usually the *fastest*, algorithm for a computer to solve a problem became a popular occupation — programming.

Then Jeannette Wing noticed that we were doing something much bigger.[157] We were in fact finding the best way to solve problems, whatever the thing doing the solving was, even if it *wasn't* a digital or electronic computer. It could be a human brain, or a group of humans, or even insects.

All the methods we have of solving problems with computers, even AI, are methods that solve problems with anything — thanks to the Church–Turing Thesis and Turing Completeness. Hence **Computational Thinking** is the way of thinking about computational problems, where "computational" takes on the very broad view that Turing realized. Almost anything "computes," so we take Computational Thinking to mean the general ways to understand problems to precisely and correctly specify how an **agent** can reliably solve all possible variations of the problems repeatedly without error[158] and without supervision.

In that definition of Computational Thinking, I've introduced the term **agent**. An agent could be a computer, and precisely specifying how it behaves might, of course, mean doing some programming. But thanks to the Church–Turing Thesis, an agent equivalently can also means a human, an organization, a team, an operating room, a bureaucracy, the legal system of a country, a robot, an autonomous AI agent, even an ant or microbe — that is, an agent is anything that can do things following rules.

An important point is that Computational Thinking involves **indirection**. It isn't just about solving a problem, but it's about solving a problem so generally so somebody else or something else — a computer, an agent, whatever — can repeatedly solve the problem in all its forms, again and again. (That's the indirection.)

For example, sorting a list of patients in front of you into alphabetical order is ordinary problem solving; but working out how to get a computer to correctly sort any number of patients into alphabetical order is a step more complicated. You can't cheat; you have to figure out a general method that always works under any circumstances thrown at it. You have to cope with patients with the same surname but different forenames; you have to cope with accents; you have to anticipate quirky variations — like sorting no patients at all, or sorting a list of patients including those with missing names because we don't know them. This is the indirection: Computational Thinking is solving every possible form of a problem so that an autonomous agent can solve any particular case of the problem without bugs.

Computational Thinking gets more fun when we realize that the agent may not be very reliable: the question arises how to block, detect, and recover from problems and errors. You can see Computational Thinking is essential in healthcare. It is how good **standard operating procedures** (SOPs) — such as the rules nurses should follow to do clinical procedures — should be devised.

Computational Thinking is best thought of as the set of methods that Computer Science uses to do its science. Other sciences have their methods, like controlled experiments, randomized controlled trials,[c] surveys, triangulation, laboratory work, or field work, and so on. Computer Science has **Computational Thinking**.

At the beginning of this book,[d] we saw how the discovery of biological bugs transformed the thinking around disease and infection — we now have methodologies that worry about and manage sterilization, cross-infection, contamination, and more. We now know that to do good science (as well as a whole host of other things, like safe cooking) you have to have reliable ways of working that take account of something you simply cannot see. Similarly, as we are maturing how we think about digital, not least learning about our own unnecessary bugs, Computational Thinking is the collection of appro-

Part II ◇ Treatment ◇ Finding solutions

---

[c] See Chapter 28: Randomized Controlled Trials, page 393 →
[d] See Chapter 2: We don't know what we don't know, page 15 ←

priate methodologies for doing good digital work. Computational Thinking helps us be successful and reliable in everything we do with digital, even though a lot of it may seem unnecessary because we can't see the real but intangible things it is sorting out for us.

In short, mature, responsible digital, programming, computer science, IT, Health IT, informatics — whatever you want to call it — should be based on doing Computational Thinking.

Computational Thinking collects together a wide range of powerful, tried-and-tested ideas, and techniques. I'll explore a few in this chapter.

First, though, why should digital healthcare worry about Computational Thinking anyway? Doesn't digital healthcare work well enough without getting "computational" or having a "methodology"? In most areas of digital, serious Computational Thinking doesn't really matter, so long as the systems work well enough. In many areas, what the computers are doing is very flexible (like graphics for movies); in many areas digital is pretty straightforward, like in banking. Even if you are richer or poorer than I am, your bank account works just like mine.

In areas like aviation, what digital has to do is complicated, but it's very well defined; for instance, aviation programmers know they have to keep the plane operating within its safety envelope. Basically, planes obey basic laws of physics, and they keep well away from each other.

In healthcare, though, things are much more complex. We don't really know what is going on, and every clinician does things differently. No two patients are the same, men and women are different, pregnant women are different, children are different — and many patients tinker with their own treatment (otherwise known as **compliance issues**). Some patients have diseases, others have injuries, some have dementia, some are unconscious on life support, and many have mixtures of problems (**comorbidities**). Each patient is unique.

Mistakes can kill or harm patients; thinking very clearly about digital healthcare is essential. Drugs have side effects, and they can interact with each other when a patient is on more than one. Computers need to keep track of them. Then there is the billing and monitoring, keeping track of equipment and use-by dates ... and much, much more. As we've seen repeatedly in this book, we are not generally thinking clearly enough about digital in healthcare. While the details may seem overwhelming, Computational Thinking is about *how* we should think; it's offering a strategic, proven, way to improve digital healthcare.

Good programmers do all sorts of things to help their computers perform quickly, efficiently, and reliably. They have developed a wide range of rigorous techniques to help. Computational Thinking says these ideas can be used for many more things than just programming digital computers.

Computational Thinking is very rich. I made a list of key insights for this book, but it quickly grew to over fifty ideas, so I've selected a few of

> **Box 13.2.** Reproducibility is essential
>
> I realized that Computer Science didn't follow standard scientific methods when I noticed some implausible articles in the respectable *Journal of Machine Learning Research* back in 2004. I noticed that many articles were not **reproducible**.[159]
>
> Reproducibility is a core part of good science, and hence of Computational Thinking: it means that the work you do should be explained fully so that others can reproduce it and check it.[160] If research in science is not reproducible, nobody can check it, and one begins to suspect whether it was accurately reported in the first place. In an exciting field like Machine Learning and digital healthcare, reproducibility is critical.
>
> Reproducibility is only just starting to be acknowledged as a very serious issue for digital healthcare. Why should we believe reports of the effectiveness of new digital healthcare ideas if nobody can check them? There are obvious conflicts of interest: people want to convince us their healthcare innovations are amazing, but they don't want to give away trade secrets. Taken together, that encourages them to exaggerate without risk of anyone being able to check their claims. If independent scientists can't reproduce a digital health report, why should any of its claims be believed to work in healthcare?
>
> Ironically, everything in digital healthcare is based on computer programs, and computer programs are very easy to share and reproduce. Every research paper on digital healthcare, those that purport to be science, should provide a web address where to get full details of what is being done. Furthermore, modern digital cryptography provides many useful techniques to help, for instance to provide certificates to ensure the website is in fact materially the same as the website that was reported in the published paper.
>
> Once we get reproducibility sorted out, digital health regulators should demand peer-reviewed evidence — publicly checkable articles in scientific journals — that proposed products work as claimed. Everything would get safer.

the more powerful and easier-to-explain ideas that have direct relevance to digital healthcare. My examples are rather "programmy," because I want to emphasize that programmers have a vast repertoire of ideas to draw on that can contribute to healthcare system design.

The first idea in my list, computational complexity, shows that digital healthcare regulation has to get involved in best practice, and start to regulate the details of programming digital systems.

Computational complexity

We know that many things that computers do, like sorting patient names into alphabetical order, are very easy to do. But there are some things, like scheduling operating rooms, that are much harder to do.

The idea from Computational Thinking is to work out a problem's **computational complexity**, and then you have a precise idea of how hard it is to do. Most things we ask computers to do have a low complexity: matching patients to their beds is easy, but scheduling operating rooms is *much* harder. In fact, scheduling operating rooms is *very* hard, especially as emergencies keep changing the schedule in real time. Since it is so hard, Computational Thinking about it suggests asking for some help: for instance, if one operating room was reserved for emergencies and never scheduled for routine operations, that would make the problem much easier to solve.[161]

Some problems have a complexity that goes up exponentially (called **combinatorial explosion**), and these are problems you really want to avoid having to solve — or you have to come to terms with imperfect solutions that can be solved more easily, but not as well.

Combinatorial explosion makes program testing hard. Very hard.

This point underlies almost every problem in digital healthcare. As programs get bigger, testing them thoroughly becomes totally impractical. If a program has one test, say testing if the patient is diabetic or not diabetic, then there are two separate outcomes to check — does the program work correctly when the patient is diabetic, and does the program work correctly when the patient is not diabetic?

Two checks doesn't sound too onerous. But as the number of program tests increases, the number of checks suffers combinatorial explosion. A lot depends on exactly how the program is structured, but basically, two more tests will need 8 checks to cover all possibilities, 3 more tests will need 16 checks ... With only 10 tests, already 1,024 checks are needed to cover every combination. The numbers start getting larger and larger very rapidly, exponentially, in fact. For 11 tests 2,048 checks are needed — now, going from 10 to 11, just one more test adds over a thousand more checks to be done.

Mersey Burns[e] is a program that has 1,125 explicit tests in its code. If we could check each case quickly, say in only a minute (assuming we knew what should happen for each test, and assuming we can work 24 hours a day, 7 days a week, and all non-stop), then doing the checks needed would take us a lot longer than the age of the universe. In other words, the complexity of even a simple app is such that we can't test it thoroughly; more precisely, we can't test it thoroughly *this way*.

Let's explain it another way, adding an important point.

Instead of thinking about a medical app like Mersey Burns, think of a game app to play chess. Of course, you would do testing to make sure that it can draw a chess board, and that the pieces move nicely. But you would *not* test it works for every possible game of chess: that's impossible, because there are far too many possible games of chess to check.

---

[e] See Chapter 10: Mersey Burns app, page 121 ←

In 1950, Claude Shannon estimated that there are 10^{120} possible chess games.[162] The number has since been revised, but the idea has become so famous that the number is now called the **Shannon Number**. The Shannon Number is a huge number — written down, the Shannon Number is $1,000,000,...,000$ except here I didn't written out in full all of its 120 zeros. In words, the Shannon Number is one million million ... million, with the word "million" repeated twenty times.

The point is, there is no way you can test a chess program thoroughly: the huge Shannon Number shows there are far, far, far too many games to be able to check each one is played correctly. And here's the important point: to check a chess program this way, would you have to know what should happen in every possible game, and nobody can play chess that well!

Chess is too hard to test, and unfortunately almost every medical app or digital system is *much* harder than chess.

The conclusion is that we cannot rely on testing. Instead, you sample a manageable number of cases to persuade you the app basically works, then you have to rely on the program being so well written that there are very few (preferably zero) bugs left that you haven't spotted. The question is: how can you write a program that you can rely on when testing is not sufficient?

David Parnas is the key character who cracked this problem.[163] If programs are broken up into independent **modules**, then the modules can be tested independently. Since they can be checked independently, the worst of the combinatorial explosion is avoided. If you write a program that includes a previously checked module, you do not need to waste much time re-checking it. Indeed, most of your "checking" will be checking whether you properly understand how the module works so you can use it reliably. Moreover, the more people use a module, the more real-world checking it will get and the more reliable you can assume it will become.

Unfortunately, Mersey Burns has no modules, and so Computational Thinking therefore tells us we cannot check it effectively.[164] Mersey Burns is a typical digital system, so this isn't a criticism of Mersey Burns, but is a weakness almost all (if not all) current digital healthcare systems suffer from: we cannot reliably check typical digital healthcare systems thoroughly enough to be sure they are free from bugs. Therefore we cannot eliminate harm caused by digital systems.

The deeper value of testing is not just that it finds mistakes in a program (which you want to understand and then fix), but that it shows that the way you made the program let some faults get through. If you fix the faults in the way you designed the program, which allowed the bugs to happen, you can now fix many bugs in one go, even ones you have not yet found. In other words, truly understanding a bug means not understanding why the program failed, but understanding how you managed to overlook the problem when designing the program. The aim, then, is to correct the *cause* of the bug, rather than be distracted into the temptation of fixing one bug at a time. It is very hard to think like this, because the main reason bugs happen bugs happen is that the programming process is not rigorous enough, and working out how to program better is very hard to do on your own. It's easier, and unfortunately distractingly satisfying, to fix bugs one at a time.

Seeing finding bugs as finding problems with the design process like this is a bit like the thinking behind Safety Two. You are interested not so much in problems, but in having a process to do better.

The important insight from this discussion is that medical device regulation will only be effective when it starts to address *how* programs are designed and built. Current digital health regulation is steeped in quality control processes (like writing documentation) and not in exactly how programs are constructed. It's a bit like having building regulations without demanding to see and check the structural engineering calculations — and if it's a hospital, it'll have all sorts of requirements for infection control, handwashing stations, ventilation, and more to make it work safely and effectively for healthcare. Buildings may look nice, but may not be safe. Likewise, under today's digital health regulations, digital systems can look nice but not be sufficiently safe.

Tony Hoare summed up the choice perfectly in his 1980 Turing Award lecture:

> There are two ways of constructing a software design. One way is to make it so simple that there are *obviously* no deficiencies. And the other way is to make it so complicated that there are no *obvious* deficiencies.[165]

Until we more tightly regulate digital healthcare to require professional methods to program safely, we'll continue to suffer from unnecessary bugs, and therefore both patients and healthcare professionals will continue to suffer preventable harms from using digital systems. To be more realistic, digital healthcare regulation needs to be more mature. In building safety, mentioned above, there are a whole range of regulations that are enforced differently in different aspects of building. The gas safety, the electric safety, the fire safety, the structural safety are all regulated, and collectively make a coherent whole.

In digital healthcare we haven't done this. It's as crazy, to my mind, as if the building industry said we can't regulate electric lighting by using gas regulations, so we won't regulate lighting then. In buildings, which we understand well, there's an obvious fallacy we can see in that suggestion. In digital healthcare, we haven't got the cultural awareness and maturity to see through the analogous fallacies.

Fortunately, though, there are ways to program better. I'll talk about them later in this book.[f]

---

[f] See Chapter 27: Stories for developers, page 367 →

Graceful degradation

When things start to go wrong (perhaps because of a bug), we don't want the computer (or infusion pump or pacemaker...) to crash and stop everything. Rather, we want the computer to keep going, perhaps more slowly, so that we can get the job done. In healthcare, losing patient data would be a disaster, so graceful degradation means working out what must be saved as things start to deteriorate — and also recognizing when things are deteriorating *before* they crash! It is very hard to ensure graceful degradation, and it requires a lot of thought. The main way is to anticipate problems, then stop taking on new work that would overwhelm the computer; another way is to use logs, so that after rebooting, the log can be re-rerun to recover everything that was being done just before the crash.

Error correction

Computer networks are often unreliable (they may be interrupted for many reasons, or simply get unplugged), so network communications always use error correction, so that errors don't matter. Although things may go more slowly, the system will recover.

One of the basic types of error correction in computer networks is **handshaking**. When I send you something, I expect you to shake my hand to confirm you've got it. If I don't get a "shake," then I need to do something to recover from the error, like send the data again. The problem I reported where 73 nurses were investigated[g] for losing patient information happened because the computer systems had no way of knowing whether data had got to its destination and had not been deleted once there. Since the computer systems didn't report any errors — they weren't checking for any errors — the managers just presumed that the loss of data must have been caused by something other than the computers, namely the nurses.

But that's digital systems. The insight of Computational Thinking is that this is a general approach to any complex system, not just digital systems (where it is obviously necessary). You go to your doctor and they test you. "If you don't hear from us, your tests are clear!" Well, if you don't hear from them, perhaps they lost the tests? Perhaps they got your address wrong? How can you be sure that no news is good news? You can't.

Mettaloka Halwala, a father of two daughters, died from chemotherapy complications in 2015.

A PET scan at Melbourne's Austin Hospital had shown signs of potentially fatal lung toxicity but the results were faxed to the wrong number. The coroner, Rosemary Carlin, said,

---

[g] See Chapter 8: Disciplinary action against 73 nurses, page 92 ←

Part II ◇ Treatment ◇ Finding solutions

> It is difficult to understand why such an antiquated and
> unreliable means of communication persists at all in the
> medical profession.[166]

Computational Thinking shows that this problem is not unique to the fax technology, whether it's antiquated or not. Faxes may be old and antiquated, but the *computational* problem of losing messages can happen with any poorly designed system, even the latest ones. The age of technology is irrelevant if it is not designed for reliability.

In this case, the fax machine also served as a printer that was shared with 20 specialities — even if the fax had been sent to the right place, somebody else might have inadvertently walked off with it. Yet there were no checks in place to detect error! The absence of checks, not the presence of faxes, is the computational problem.

In another case, a young mother died after referral letters were sent to house number 16 rather than to house number 1b. Unless there is some error-checking, nobody knows anything has gone wrong until after an investigation — which is far too late. In this case, perhaps the letters should have said, "Please ring and confirm your appointment. If we don't hear from you in a week, we will …" … do something appropriate for the seriousness of your condition.[167]

We've known for centuries that b and 6 are readily confusable, as are 5 and S, 0 and O, I and 1, and more. There isn't really any excuse for unwittingly confusing them; there certainly isn't any excuse for computer programs not being designed to help users avoid input errors caused by these well-known confusions. Indeed, there are many easy solutions. In the present case, the most strategic thing would be to tell the patient when they first register: "You have a house number that can be misread. Why not also give your house a name to help avoid problems? Perhaps you'd like to nominate a friend's address we can also send copies to?" Writing the house number as 1-b not as 1b would have helped, as would using a post code, patient's name, house name. Having a box on the envelope that says, "If incorrectly sent, please return to sender so that we can sort out the error." A copy of the letter could have gone to the patient's GP and to the nominated friend. And so on. It's not hard to think of solutions *if* you want to make healthcare safer, and with digital it's not hard to implement solutions without having to retrain everybody and expecting them to remember all the new rules.

Check checking

Programming is difficult, so programs end up with bugs because we either make slips or because we don't quite understand the problem we are trying to solve with the program. At least when we pause to think we know our limitations, the obvious insight is this: we should program in a way that *ex-*

pects and therefore defends against problems. Not only should the programming process and the programs themselves be designed to detect many errors (whether bugs, errors in data or use errors), but we also need to thoughtfully learn from the checking process itself how to make the next version of the programs even better and more reliable.

The next level insight is that the checking process itself may have bugs, and therefore we should design it to detect its own bugs.

So, not only should we design programs to be testable (because they are rarely totally correct), but, also, we should design the testing *process*, for instance to plot discrepancies, so that we can more easily learn to do better next time. Build tools to help testing, and make those tools better by *their* better testing — and so on.

Unfortunately, programming is so much fun, we often get so excited that we forget our programming may be buggy. This, of course, is standard loss of situational awareness.[h] The main solution is to use software engineering tools that give us broader awareness, Formal Methods, testing tools, code review, decent programming languages, and so on.

The Computational Thinking insight is that many activities — say, planning the activity of introducing a digital system to help improve some work in a hospital — are pretty much as complex as programming, and we should do those activities with the same cautious attitude we properly bring to programming. We may be wrong, but, if so, how will we find out, and how can we do better?

Expect bugs; check for bugs; find bugs; fix bugs; fix the causes of bugs. I can't resist repeating what I said earlier:

> In other words, truly understanding a bug means not understanding why the program failed, but understanding how you managed to overlook the problem when designing the program. The aim, then, is to correct the *cause* of the bug, rather than be distracted into the temptation of fixing one bug at a time.

Abstraction

Abstraction means finding a simpler way of thinking about a problem that will still solve the problem you are worried about. I have one egg in the kitchen. It may be white, brown, in a plastic tray, or in a paper tray, it may be in the fridge or on the worktop — those are all distracting concrete details — but with the abstraction "one" I know I need two more eggs for my three-egg recipe. The abstraction of number doesn't tell us everything about eggs, but

---

[h] See Chapter 20: Situational Awareness, page 261 →

it tells us everything we need to know about the quantity — in this case, of eggs.

Pulling out the core parts of a solution so that it will work with many problems is abstraction. One of the clever results of abstraction is that if you test the abstraction, you know it should work on all the specific problems it works for. Generally, working out exactly what the "core parts of a solution" are helps create much better solutions.

First-class objects

Computers handle objects and data, from simple keystrokes to complex patient data, but it is not all handled the same way. For example, you can often copy a small piece of text from the screen, but you can't copy several bits of text. Or when using a calculator, you can type $4 + 5$ (to get 9, of course) but almost everywhere else the computer wants a number, you can't type a formula to work out the answer directly — you have to do it yourself, and perhaps you'll make a mistake. Or you can email a text document, but you may not be able to email an X-ray — if so, X-rays are not first-class. The idea of a **first-class object** is that you can do anything with it.

A special case of being first-class is **equal opportunity**: there being no difference between what the user can do and what the computer can do.[168] For instance, can you copy everything any text computer generates, as if you had been typing it yourself? Often the system displays something, like the patient's name, but it's second-class text you can't in some circumstances copy. Computational Thinking asks why: editing and other operations are computational, so why are they not implemented uniformly? There may be good reasons (such as confidentiality), but often it's just an oversight or a bug.

The advantage of something being first-class is that the user is not disappointed that they can't do something; or, equally, that what they learned in one part of the user interface works elsewhere.

Generally, being first-class is an ideal (because it's difficult to do perfectly), but the idea suggests making a list of the operations that can be done with objects and data, and then checking whether some features have been accidentally missed or incompletely implemented out in some contexts.

The idea of first-class objects is very powerful for programming language design, as completeness is important, but programming languages are in many ways much simpler than user interfaces, so being first-class doesn't make everything terribly complicated. There are many other design principles for programming languages that would be fruitful for user interface design development.[169]

Optimization

Solutions generally aren't fast enough, or they aren't as fast as you'd want, so profile and monitor them to see how to improve them.

Early computers were very slow and limited, so from the earliest days Computer Science worried a lot about how to make programs small and fast. We'd write a program, and see where all the time went when it was run, then we'd experiment and improve it until it ran faster. You can always improve something.

Optimization is Computational Thinking because so many people accept slow solutions. Computational Thinking means deliberately finding out why things are slow, and then seeing how to improve them — or finding out, if so, why they *have* to be slow. Often, things are slow because they are wrong! However, it's possible to get too keen on optimization and impose it too soon; this just makes things go wrong faster.[i]

Separation of concerns

To make it possible to write complex programs and get them right, ideas and actions are carefully separated so that they do not influence each other. Then we can think about them separately, one at a time.

For example, you might want to sort a list of patient names into alphabetical order. This is a complex problem because to sort people's names you need to pick out the surname. Rather than make a complex program, we split oof — we separate — sorting into a generic problem. We write a program that can sort *anything*.

Separately, we work out what we want to sort: in this case, patient surnames. Doing both together would be a recipe for the problems to get intractably mixed up and become very hard to debug. The code for sorting (which is hard enough to get right) would be all mixed up with stuff about surnames (which are hard enough to get right). Mixing two hard problems together makes solving them both correctly at the same time very unlikely. It's better to separate concerns.

Separation of concerns is closely related to **decomposition** — splitting problems into simpler parts — but it then keeps those parts separate so they can be solved independently, which also controls the possible combinatorial explosion.

Things go wrong, computers crash or get attacked by hackers, so we log everything they do so that later we can work out exactly what went wrong.[170] Often logs are also used to recover everything that would otherwise have been lost. Good logs will include listings of routine tests passed by the program, to confirm it is working correctly.

---

[i] See Chapter 21: Premature optimization, page 280 $\rightarrow$

There is a whole world of new digital techniques that can provide secure signatures, stop information being tampered with, and *much* more. This is an example of Computational Thinking that doesn't just help solve a problem well, but completely transforms what can be done. (Digital currencies, like Bitcoin, are a financial innovation on a par with the invention of coinage, or when the Romans invented the predecessor of our modern check, the *præscriptiones*.)

Avoid thinking

A chapter on Computational Thinking says *avoid* thinking!? I mean, of course, get the computer to do your thinking for you. Human thinking is slow, easily distracted, and unreliable.[j,k] Computer thinking is fast, tireless, and repeatable.

Computer thinking is no more reliable than the human thinking that went into programming it, but you can win by using several programs — if they agree, you are very likely to have understood the problem and programmed it correctly. In contrast, when several humans agree, it may be because of group think or peer pressure, or just idleness — agreeing is simpler than working out your own opinions.

Here's an example. You've built a digital health system, maybe a medical app, and the question is: does it work correctly? This is actually such a hard question, and most developers would rather not go there; they'd rather rely on hope. As we've seen throughout this book, that strategy isn't very reliable.

Instead, computational thinking says: how could a computer save you doing all the work of answering the question? At its simplest, why not program a computer to simulate all the ways of using your system? Then, instead of taking weeks to test the system on people, you can do all the tests in a few minutes. Moreover, when the system is debugged, it will only take a few more minutes to rerun the tests — it's really no more effort. Of course, this efficient process doesn't answer all the questions — you can still use people to help answer the question, doing UCD[l] — but the computer testing has very efficiently answered 90% of the question.

There's a nice twist. If you can't think of a way that a computer could help solve your problem, *you don't really know what the problem is.* You need to tighten up the problem specification (or do something else).

———————————————— ■ ————————————————

Computational Thinking, then, is thinking in a clear way to solve problems efficiently and correctly with as little hassle as possible. Donald Knuth takes it a stage further: science in general (not just Computational Think-

---

[j] See Chapter 3: Cat Thinking, page 25 ←
[k] See Chapter 20: Human Factors, page 259 →
[l] See Chapter 22: User Centered Design, page 301 →

ing) is what we understand well enough to explain to a computer.[171] In other words, anything that is too vague to be explained to a computer is not science. We would like everything in digital healthcare to be evidence based, to be based in science. That means we must use Computational Thinking, otherwise we are being too vague — and probably, in a Cat Thinking way,[m] letting hormones win over evidence.

Computers do exactly what they are told, and Computational Thinking has to be precise and correct; there is no scope for cheating and workarounds that humans intuitively do quietly — even secretly — to make rules work. There is a lot of science about programming computers efficiently and correctly.

Because of the Church–Turing Thesis, Computational Thinking doesn't just apply to digital computers. Computational Thinking also applies to anything we humans can think of that "computes." That includes any ideas of health, digital or not, hospitals, hospices, general practices, ambulance services, and more.

Imagine we've spotted that a hospital ward is being run on paper, and we want to computerize it. The standard approach would be to ask managers what is going on, and draft a specification of what they want the computer system to do to help. We then implement the system, debug it, and in an ideal world we would then do User Centered Design (UCD)[n] to make the system better match what people on the ground needed. Then the system would be delivered.

A more mature view is to consider: what is the hospital ward *already* computing (that is, doing things a computer could do) and trying to compute, and how can we re-specify or debug it so that it can be done better? We do not need to computerize the bits of paper; we need to computerize what the bits of paper were trying to *do*.[95] In turn, the bits of paper are probably a historical solution to problems, and we should try to work out what computation is going on that is worth supporting. The paper, the notes and forms, *were* the best way of solving the problem before we had digital, but now there are better ways of doing things using computers. Simulating an old paper solution is not likely to be a good idea.

Gradually, looking at the ward as a computer, we begin to see many things that can be improved — before anything specifically digital is attempted. Before we get distracted by touch screens or blockchains. And then, when we look more computationally, the digital computer system is going to end up being a much better fit, aligning to the improved work practices.

Although AI is often stunning, throwing in AI to solve a problem can often make things worse. AI allows you to rush in with a computer system that will learn how to make things work. That means nobody needs to seriously think through what's needed, as the AI will sort it out as it goes along. In

---

[m] See Chapter 3: Cat Thinking, page 25 ←
[n] See Chapter 22: User Centered Design, page 301 →

Part II ◇ Treatment ◇ Finding solutions

other words, AI can be a lazy way to skip doing the Computational Thinking. AI will reinforce any inefficient and error-prone procedures, because it can learn how to work with them. There will be no critical Computational Thinking. Any bugs in what it is learning to do will now just happen faster — and without the oversight humans used to have to stop bad things happening. A special case of AI reinforcing existing problems occurs in bias — if existing procedures are racially or biased in other ways, the AI will just continue the problems. In fact, AI will probably make the ethical problems harder to spot as nobody will really know what the AI is doing. I'll talk more about this serious problem later.[o]

———————— ■ ————————

Take the story about Denise Melanson:[p] I described some ideas to help make prescribing drug doses more reliable, but I didn't explain where my ideas came from.

One of the key bits of the story that had been computerized were printing the drug bag label, and controlling the motor inside the infusion pump to deliver a set rate of drug. But the larger computational story should also involve what computing went on inside the nurses' heads: why were they working out the drug dose calculation, when digital computers are much better at doing that sort of work? If the infusion pump could have read the drug bag label (say, using a barcode, or even using Near-Field Communication, NFC, a basic sort of Wi-Fi), then the calculation error would never have happened. And so on.

Indeed, why did the drug bag label present all the data to do the drug dose calculation so the nurses had to work out how to do it and then had to do it? We know that computers are better at sums than people. Why didn't the pharmacy label printing computer do the calculation itself? Actually, it did, but it buried it amongst a lot of confusing information that was not needed — because nobody had done the Computational Thinking to work out what was *actually* needed.

———————— ■ ————————

Charlene Murphey died at Vanderbilt University Medical Center in December 2017 during preparation for a body scan. She had an erroneous dose of vecuronium, which is a muscle relaxant, so Charlene suffocated, unable to breath. Her nurse, RaDonda Leanne Vaught, had intended to give her versed, a curiously named tradename for midazolam, a standard anti-anxiety drug.

There is a longer story here, but put very briefly: the nurse tried to find the drug called versed in the automated drug dispensing cabinet (ADC). She typed its first two letters, VE, into the computer, and then took out the drug the computer offered her — which unfortunately was vecuronium.[172]

This is drug name confusion, and it is not a new or unexpected problem.

---

[o] See Chapter 18: AI and ethics, page 230 →
[p] See Chapter 5: Denise Melanson's fatal overdose, page 49 ←

> **Box 13.3.** Medical "algorithms" aren't digital algorithms
>
> Naturally we want all digital systems to use best practice, and that would include being properly based in the medical literature. It seems elementary to require digital systems to be based at least on the best quality peer-reviewed medical literature.
>
> Take **body mass index**, BMI. We make an app that works out BMI for you and, as it is based on the medical literature, it must be right.
>
> No. The medical literature does *not* provide algorithms, clear specifications for basing computer programs on. It provides, at best, basic formulas and, usually, some statistical testing of clinical outcomes.
>
> The usual formula for BMI, the Quetelet index,[173] is your body weight divided by the square of your height.
>
> To be an algorithm for a computer, the computer must also know that body mass and height are both positive, and that they fall in reasonable range. You have to decide what to do with units; for example, in Europe, kilograms and meters make sense, but in the US, pounds and feet make sense (box 25.1 talks more about internationalization). An algorithm, unlike a clinical formula, needs to know what to do when the numbers entered by the user do not fall within valid ranges, or even what to do when some of the input is missing or is syntactically invalid. Are these the right numbers for the patient in the room, or do they refer to some other patient? If the numbers come out of a database, then there need to be more checks. And so on. In other words, a clinical algorithm is only one part of the story.
>
> Healthy 32-year-old Liam Thorp was called up for an urgent COVID-19 vaccination.[174] He phoned his doctor to ask why he'd been called up, and found out he was recorded as being 6.2 cm high (not 6 foot 2), which led to an *enormous* BMI of about 28,000. For comparison, a BMI of 40 or over is considered morbidly obese. So, the developers had followed the BMI clinical algorithm to the letter, but they had totally failed to check any data for validity, let alone common sense.

The Computational Thinking that should have gone on much earlier when the ADC was designed should at least have included this simple precaution:

- 🐦 We are creating a program that allows the user to enter abbreviations of drug names. What errors might this induce? To find out, let's list the equivalence classes [a standard Computer Science problem] of drugs so that we can check that different classes of drug are never confusable, cannot be stored together in one machine, or at least always get additional user confirmations. When a drug is stored in the cabinet, the equivalence class tests must be run again to stop unexpected confusions, with new drug names added after we've delivered the system. We will put all these tests in a **test suite** so that they can be automatically checked again whenever any part of the system is updated.

I've used the standard technical term here (equivalence class) to emphasize that this is routine stuff for computational thinkers. If you are going to program computers, this changes how the world works, and you have a moral duty to explore the world you have created to ensure it is as safe as possible, and stays as safe as possible even after modifications, routine updates, and future developers overriding your original design decisions. Equivalence class algorithms are routinely taught to undergraduate students.

One wonders why the manufacturers of drugs do not do this sort of thinking when drugs are named. Why are different classes of drugs even given confusable names in the first place? Why is a drug even called versed, which is already a common word meaning something completely different? You don't even need to be well-versed in English to know this!

One wonders why there aren't more slices of cheese[q] in the story. If the drug cabinet has dangerous drugs in it, why aren't two nurses always required to confirm the correct drug has been chosen? Why doesn't the drug cabinet ask for independent confirmation? Or, why doesn't a syringe driver or infusion pump use an alarm when a different sort of drug is used? (Here's one case: imagine that a patient has already had some drug; if the patient's infusion pump is now given a different type of drug, why not ask for confirmation?) And so on.

There is an important twist to Charlene Murphey's tragic story. Her nurse, Vaught, did not at first find any drugs after searching for VE, so she entered the override function. Then vecuronium was matched. Using the override is routine at many hospitals, as it's so often needed just to get your job done. Previously, override must have been used countless times without any problems. Vaught has been charged with a criminal offense, but the patient safety community has rallied behind her.[175] Certainly, criminalizing Vaught for exposing a design problem is not going to help improve any digital systems.

After something goes wrong, you naturally want to find out why it went wrong. **Incident analysis** — not just doing an investigation, but working out the causes of whatever went wrong — can benefit enormously from Computational Thinking, including an awareness of how digital systems may have contributed to the incident.

When something goes wrong with a computer, you immediately think of bugs, things wrong with the design of the program. You don't blame the computer; you look for bugs and wonder whether it was properly programmed. So when something seems to go wrong with a nurse, you should not blame the nurse, but wonder what has gone wrong with the system they are working in — what's gone wrong with their "program." If their program, their set of rules or standard operating procedure, was not designed understanding Human Factors,[r] then that's like writing a computer program with-

---

[q] See Chapter 6: Swiss Cheese Model, page 61 ←
[r] See Chapter 20: Human Factors, page 259 →

out worrying about how the computer will run it, without understanding Computer Factors.[s]

When a computer program doesn't work, it will be the designer's fault for not finding out enough about the computer (and the algorithm the program is trying to run), just as the nurse "crashing" is the fault of the system for not creating a program or set of rules that works properly *given* everything we know about humans.

Putting the insights of this chapter another way: worrying about and avoiding bugs is Safety One thinking, but Computational Thinking is Safety Two thinking. Design and develop digital healthcare properly, and avoid the problems.

Part II ◇ Treatment ◇ Finding solutions

---

[s] See Chapter 21: Computer Factors, page 277 →

Drug doses and other forms of patient treatment require detailed calculations. Calculation errors are one of the most common types of error and they could be reduced in many ways. Calculators themselves ignore errors, and they should be fixed if they are going to be used in healthcare.

14

Risky calculations

Kimberly Hiatt was a pediatric nurse in the Seattle Children's Hospital, USA. She somehow made a calculation mistake. We don't know all the details, but on 14 September 2010, instead of 140 milligrams of calcium chloride for eight-month-old Kaia Zautner, she drew up 1.4 grams. She immediately reported the error to staff at the Cardiac Intensive Care Unit at the hospital,[176] and reported the error on the hospital computer:

> I messed up. I've been giving $CaCl_2$ [calcium chloride] for years. I was talking to someone while drawing it up. Miscalculated in my head the correct mLs according to the mg/mL. First med error in 25 years of working here. I am simply sick about it. Will be more careful in the future.[177]

The hospital escorted her from the hospital, put her on administrative leave, then fired her. The Nursing Commission gave her a $3,000 fine and 80 hours of coursework, and 4 years of probation. The baby, Kaia Zautner, died. A statement by a cardiologist said it was not clear whether the mistake caused the death of the child, as the baby was already critically ill, but that it would have exacerbated cardiac dysfunction.

Sadly, Kimberly Hiatt committed suicide. As a result, the Nursing Commission closed its investigation.

Hiatt was a tragic **second victim**.[67]

If the hospital had decided to support Hiatt, she could have been one of the safest nurses in the hospital, and she would have been able to contribute to making hospital systems safer — improving drug labels, changing procedures, changing calculators, who knows what? Even if there were reasons to separate her from direct clinical duties, she could have been a fantastic mentor or trainer. We shall never know. We shall never know what patient safety insights have gone to her grave.

Fix It: See and solve the problems of digital healthcare. Harold Thimbleby, Oxford University Press. © Harold Thimbleby 2021.
DOI: 10.1093/oso/9780198861270.003.0014

> **Box 14.1.** Handheld devices may have real bugs
>
> How often do you disinfect your handheld devices?
> Over two thirds of nursing students' mobile phones are contaminated with the "superbug" methicillin-resistant *Staphylococcus aureus* (widely known as MRSA).[178] This means that student nurses — in fact, probably everyone — carry drug resistant infections around hospitals, to their homes, and plausibly infect other people.
> The authors of the paper say more research is needed on how to address the problem; for instance, although their research showed the bugs were present on phones, the research did not explore whether cleaning mobile phones would be linked with a reduction in healthcare-associated infections. It seems obvious it would, especially given all the evidence for the effectiveness of handwashing.
> The infection problem shows that just testing new digital applications in the lab or in simulation studies is not sufficient — these are *medical* devices, and they can have direct medical impact. The new applications may introduce more infections that offset the clinical benefits of the applications — especially when working with immuno-compromised patients.

The suicide of healthcare workers is a taboo subject. I wonder what Seattle Children's Hospital's approach to mental health is — if it has a process, inevitably it'll be computerized, so this, too, is a digital health issue in itself. As Clare Gerada points out, there's a doctor's suicide every three weeks in the NHS, and the fact barely registers.[179]

One insight is that, despite all the computers and digital things in the Seattle Children's Hospital, none intercepted or stopped the error. None apparently even noticed it.

Hiatt did the calculation in her head. Calculations are all over healthcare, and calculators are the natural response to them. Calculators are digital, and surely (you'd think) it's better to use one than doing calculations in your head or by hand? Calculators must be the most common form of digital healthcare. We take them for granted.

So let's have a closer look.

Calculators have a very long history, starting with counting in sand, and on counting boards, and then the abacus, which was already in use by the Sumerians by around 2700 BC. Blaise Pascal invented the first real digital calculator in the 1640s to help with his father's tax returns, but what we recognize today as modern handheld calculators were developed in the late 1970s. Manufacturers have now had half a century of experience with them. Today, of course, mobile phones can run apps that turn them into simulations of handheld calculators.

With all this experience, we would expect today's calculators to be very reliable, and certainly adequate for use in hospitals.

Well, let's see how well modern calculators work …

Here's a very simple calculation: What percentage of the world is British?

This calculation is going to be much easier to do than a typical drug dose calculation, but going through it will show some of the issues — and it'll show up some worrying surprises.

In August 2019 the British population was just over 66 million. The world's population was just over 7.5 billion.[5] To find out the percentage of British people in the world, we divide 66 million by 7.5 billion, then multiply by 100 to turn the fraction into a percentage. It sounds easy enough …

On most calculators, we need to do something like pressing `AC`, to clear the calculator and make sure no previous numbers interfere with our calculation; then we need to press 66000000 `÷` 7500000000 `×` 100 `=` to get the answer. It would have been more reliable to enter 7,500,000,000 using separators (a number that's now clearly in the billions), but calculators don't like you typing commas! Interestingly, the iPhone (but not the Casio) displays commas, so large numbers are at least easier to read correctly on the iPhone.

If we do this sum on the Casio HS-8V, currently one of the most popular handheld calculators, we'll get the answer 88%.

Surely Britain isn't 88% of the world's population?!

Let's try the iPhone (running Apple's iOS operating system). That gets 8.8%. Closer, but still nowhere near right.

Let's try the iPhone in landscape mode, which makes the calculator turn into a scientific calculator. In scientific mode the iPhone gets 0.88%. Which is right at last.

Pictures of these calculators getting *different* results for *exactly the same* calculation are shown in figure 14.1.

There is no trick here. Try it yourself — but remember that different calculators do different things and you may not at first get the results I found. Also, Apple may have updated their calculator before you read this. I was running iOS version 13.2.2 in November 2019, but their calculator has had this bug ever since the iPhone came out in 2007.

When I was at primary school, I was taught to do sums in two different ways. For example, add up a column of numbers from the top, then add up from the bottom to the top. If I get different answers, at least one of them must be wrong, and I should try again.

The Casio is just wrong, but the iPhone has two ways of doing the calculation, and it gets different answers. So the iPhone is wrong *and* it could have worked out that it was wrong, at least if it did sums the way I was taught to at school.[180]

None of these calculators tell the user a mistake has happened. The user will remain oblivious. All of the problems could have raised warning flags and alerted the user that something was awry. It would have been easy for all the calculators to have been designed to detect errors and warn the user.

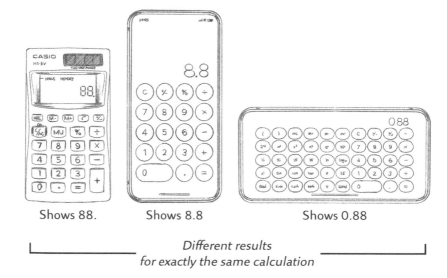

Shows 88.   Shows 8.8   Shows 0.88

Different results
for exactly the same calculation

Figure 14.1. What percentage of the world is British? We get three different answers doing the same calculation on two calculators. Worse, there are no error messages or any warnings of the bugs and incorrect results. In landscape mode, the iPhone can handle larger numbers, and in this mode it gets the right answer.

There are more problems with calculators.

If you make a keying mistake that you do notice, most calculators make correcting it very difficult.

For example, if you press ■✕ instead of ■÷, there's not a lot you can do on most calculators but to start all over again.

Some calculators do have delete keys. The whole point of a delete key, surely, is to correct errors? But it isn't so simple.

Let's say you accidentally press two decimal points, and try to delete the second one. This should correct your error, but:

◑ On the iPhone and on many popular calculators, you aren't allowed to have two decimal points in the first place. So the delete key, if you do press it, will delete the only decimal point you have, and will therefore create a new error of having no decimal point at all.[181]

◑ On some calculators, like the Casio HR-150TEC calculator, the delete key only deletes digits and nothing else. So if you keyed ▪4▪ ▪5▪ ▪.▪ ▪.▪ ▪5▪ ▪7▪ and tried to correct that extra decimal point, you'd lose the digit before the decimal point, and be left with 4.57.

Both cases are wrong, and, worse, get no error warnings from the calculator when they occur. So the user may well be oblivious. You only do a calculation with a calculator because you don't know the answer, so it is unlikely that you know the answer is wrong.

- ◗ It's very easy to find bugs like these problems with decimal points and delete keys, as well as many other bugs, completely automatically using computer tools.[182] It's surprising that major manufacturers do not use computer tools to help them find *and fix* bugs.

- ◗ But we can't blame manufacturers, because we all buy these things, so in principle the manufacturers are selling us stuff we want. The problem is, we can't see the bugs, so we have no idea which products are safe and which are dangerous. A solution to this problem is to have safety ratings, which we'll discuss later.[a]

The calculators are CE-marked, which makes it look like they are certified as "safe." The rules for CE marking are strange; since calculators are generic "office equipment," they are certified as appropriate for use *in offices.* Yet they are regularly used in hospitals for life-critical calculations. Surely the CE marking for hospital calculators should be appropriate for *that* use?

Nobody is going to die over arguing what proportion of the world is British. My population example was not a medical calculation that any lives directly depend on, but it's a clear example of how unreliable calculators are — even when doing very simple things.

Not only are calculators unreliable, but they don't do anything about the errors they cause.

Why did the calculators go wrong on such a simple problem as answering "what percentage of the world is British?" (If you prefer, you can do this calculation using the population of your own country.[183])

My "trick" — showing you a deliberate error, but which could have happened accidentally — was that the population of the world is too big for the calculators to display. The display throws away digits when there are too many for it to handle. So the calculators end up getting numbers that are too small, *they have no idea*, and things go awry. The problem is that nothing in the calculator notices or warns that there is a discrepancy between what the user has done and what the program is working on.

I chose this problem because it is easy to show you, but calculators have plenty of other problems that are equally if not more worrying — especially as calculators are used throughout hospitals to do things like working out critical drug doses. I published a major critique of calculators in 2000, and Will Thimbleby and I did research that developed a novel design that considerably improved on them, showing how to make them much safer.[184]

The point is that the problems are easy to fix if anybody wants to fix them. The calculator problem is not a curiosity, but is a symptom of lax program-

---

[a] See Chapter 29: Safety ratings will improve healthcare, page 401 →

ming that did not handle user input correctly — in fact, these dangerous number bugs are ubiquitous.[55]

I've told many people (including Apple, Casio, and HP) about these sorts of bugs, but most people argue "*but* that's what calculators do." Which is true, of course. But surely they could be safer? When a calculator *causes* a mistake, it would make things much safer if at least it warned the user.

———————————◼———————————

Spreadsheets are used everywhere, and they are used throughout healthcare. Microsoft's Excel spreadsheet application is the most well known, and I'll use it for the next story.

Excel can trace its history back to an early spreadsheet that Microsoft marketed in 1982 called Multiplan; the first version of Microsoft's Excel was released in 1985 (for the Apple Mac) and then in 1987 for the PC. Excel is now available for Windows, Mac OS, and iOS (iPhones and iPads). The various versions are all compatible with each other, but to be specific — and in case you want to double-check — I'll take my examples below from the Apple Mac version 16.47, as updated in 2021.

In short: Microsoft have been developing and improving Excel for over thirty years. They have had ample time to fix bugs — but they have the problem of any successful software that they have had to stay backward compatible so that users' spreadsheets continue to work as Microsoft continually upgrade their software. Some of the "deliberate bugs" in today's Excel may be hang-overs from accidental bugs in earlier versions. From a commercial point of view, keeping existing customers is important. From a digital healthcare point of view, eliminating any bug that could cause patient harm is a priority.

It would be possible, at least in principle, for Excel to have two modes. One is a backwards-compatible mode, the other is a safe mode, perhaps especially for healthcare use. Unlike Microsoft Word, Excel does not have any preferences, but it already has permissions and properties that could be extended to help. One current property, for instance, is "Checked by" and maybe this idea could be extended to cover "Checked by Excel Digital Health Safety Mode"? We'll soon see why I think this (or something like it) would be a really good idea.

So, let's start off with the top-left of an empty spreadsheet. I've numbered a series of spreadsheet pictures to make it easier to follow the step-by-step changes I make to the spreadsheet. (For copyright reasons, I need to make clear that these are not actual screenshots, but my own diagrams to reproduce the exact behavior of Microsoft Excel Apple Mac version 16.47.)

Here's picture 1, the top-left of an empty spreadsheet:

Microsoft Excel Apple Mac version 16.47

1.

	A	B	...
1			
2			
3			
...	...	...	

Now type 1 and 10 into the empty cells A1 and A2. We will get this:

Microsoft Excel Apple Mac version 16.47

2.

	A	B	...
1	1		
2	10		
3			
...	...	...	

Although we'd usually want to do far more interesting things, a simple thing to start off with would be to add up these two numbers.

Of course, in this simple case, we already know the answer will be $1 + 10 = 11$, so we don't expect anything exciting. In general, spreadsheets are much bigger and much more complicated, and we won't always know the answer — in fact, the whole point of using Excel is to help us when we don't know the answers we want. It's always a good idea to do some sums where you do know the answers as part of your checking that the spreadsheet is doing what you want it to do.

Excel provides two main ways to add up numbers: using the + operator, and using the SUM() function. We'll put SUM(A1:A2) as a formula in cell A3, and as a reminder, I'll write it out in full in cell B3 so it's easy to keep track of what's going on when I start editing the spreadsheet further. (If you want to do this too, just write ="= SUM(A1:A2)" into cell B3, which will make everything work exactly as shown.)

Microsoft Excel Apple Mac version 16.47

3.

	A	B	...
1	1		
2	10		
3	11	= SUM(A1:A2)	
...	...	...	

Nothing exciting is happening so far. We have two cells, containing 1 and 10; their sum (shown in cell B3) is 11.

Let's edit cell A1 to be 70 kg, maybe representing a patient's weight. Now hit return, so Excel recalculates the sum. Picture 4, below, shows what happens:

Part II ◇ Treatment ◇ Finding solutions

4.

Microsoft Excel Apple Mac version 16.47

	A	B	...
1	70 kg		
2	10		
3	10	= SUM(A1:A2)	
...	...		...

The sum of 70 kg and 10 is *not* 10. Something has gone wrong.

Similar strange results would be given if we'd tried PRODUCT, MIN, MAX, MEAN, IF, or many other functions instead of SUM. In fact, the problem is Excel itself.

What's happening is that Excel treats 70 kg as zero.

There's a reason for this apparently strange behavior.

Imagine you want to add up a column of hundreds of numbers. You'd use SUM to do that easily, say, by writing =SUM(A1:A100). In a long column of numbers you *might* want missing numbers to be treated as zero, you might break up the column with blank lines to make the spreadsheet more readable, you might have missing numbers, or you might want headings. In all these cases, "anything not a number is zero" seems to be what you want. This is a deliberate feature of Excel. It's intentional. Since it probably isn't a feature you want, programmers prefer to use the more accurate word **misfeature** for a "feature" that is more often a bug.

Unfortunately, if something is meant to be a number, but has an error in it, then Excel will *silently* take it to be zero. That's why my example of 70 kg is treated as zero. Indeed, if you typed 70 followed by a "non-breaking space," which you can't see at all, the Excel cell would look exactly like 70, but Excel would still treat it as zero. There might be "a reason," but it's not a good enough reason for healthcare where safety ought to be more important than the occasional convenience for Excel programmers.

I want to emphasize again that I've made up these simple examples to make the problems obvious. In a real use of Excel, you might be busy trying to treat a patient, and you'd be doing a far more complicated calculation, for which you might not know the right answer. Of course you might have an idea what the right sort of answer would be, but there's no guarantee that Excel's errors won't give you an answer close to what looks OK but is still wrong enough to harm your patient.

Excel is actually perfectly good at recognizing errors when it wants to. For example, if you do a division by zero sum, say =1/0, Excel's answer is #DIV/0!, and the error of writing =bad in a cell is #NAME?, and so on.

In all such errors that Excel recognizes, there's a little pop-up that gives you further insights and help. Why doesn't Excel do this for errors with SUM, like the ones I've just been talking about? Well, this would make the improved version of Excel incompatible with earlier versions, which is a knock-on problem. Instead, perhaps cells could have a new cell feature — features like formatting (which is already widely used) are easy enough to

---

Box 14.2. Austerity by spreadsheet

No discussion of spreadsheet errors would be complete without a mention of the Reinhart and Rogoff story.

Without a doubt, austerity (that is, governments cutting back on public funding) has killed many people. In the UK, the Government policy of austerity reduced state funding for health and social services, and resulted in about 22,000 excess deaths per year (in a population of 66 million).[185] The austerity policy was at least partly due to a buggy spreadsheet.

In brief, two Harvard University economists, Carmen Reinhart and Kenneth Rogoff, published a paper in 2010 called "Growth in a Time of Debt," where they showed that high debt slows down growth. Their influential paper was used to justify government austerity programs worldwide. For example, Olli Rehn, the EU Commissioner for Economic Affairs, and George Osborne, who became the UK Chancellor of the Exchequer, both relied on the paper to argue that national debt was the universal cause of financial crises.[186]

Then, in 2013, Thomas Herndon, Michael Ash, and Robert Pollin revealed numerous errors in the Reinhart-Rogoff spreadsheet.[187] They showed, in their words, that "exclusion of available data, coding errors and inappropriate weighting of summary statistics led to serious miscalculations that inaccurately represent the relationship between public debt and GDP growth."

It's a high-profile example of one buggy spreadsheet causing problems affecting millions of people.[188]

Reinhart and Rogoff's problem was that their spreadsheet calculated something complicated, and they didn't notice they'd made some serious errors.

---

add without breaking anything else — to mean something like, "This is not a number, but it is being deliberately used in a SUM calculation." That would preserve backward compatibility — you'd be warned about potential problems, but you could override each one if you approved of it.

I haven't covered all the possible responses to this problem of Excel in this brief discussion, but I've certainly shown that Excel unnecessarily, and dangerously (certainly when it's used in healthcare), ignores use errors.

Another approach[189] is to use Excel's built-in data validation. You can program Excel so that a user making a mistake, like we did in our example above, will result in a warning dialog box popping up. This might be a good idea ... you might think.

You've successfully got an error warning dialog box to pop up, but this isn't the end of your problems. There's a button in Excel's dialog box, Retry. Curiously, if the user clicks Retry, Excel will carry on, ignoring the error. There will be no further warnings, and Excel *still* treats the bad number incorrectly.

With lots of warnings, anyway, many users understandably get **alarm automation** or **alarm fatigue** — they'll just hit return whenever a message pops up. Why read it? These pesky messages happen all the time! So, Excel might have warned the user, but it hasn't ensured the user doesn't carry on and make the horrible mistake of relying on the bad results that are about to happen.

I understand Microsoft wants to keep Excel backward compatible with earlier versions, but I think it needs a feature (perhaps a bit like some we suggested above) that can be used to force it to report errors *and* stop the user progressing without correcting the error (so that alarm fatigue is managed). Any hospital would then configure Excel so that all use of it in the hospital was safer. Maybe there should be a special designed-for-healthcare spreadsheet: it could be close enough to Excel to have all its advantages, but it could be much safer.

One problem undermining this dream is that if anyone made a healthcare spreadsheet like this, I think it would need to be regulated as a healthcare device — which manufacturer wants to do that while there is a huge market for unregulated software? In the meantime, manufacturers are selling unsuitable digital systems into healthcare without restriction.

To summarize: calculators and spreadsheets are used all over healthcare, yet they ignore errors that are likely to be critical in patient treatment. Many "little" digital systems, from printers to Excel, are not regulated for use in healthcare. They are treated like office equipment and are just assumed to be good enough. I've shown this just isn't the case. *All* digital systems used in healthcare need thorough regulation; digital regulation needs a serious rethink as part of improving safety across healthcare.

———————————■———————————

There's a similar problem with Europe's most popular infusion pump, the B-Braun Infusomat (figure 14.2). Now, because it's an infusion pump, we can't deny that the user, typically a nurse, has better things to do than notice and fix unnecessary bugs. They have a patient to look after.

I am now going to spell out the steps taken to show a bug in the B-Braun Infusomat that could trip up a nurse. Worse, the bug could trip up a nurse and mislead any investigation into the error, because the bug also means that the B-Braun records the wrong details in its logs. I emphasize this is not the only bug I've found with the Infusomat, but it's one of the easiest to explain.

The Infusomat can be programmed to deliver drugs into a patient, and it can do so at various rates as set by the user. The four arrow keys on it let you enter numbers; the idea is that the left and right arrows choose a digit, and the up and down arrow keys adjust the chosen digit.

Here's an example, showing how a display of zero changes when the up arrow is pressed:

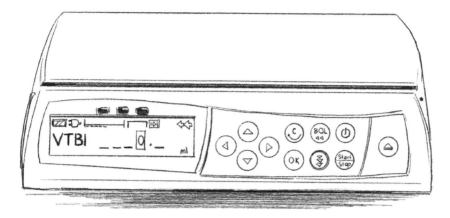

Figure 14.2. This drawing is based on a simulation I programmed of the B-Braun Infusomat infusion pump, so I could carefully explore the Infusomat's design and engineering in detail. You can move the mouse around and click on buttons and they do what they do on the real Infusomat. I ran my simulation in parallel with using a real Infusomat (software version 686E), and continually updated my simulation with everything I learned from the real Infusomat to ensure my simulation was accurate.

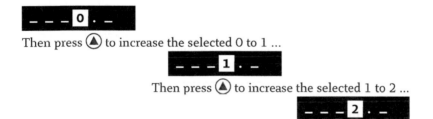

It seems very straightforward: pressing the "up" button, (▲), increases the selected digit 0 to become 1, and pressing it again increases 1 to 2. Of course, if we carry on pressing it, 2 increases to 3, and so on, so we can easily set any digit we like.

Our research has shown this to be a reliable way of entering numbers, *provided that there are no bugs.*[190]

Each time any button is pressed, the Infusomat clicks, providing audible confirmation that the button has been pressed hard enough and is working properly. This might be what you think, but if you press a button twice quickly, it may click twice but nothing at all will happen, or it may happen just once. These bugs could be serious problems if a nurse urgently needs to change the dose, and presses buttons quickly. It will sound like the number has changed each time the button is pressed, but the clicks are misleading.

> **Box 14.3.** Solving a hindsight problem
>
> A knee-jerk reaction to the Infusomat problems would be that the Infusomat should have been formally specified and shown to comply with some standard theorems, like "only the highlighted digit changes" (which is easily turned into a precise mathematical statement). Unfortunately, this is **hindsight bias**: we now know this is a problem, but at the time of design, it'd have been very hard to specify the millions of critical design ideas, let alone include this one.
>
> Instead, we can get a computer to find them. In principle, there are an infinite number of mathematical theorems describing a system, so we need some constraints such as: find small theorems; or find **partial theorems**[191] — theorems that are *often but not always* true.
>
> The "only the highlighted digit changes" is, on the *actual* Infusomat, a partial theorem. It's usually true, but the Infusomat's bugs make it fail. In other words, we can find bugs like this automatically.
>
> A really important insight with partial theorems is that they indicate likely problems for users. Most of the time, a partial theorem is true — so the user will come to believe it is *actually* true. One day they will be misled.
>
> So, we get the computer to list partial theorems, and then go over them. Some indicate bugs, some indicate strange design decisions, and some — given the complexity of clinical tasks — might actually make sense.
>
> For example, when we tried automatically looking for partial theorems, our tool found theorems that failed when a device was switched off. Well, most users know that when a device is switched off, it doesn't work! Also, when a device is switched off, it is usually safe. So we tell the tool: find partial theorems, but ignore those caused by "Off." We then get a tighter list, and repeat the process, gradually either improving our list of theorems, or improving the design by fixing its bugs.

I'll now run through how to set a drug dose of 0.01 mL, as a simple example. Let's see what happens, and *how* it happens.

We'll start from the display showing zero as before, and press ▶ a couple of times to move the cursor to the right. The number shown "expands" nicely, creating two extra 0 digits, so the displayed value is 0.00, with the third zero being selected. We now have the cursor selecting the digit we want to change. To increase the 0.00 to 0.01, we press ▲, expecting, of course, to increase that digit. Here's exactly what happens:

$$ \_ \_ \_ 0 . 0 \boxed{0} $$

Then press ▲ to increase the selected 0 to 1 ...

$$ \_ \_ \_ 0 . 1 \boxed{0} $$

Oops! The wrong digit, not the one under the cursor, has changed!

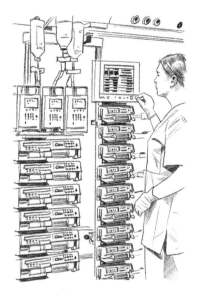

Figure 14.3. Sometimes patients need lots of different drugs. Here, many infusion pumps and syringe drivers are being used for one patient.

Like many of the bugs we've encountered, the device has let the user do something that it doesn't cope with correctly. The dose the pump is going to give the patient is apparently ten times higher than what was intended, but the pump doesn't warn the user that anything unexpected has happened. It's possible that the Infusomat can't physically deliver such a small dose, so it's just made the number larger. That's a possible explanation, but it isn't an excuse for silently changing the dose by a factor of ten — it's a bug.

There will normally be an investigation if harm happens to a patient. The Infusomat keeps a log of what it does, and the log will show that the user entered 0.1. If investigated, the user will say they entered 0.01; they don't understand how they could possibly have made a mistake. In fact, they didn't. The Infusomat made a mistake. Unfortunately, the investigators are more likely to believe the logs, and blame the nurse's dishonesty or their faulty memory.

I've seen sick babies in intensive care connected to 18 Infusomats (figure 14.3), stacked one above another. Multiplying up a "tiny" risk like being caught out by a bug will potentially harm thousands of people worldwide, and probably incriminate thousands of nurses along the way. One might argue that the bug is unlikely to happen in practice, and that a professional nurse should check. But why should a nurse have to check there are no bugs affecting their patient care?

This chapter has been a list of problems, but I put it in Part II (finding solutions), rather than in Part I (riskier than you think), because the key to finding solutions is to realize that there *is* a problem to solve.

The problem with numbers in healthcare is ubiquitous, and once it's recognized as a problem it will be really easy to fix. Ironically, computers were invented to handle numbers; numbers are easy. There is no excuse not to solve these problems now before more people are harmed.[55]

Software warranties generally deny all liability for problems. Manufacturers and developers should be required to be more accountable. Everyone needs to be constantly curious about improving systems and reporting problems.

15

Who's accountable?

To use the Mersey Burns app[a] you first have to agree to its terms and conditions. Here's an extract taken directly from the app's terms itself:[192]

> **No warranties** The app is provided on an "as is" basis without any representations or warranties ...
>
> **Liability** Under no circumstances will St Helens and Knowsley Teaching Hospitals NHS Trust [the legal owners of the app] be liable ...
>
> **Indemnification** You agree to indemnify and hold St Helens and Knowsley Teaching Hospitals NHS Trust harmless from any claim ...
>
> **Modification** You must promptly download any update to the App from the 'App store' upon such update becoming available, and you must check the disclaimer page of the App prior to each use of the App ...[193]

And to rub it in, they add that they can modify the terms and conditions or the software at any time without giving you any notice.

I imagine — I don't know — that the Mersey Burns developers were told by their lawyers that this is what they had to say, whatever they thought. If these terms and conditions are legal and binding, I'd like us to change the law so that developers and resellers take some responsibility, as they have to with almost everything else in the world.

This problem is not unique to Mersey Burns by any means. Here is an extract from the terms from another medical app, with its original capital letters (I've lightly edited it to make it briefer and easier to read):

---

[a] See Chapter 10: Mersey Burns app, page 121 ←

Fix It: See and solve the problems of digital healthcare. Harold Thimbleby, Oxford University Press. © Harold Thimbleby 2021.
DOI: 10.1093/oso/9780198861270.003.0015

BY ACCESSING OR USING THIS APP YOU AGREE TO BE BOUND BY THE TERMS AND CONDITIONS

THE SERVICE IS PROVIDED ON AN "AS IS, AS AVAILABLE" BASIS. NONE OF THE DEVELOPERS OR THEIR AGENTS MAKES ANY WARRANTIES OF ANY KIND, EITHER EXPRESS OR IMPLIED, WITHOUT LIMITATION, FOR ANY PARTICULAR PURPOSE.

The company aims to keep the Site available to maintain saved information. However, we shall not be liable for lost altered, or corrupted information. We do not warrant that the Service will be uninterrupted or error-free or that defects will be corrected.

YOU ASSUME TOTAL RESPONSIBILITY AND RISK FOR YOUR USE OF THE SITE AND THE INTERNET.

You agree to indemnify, defend and hold the company and information providers harmless from and against any and all claims, legal action, liability, losses, damages, costs and expenses (including accounting and attorneys' fees).

Your sole remedy for dissatisfaction is to stop using the application.[194]

There is, unfortunately, nothing unusual about such warranties for digital systems.

If you use an iPad or iPhone (I'm mentioning them because I have these; I am familiar with them, and I think they are great), you've *already* agreed to Apple's own terms, which apply to everything you do on them:

YOU FURTHER ACKNOWLEDGE THAT THE iOS SOFTWARE AND SERVICES ARE NOT INTENDED OR SUITABLE FOR USE IN SITUATIONS OR ENVIRONMENTS WHERE THE FAILURE OR TIME DELAYS OF, OR ERRORS OR INACCURACIES IN, THE CONTENT, DATA OR INFORMATION PROVIDED BY THE iOS SOFTWARE OR SERVICES COULD LEAD TO DEATH, PERSONAL INJURY, OR SEVERE PHYSICAL OR ENVIRONMENTAL DAMAGE, INCLUDING WITHOUT LIMITATION THE OPERATION OF NUCLEAR FACILITIES, AIRCRAFT NAVIGATION OR COMMUNICATION SYSTEMS, AIR TRAFFIC CONTROL, LIFE SUPPORT OR WEAPONS SYSTEMS.[195]

Apple is a world leader, no question. Their warning is normal, standard practice across the digital industry. Apple wants you to be clear that their software is unsuitable for running medical apps: failure of many medical apps could lead to personal injury. It certainly undermines any safe medical app use, especially in the radiology department.

Under British Law, the Unfair Contract Terms Act 1977 (UCTA) prohibits excluding liability for causing personal injury or death. As it says,

> **Section 2(1)** A person cannot by reference to any contract term [...] exclude or restrict his liability for death or personal injury resulting from negligence.

> **Section 2(2)** In the case of other loss or damage (i.e., other than death or personal injury), a person cannot so exclude or restrict his liability for negligence except in so far as satisfies the requirement of reasonableness.

The clash between the warranty and the law (and any contractual arrangements made when the product or service was purchased) means that a court case balancing the issues could be interesting and expensive. So far, there are no precedents, since so few people are aware of the pervasive nature of bugs and their impact on the reliability of healthcare systems.

I think, at root, there is a serious regulatory problem: it's understandable that manufacturers don't want to say "feel free to sue us for anything and everything!" but equally it's unfortunate they revert to denying *all* liability as strongly as they possibly can. Regulation could step in and provide a lot of the missing clarity. Clarity would also help make problems easier to solve. With clarity, insurers would be clearer about their liabilities, as would patients and staff caught up in incidents. Everything would be easier to solve amicably. And, if the regulations were sensible, then there would be fewer bugs and software failures, because manufacturers would prefer to — or would have to — improve quality rather than seek refuge behind restrictive warranties.

Warranties for big systems, such as hospital systems, go further than the app warranties consumers are familiar with. They usually add confidentiality clauses (**gag clauses**), so they are much harder to get access to and discuss freely. Often manufacturers further add **DeWitt clauses**, named after the man who fought for the right to publish his research on database systems (and to stay employed at his university when Oracle, a disappointed company, complained) — if the agreement includes a prohibition to name or publish clear research about a system, it's now called a DeWitt clause.[196] Many digital health systems forbid researchers from publishing screenshots.

The manufacturers argue that the research might be wrong or even vexatious. My view is that if scientists make errors, they are pleased to be corrected; that is the way science works. Otherwise, publishing specific details enables other researchers to test and duplicate the claims rigorously. In this book, I've taken that view: I've certainly criticized systems, but I have given you enough information to check what I've said. Manufacturers may make changes as a result of what I've said, in a sense invalidating it, but that would be good — patients would benefit. On the other hand, if I'd anonymized everything, you probably wouldn't believe me, and manufacturers would have had no incentive to improve.

Part II ◇ Treatment ◇ Finding solutions

We'd think it very strange indeed if car manufacturers or even smart phone manufacturers prohibited people publishing reports of their products' performance and handling. We rightly expect the media to regularly report details of the latest cars and phones to inform us. It helps us choose which to buy. It's ironic that when it really matters — when it comes to healthcare — the manufacturers on the whole don't want us to know.

In the US, manufacturers can also appeal to the **learned intermediary** doctrine in law: the manufacturer informs the clinician, who then acts as a learned intermediary with the patient. The idea is that with drugs, the doctor knows more about the various effects of the drug and the particular patient's condition, so they are advised by the manufacturer, but take responsibility for their advice to the patient.

The learned intermediary doctrine (or variations in other countries) is also used, I think mischievously, to protect manufacturers of patient data systems. The idea here is that the patient record system, heart monitor, or whatever, presents data to the clinician, and the clinician uses their professional expertise to determine what to do. The problem is that, used liberally, the doctrine allows the manufacturer to evade responsibility for debugging their system: the data is described as "advisory" rather than as "correct."

In the Lisa Norris radiotherapy overdose case, we saw that manufacturers changed the specification of their system and the radiotherapists didn't know they had.[b] With the Graseby syringe drivers used in Gosport,[c] Smiths Medical, their makers, have taken this further. Their operator's manual says:

> All possible care has been taken in the preparation of this publication, but Smiths Medical accepts no liability for any inaccuracies that may be found.
>
> Smiths Medical reserves the right to make changes without notice both to this publication and to the product which it describes.

Why would you not want to be responsible for inaccuracies? Why would you want to make changes but notify nobody? Surely good practice is to notify all relevant parties when changes are made, and thus avoid some of the problems that undermined the safety of Lisa Norris's treatment plan.

Smiths could have said they put all reasonable efforts into the system and its manual, maybe mentioned using state-of-the-art methods, and also stated that they'd like to hear from anybody who found errors so they can correct them speedily.[197]

More contractual problems arise as healthcare organizations walk into contracts that tie them up for years. Hospedia tied the NHS into long-term contracts to provide patients with pay TV. A service like that *might* have

---

[b] See Chapter 7: Beatson Oncology Centre, page 69 ←
[c] See Chapter 8: Gosport War Memorial Hospital tragedy, page 84 ←

seemed sensible a long time ago, but now hospital Wi-Fi makes streaming free — except some NHS regions signed an exclusive contract with Hospedia to provide video at cost to patients until 2027. How could the NHS's procurement be so naïve about the rate of change of digital technology as to lock themselves up for over twenty years? (They signed up in 2004 and the contract runs to 2027.) Well, Hospedia must have had a very good story to sell, and they must have sold it to procurement people who didn't understand digital technology.[198]

Manufacturers resist calls for stricter regulation because, as they say, it would stifle innovation, slow the development of new treatments, and cost a lot of money, and by the time something was approved it'd already be obsolete. None of these claims holds water. Airplanes have to go through rigorous testing and test flights, and can take over five years to get airworthiness certificates. Plane manufacturers understand this, and it doesn't limit the innovation (the Boeing 737 MAX tragedies mark a recent exception I'll discuss in more detail later).[d] People's lives depend on safe aircraft. As I'll soon argue, manufacturers could improve their devices in the time it takes to get them certified — it isn't wasted time; why rush to market with unreliable digital healthcare? Unfortunately, digital encourages this, because you can rush to market, for all the usual commercial reasons, and then sort out the software over the lifetime of the product (for instance, continually developing bug fixes and upgrades, taking advantage of the internet to deliver them). It is of course a good idea to fix bugs, but *planning* product development so the manufacturers needn't worry about the bugs in their products is unhelpful.

Until the law is changed, there is little incentive to improve digital systems, in hospitals or anywhere else. Gag clauses and lack of accountability have nothing to do with safe and effective healthcare. Indeed, both increase costs as well as compromising safety.[199]

I went to the website of the UK's MHRA, the Medicines and Healthcare Products Regulatory Agency. They say:

> The MHRA does not accept liability for any errors, omissions, misleading or other statements whether negligent or otherwise.

Even when they are negligent? I thought the MHRA enforced the law to make healthcare safer. Wouldn't it be more reassuring if the MHRA felt able to say something like,

> The MHRA defines and enforces the standards to which all medical devices and manufacturers must comply. We require manufacturers to accept liability for their products, as we accept liability for our own publications and regulations.

---

[d] See Chapter 26: Boeing 737 MAX crashes, page 352 →

The MHRA could be the world's leading medical regulator, making all the UK's medical and digital healthcare products the safest and most highly competitive internationally. Of course, by being similarly proactive, the same could be said of the US FDA, the Australian Health Practitioner Regulation Agency (AHPRA), or the Nigerian National Agency for Food & Drug Administration & Control (NAFDAC) too. Size is no barrier; the Nepal Department of Drug Administration has some ideas ...

The point is, *any* regulator, so motivated, could improve digital accountability and hence drive improvement in the quality of digital health and health more widely. Besides, safer digital healthcare would be more profitable and more competitive.

Until that time, why do we use any digital healthcare systems and medical apps when the manufacturers, developers, and regulators take so little responsibility for their safety?

Some programmers like to call themselves software architects. A real architect (somebody who designs and assesses buildings) in the UK is required to have professional indemnity insurance, at a minimum (as of 2018) of £250,000 — a very small figure compared to clinicians! As the Architects Registration Board says,[200] anyone who is carrying out professional work (even if they do it for free) may face liabilities, and they may continue to face costly cases even after their own death, so their insurance plans should cover this too.

It is the nature of building projects that faults and defects caused by failures in architectural design may not be visible for years, so the architect remains liable (in the UK) for 15 years for such liabilities. One wonders what manufacturers and software vendors will do another 15 years later — when the systems for which they should have been liable are no longer supported, no longer run, and, anyway, the original programmers have long since left. What a difference between real architecture and software architecture.

That's regulation for architects, but I could make similar arguments based on the regulation of nursing, allied health professionals, even rehabilitation engineers. Programmers, especially programmers developing and programming digital healthcare, need to become accountable, just like other professionals. Indeed, as I'll argue again and again, programmers build the systems that care for patients (often being the last stage of delivering critical care, like drugs and radiotherapy), so their regulation should surely be comparable to the regulations of the people qualified to use their devices and systems.

Part II ◇ Treatment ◇ Finding solutions

Digital healthcare needs much better regulation — and regulation needs to keep up with the unique issues of digital healthcare. Better regulation is a Safety Two approach: regulate for better processes to stop things going wrong.

16

Regulation needs fixing

Regulation is always in flux, and there are always proposals to change it. No doubt some of this chapter will soon be out of date on some technicalities, but it won't go out of date on the *attitudes* that underlie regulation. Regulation needs tightening, and it urgently needs to stay up-to-date with the unique issues raised by digital healthcare.

The US regulator, the FDA, has a regulatory shortcut called 510(k) that allows devices to be approved if they are substantially similar to some previous device that has previously been approved. This is supposed to encourage innovation, and it's a light-touch approach that industry supports — as, it must be said, do many patients eager to get help from new promises, like rapid treatments for their diseases.

The 510(k) process creates a daisy chain of products, each being justified by an earlier one that had been approved. It's possible for earlier products in the chain to be withdrawn from the market because they are obsolete or unsafe, yet industry can keep adding new approved products onto the end of the chain.

In the UK and across the EU the situation is similar.

CE marking is an EU idea used to regulate almost every product, from children's toys to hot water boilers and explosives. It allows approved products to be marketed in the EU. In particular, medical devices, and digital systems, like medical apps, must be certified with the CE marking in order to be legally used.[201]

To be legal, CE marking has to be printed precisely (figure 16.1). A correctly printed CE marking is supposed to mean that an "authority" claims that the marked product meets the relevant European standards. A CE-marked product can therefore probably be used safely. CE marking and what it really means is terribly complicated,[202] and I'd argue that if the aim is to ensure safety, then the law should be a lot simpler and work as we all expect it to — which it doesn't.

Fix It: See and solve the problems of digital healthcare. Harold Thimbleby,
Oxford University Press. © Harold Thimbleby 2021.
DOI: 10.1093/oso/9780198861270.003.0016

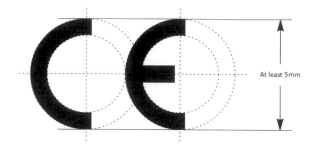

At least 5mm

Figure 16.1. The required dimensions for the CE mark are stricter than what it stands for. The pedantry in what a CE mark looks like and what it actually means for patient safety make a surprising contrast.

One of the important aspects of safety regulation is finding the right balance for proportionate regulation: not too much, and not too little, *given* what you are trying to achieve. In healthcare, products range from bed sheets to heart pacemakers, from cancer drugs to water jugs, from sheets of note paper to ECT machines. Medical device regulation is unavoidably complex.

In Europe devices are classified, and cover a range from unclassified, to classified as Class I, Class II or Class III, depending on the risk to the patient or member of staff. Class I is the least risky, and includes devices like thermometers and weighing scales; Class II is more risky including devices like ultrasound machines; finally, Class III is the most risky, including devices like brain implants for controlling Parkinson's. In the US, the classification system follows the same general idea, but is completely different in details. In all areas of the world, the classification strategy predates thinking about digital, and it is now being tweaked to fit.

A European Class I medical device can be self-certified *by the manufacturer* themselves.[203] When CE marking of medical devices is self-assessed, the developers who overlooked bugs in the first place may be the same team that self-assess to certify the software is safe. This is clearly an unsafe process. It's marking your own homework. It matters because digital crosses the conventional classifications. Microsoft Excel is not a medical device (according to the rules), but it is used for doing radiotherapy calculations that are a matter of life and death. Excel, seen like that, has uses as risky as any Class III device, yet it needs no regulation.

In more complex cases the certifying authority in the EU will need to be a **Notified Body**, which are themselves regulated. If a Notified Body declines to award a CE marking, the manufacturer can shop around Europe to find one that will. There are over 50 Notified Bodies, and they vie for the lucrative business of awarding CE markings.[204]

Strangely, some critical devices don't need approval to use in healthcare.

Calculators, which are widely used for critical drug calculations, are considered to be "office" products, so their CE marking means they are fine for offices. It says nothing about their safety or appropriateness for use in healthcare, and we've already seen that they have faults.[a]

The CE marking system is confidential, so it's impossible for third parties (like hospitals considering buying and using a CE-marked product) to find out what's going on. CE marking, then, doesn't do much to make digital healthcare any less risky.

Devices with higher classifications need to be certified by independent Notified Bodies *but* they aren't required to see the programs. It's like your teacher giving your homework a mark without them ever reading it, and, moreover, in a world where you pay them to pass you. And if you don't like the mark you get, you can go find another teacher who's nicer to you.

The existing regulatory approaches don't make sense for digital healthcare. For a start, the FDA's 510(k) idea of substantial equivalence requires arguing that two digital systems — the old one and the new one being approved — are equivalent. Yet equivalence is a well-known unsolvable problem in computer science; that is, you might build programs to be equivalent, but you *cannot* check whether two programs do the same thing after they've been built.[205] It is mathematically impossible. Therefore, you cannot regulate for substantial digital equivalence afterwards, unless you know all the math behind the construction of the two products, and even then it will often be impractical. Then, if you think of 5010(k), CE markings, and other regulatory ideas, they were developed before digital issues were relevant to healthcare. The current and future regulation of digital healthcare so far still doesn't take account of the power of digital, which means, for instance, that computers can do anything and can mislead clinical practice.[b]

Internationally, regulators have started to explore the issues of digital systems. It is now recognized in principle by regulators — but not yet in any regulations — that software is critically used across healthcare in different ways. Three main classes have been identified:

1. Software that on its own is effectively a medical device — **Software as a Medical Device**, SaMD;

2. Software that is part of a physical medical device — **Software in a Medical Device**, SiMD;

3. Software used in the manufacture or maintenance of a medical device.

The last category covers the case that software may be used in the design of conventional medical devices, like hip implants. If there were any bugs

---

[a] See Chapter 14: Risky calculations, page 177 ←
[b] See Chapter 13: Computational Thinking, page 151 ←

in the software, the medical device would be compromised. Bugs in any healthcare software are critical, wherever the software is used in the process.

For example, you could have a spreadsheet full of numbers. This is obviously data. But the data could have been generated from a software formula. Now the data is obviously program! The program might be AI; then the program itself has been generated by learning something from its training data. Is it data or program? Or print the spreadsheet onto paper; now it's *obviously* just numbers and not software. Yet from a regulatory perspective, that data should have been at least checked by software, so the data and its correctness depends totally on the quality of the software used in its production.

The problem for regulators is that historically medical devices were obviously physical, and the regulatory frameworks matured around that assumption. Then software become pervasive across healthcare, and changed the rules. Unfortunately, software has got to its present position with no real regulation. Even if we work out how to regulate digital perfectly, there is a huge backlog of unregulated and hardly regulated software that patient health depends on, and it will take ages to sort things out.

An area that is missed in the three-point classification above is **emergent behavior**. Things happen when software is joined with other things (including other software) that cannot be anticipated just by examining the software alone. The new things "emerge" — meaning the problems cannot be seen in the digital systems considered separately. For example, cybersecurity problems aren't caused by *one* system, but by connected systems, possible failing firewalls, and more. In a famous example, a single employee in the NHS managed to email 1.2 million staff; which was exacerbated by many staff using "reply to all" to complain about it.[206] Considered alone, email is wonderful, but its features have unexpected emergent features when used, which become painfully obvious in large organizations. Indeed, this email chaos is a bug: this reply-to-all problem is not a new emergent problem that should have caught anyone by surprise. It's a well-known bug that the NHS uses email with anything like a reply-to-all feature without a check on the number of emails that are going to be sent.

The same sort of buggy email features are still being used to accidentally, and quite inappropriately, mail confidential patient information. One case had a "horrendous breach of privacy," emailing identity details of 2,000 patients at a gender identity clinic.[207] This serious unlawful incident will likely cost the NHS many millions of pounds in compensation. It's important to fix well-known bugs, and certainly not just use standard digital systems, like "common off the shelf" (COTS) office email systems, assuming them to be immediately suitable for use in healthcare. There have been enough healthcare email fiascos for this not to be an unexpected problem.

I ordered a brand new Cardinal Health Alaris GP infusion pump after I visited one of their factories. I waited to get one of the first on the market.

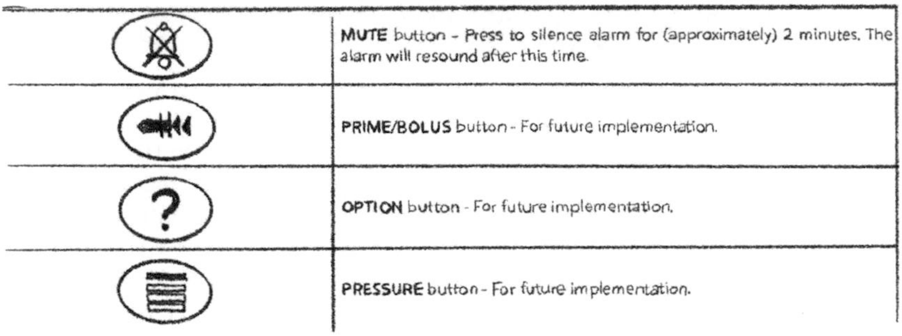

(icon)	**MUTE** button - Press to silence alarm for (approximately) 2 minutes. The alarm will resound after this time.
(icon)	**PRIME/BOLUS** button - For future implementation.
(?)	**OPTION** button - For future implementation.
(icon)	**PRESSURE** button - For future implementation.

Figure 16.2. A drawing showing part of the Alaris GP pump's operator manual. Since the missing features, "For future implementaton," are clearly written into the user manual, this can be no accident. The device's computer program is not finished.

When my new infusion pump turned up, it had very few features that worked. A small part of the user manual that came with it has been redrawn in figure 16.2.[208] Notice that three buttons on the front panel have not yet been implemented. They do nothing. The device is approved, but when the software is upgraded later, then these buttons can be programmed by the manufacturer to do anything. Whatever the buttons then do, the regulators won't have seen it, since the pump has already been approved without the functionality being implemented. Since it's a digital device, new features could do almost anything and change the behavior — and safety — of the approved Alaris GP.

An infusion pump (like the Alaris GP) is no longer a pump — it's more like an iPad. You can download apps to make your iPad do practically anything, and its behavior can change from being a novel to a virtual reality enhancer to a fitness monitor. Similarly, the software downloaded to upgrade an infusion pump can change it beyond recognition.

I used the Alaris GP in my postgraduate lectures as a case study of medical device design. It prompted some interesting discussion, and I put it away until I ran the course again the following year. The next year, the Alaris GP did not work. The battery had gone flat over the year, so I plugged it in and waited for it to charge back up. It didn't. It never worked again. The Alaris GP has a bug: the software it runs on requires battery backup, and when the battery goes flat, the software disappears and the device becomes unusable. This is not a helpful bug for hospital equipment that may be stored in cupboards, and is relied on to work when it's brought out to be used.

To be clear: the flat battery itself is a hardware problem (you need to recharge it or get a new battery), but a device unable to cope with a flat battery is a software problem: it's a bug that the digital features cannot cope with normal and expected conditions, like a battery going flat. Most likely, the

Part II ◇ Treatment ◇ Finding solutions

> **Box 16.1.** Drug regulation and fake drugs
>
> In just one submission to NICE, the UK's organization that reviews NHS treatments, a drug company provided 151 pages documenting rigorous evidence of clinical trials, modeling, and the economic value of their treatment for cystic fibrosis.[209] Cystic fibrosis is a nasty genetic disease that affects about 0.07% of the population in Ireland, the worst affected country in the world. Just one of the relevant cystic fibrosis drug trials involved 1,030 patients in 191 sites across 15 countries and took over 96 weeks — the trial was rigorously designed and registered in a national database and has rigorous peer-reviewed papers where more details can be found.[210] Why do digital systems that affect 100% of patients not require a comparable approach?
>
> Then there's the huge problem of fake medicines. The European Union (EU) Falsified Medicines Directive (Directive 2011/62/EU) has measures requiring obligatory safety features, including anti-tampering devices; rules on the import of pharmaceutical ingredients; and rigorous record-keeping requirements. If medicines can be faked, why not digital systems? Just consider cybersecurity hacks: faking digital systems is *very* common. Where, then, are the special regulations for fake digital healthcare?
>
> A typical cystic fibrosis treatment can cost the NHS £100,000 a year per patient. A typical medical app is free. No wonder medical device companies can't afford to develop safer software.

Alaris GP software is stored in "volatile memory," which requires battery power to work; when the battery goes flat, the memory fails. Clearly, at least some of the software ought to be stored in non-volatile memory so nothing essential disappears when the battery goes flat. Some people might want to argue that this problem is a hardware fault and not a bug, but the fact is, the Alaris no longer works because the software doesn't work. I call that a bug.

The FDA reviews the documentation (but not the software) that the manufacturer provides to justify their device being approved. In 2011 the US National Academy of Sciences reviewed the FDA's 35-year-old 510(k) regulatory process, and found it to be ineffective in assuring safety or clinical effectiveness.

The National Academy of Sciences concluded:

> Manufacturers are increasingly using software in devices, software as devices, and software as a tool in producing devices. That trend is expected to continue. The committee found that current guidance on software validation is insufficient for preventing serious software-based device failures.[211]

More defensive people will say that was written way back in 2011, and that much has changed since then.

Take one example: Europe has revised its Medical Device Regulations (MDR),[212] saying "a fundamental revision of those Directives is needed to establish a robust, transparent, predictable, and sustainable regulatory framework for medical devices which ensures a high level of safety and health whilst supporting innovation." While the new regulations are stricter, they are not stricter *for digital systems*. AI and ML are not mentioned, safer programming techniques are not mentioned, the internet isn't mentioned, and so on. Fortunately, the MDR specifies *minimum* standards, and countries are free to enforce higher standards, for instance in developer qualifications.

I find it interesting to contrast medical device regulations with, say, electrical or gas regulations. Electrical regulations, gas regulations, and many other regulations are very specific on technical details and on the qualifications and the certificates practitioners require to operate. People go to prison for flouting the rules.[213] In medical devices, the regulations (so far) are very vague. The MDR, for instance, does not specify that manufacturers need a specific level of digital qualifications. The gap between medical regulation and digital practice is huge, and is increasing. Digital isn't stopping to let regulation catch up.

If the lax regulation of digital healthcare is astonishing, the Netflix documentary, *The Bleeding Edge*,[214] about more conventional non-digital medical devices, such as hip implants and vaginal meshes, is utterly sobering. The 99-minute documentary interleaves facts about the $400 billion[5] US medical device industry, ineffective regulations, and cover ups, underpinned by powerful personal stories of people harmed, many horribly and irrevocably.

The UK's Health and Safety at Work Act, 1974,[215] is arguably the most important piece of health and safety legislation in UK history. The Act says of itself that it is

> An Act to make further provision for securing the health, safety, and welfare of persons at work, for protecting others [which includes patients] against risks to health or safety in connection with the activities of persons at work.

The Act's important Section 6 is a really good summary of what needs to be done to fix risky digital healthcare, and, at least in the UK, *it's the law*. Here's some of what it says:

(1) It shall be the duty of any person who designs, manufactures, imports or supplies any article for use at work [...]

    (a) to ensure, so far as is reasonably practicable, that the article is so designed and constructed that it will be safe and without risks to health at all times when it is being set, used, cleaned or maintained by a person at work;

    (b) to carry out or arrange for the carrying out of such testing and examination as may be necessary for the performance of the duty imposed on him by the preceding paragraph;

Part II ◇ Treatment ◇ Finding solutions

(c) to take such steps as are necessary to secure that persons supplied by that person with the article are provided with adequate information about the use for which the article is designed or has been tested and about any conditions necessary to ensure that it will be safe and without risks to health at all such times as are mentioned in paragraph (a) above and when it is being dismantled or disposed of; and

(d) to take such steps as are necessary to secure, so far as is reasonably practicable, that persons so supplied are provided with all such revisions of information provided to them by virtue of the preceding paragraph as are necessary by reason of its becoming known that anything gives rise to a serious risk to health or safety. [...]

(2) It shall be the duty of any person who undertakes the design or manufacture of any article for use at work [...] to carry out or arrange for the carrying out of any necessary research with a view to the discovery and, so far as is reasonably practicable, the elimination or minimization of any risks to health or safety to which the design or article may give rise.

It seems, then, that a lot of people in healthcare are breaking the law! However, the UK Health and Safety Executive (HSE) has decided to *exclude* situations where

> The error was due to design failure of medical equipment, which was unknown or had not been made known to the organization through appropriate channels such as MHRA [the UK medical devices regulator] or other safety alerts.

There is a widespread view that regulating digital healthcare should be relaxed, otherwise innovation will not flourish. Yet pharmaceuticals have a rigorous regulatory environment, and drug manufacturers don't complain much — thanks to thalidomide,[c] we'd all be very alarmed if they wanted to undermine the safety and regulatory environment that has been so carefully built up.

Ironically, digital regulation is in principle much easier to enforce and comply with than pharmaceutical regulation. It is much easier to comply and document everything you do when programming.

Everything computers do is written down, so it is easy to store in controlled documents and hand over to regulators, and everything the computers do is digital and can be automatically recorded. If things weren't written down, then the computer programs wouldn't even work. In contrast, most things pharmacists and chemists do are not automatically written down, so recording things for regulatory purposes is a lot more work in addition to what they are doing in their laboratories. What are digital innovators complaining about? I think they're just complaining about the costs of having to do a good job.

---

[c] See Chapter 8: The thalidomide story, page 81 ←

Cybersecurity is a serious problem for all computers and digital systems. In healthcare, patient safety is paramount, but in the wider world, security has a higher profile than safety. Both have problems caused by poor programming and all the design and development processes that precede actual coding.

17

Safe and secure

WannaCry was a worldwide cyberattack that happened in 2017. WannaCry quickly brought healthcare services worldwide to their knees. WannaCry sounds like an exotic and highly technical attack that only nerds or malicious countries would have the skills to understand and unleash. In fact, WannaCry was completely unsophisticated. The scary thing is that something so simple was so disruptive to an unprepared world.

Kits are readily available that enable unskilled hackers to build attack systems like WannaCry. Why they want to do this is another matter.

The WannaCry attack affected some 200,000 computers running Microsoft Windows, including many computers in the NHS and other health services worldwide. Fortunately, the objective of the criminals who wrote WannaCry seems to have been criminal extortion rather than terrorism, as the attack announced itself with a computer screen that informed the users that all their data had been encrypted and that the way to recover it was to pay a ransom. The disruption would have been worse had WannaCry not been quickly stopped by a cybersecurity researcher, Marcus Hutchins, who also goes under the name MalwareTech, activating a "kill-switch," albeit largely by chance.

Even though healthcare was not a specific target of the WannaCry attack, in the UK NHS alone 37 hospital trusts, including 27 acute trusts, were infected and locked out of devices. Almost 20,000 hospital patient appointments were canceled. Some 44 hospital trusts were not infected but experienced disruption, 21 trusts and 71 doctor (GP) practices had systems trying to contact the WannaCry command server, 595 GP practices were infected and locked out of devices. There would have been an unknown amount of further NHS disruption that was not reported — not least because computer systems and email were shut down to try to limit the problems.

Disruption to healthcare in other countries worldwide was on a similar scale.

Fix It: See and solve the problems of digital healthcare. Harold Thimbleby, Oxford University Press. © Harold Thimbleby 2021. DOI: 10.1093/oso/9780198861270.003.0017

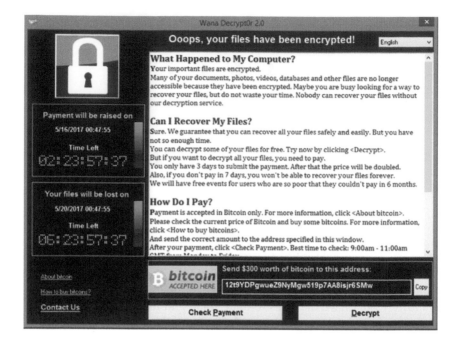

Figure 17.1. The WannaCry malware announces itself. The attack would have been much worse had it stayed silent, and just corrupted patient data without anyone noticing.

WannaCry caused huge disruption, and trying to avoid disruption caused more disruption. Queensland Health, Australia, in its attempt to protect its digital systems from WannaCry, managed to accidentally shut down the systems at five of its key hospitals. The affected hospitals were driven back to pencil and paper.[216]

The WannaCry attack just stopped things working, but it could easily have been designed to make changes to data instead of just encrypting it, because if files can be read and encrypted, then, clearly, they can be changed in arbitrary ways. WannaCry was not specifically aimed at healthcare, but imagine what the effect would have been if it had instead been designed to *change* critical medical data and, rather than blatantly announcing itself with a ransom screen (figure 17.1), and had remained hidden until several backup cycles had passed. How quickly could a hospital recover if blood groups, allergies, and other life-critical fields in medical records could no longer be trusted? Things might have gone horribly wrong long before anybody tracked down the cause.

WannaCry hit the headlines, but similar cybersecurity problems are rife.

It is sobering to search the US National Cybersecurity and Communications Integration Center's (NCCIC) database. Here's one example: Advi-

> **Box 17.1.** Ransomware and cyber extortion
>
> Cyberattacks take control of your digital systems. They can then do almost anything. Making money is easy. With **ransomware**, the cyberattack encrypts your data so you can't use it, and then holds you to ransom. Pay them thousands, and they "promise" to decrypt your data so you can use it again.
>
> In 2019, Riviera Beach, a small city of 35,000 people in Florida, paid up to a demand of $600,000.[217] The Riviera Beach cyberattack happened, ironically, after a police officer opened an email with a malware attachment.
>
> It's very good business when hackers can make so much money. Their techniques develop and they become more adept, and they stay well ahead of healthcare organizations that are already struggling with old IT infrastructure.
>
> Unfortunately, giving in to any ransom just encourages them. Worse, once a ransom is paid, the hackers have no incentive to bother to sort out the mess they've created. Recovering from a cyberattack, even when the hackers decrypt the information, can be hugely costly. The best insurance is to have safe backups from which an organization can recover. After all, you need backups in case the primary systems have a fire or other outage. Backups are intended to sort this sort of thing out, though to recover from a cyberattack it is of course essential to ensure the backup is not attacked as well.
>
> Best is not to get attacked in the first place (which requires fewer bugs). Most importantly, "IT literacy" or "digital literacy" — all staff knowing how to avoid attacks in the first place — is a good protection. Like not opening emails from strangers, and recognizing when emails spoof the people you think you know. Many years ago, I had my email account hacked because of an email that seemed to have come from a reliable colleague. Unfortunately *he* had been attacked: the hacker had already taken over his account. I was fooled. I now use **two-step authentication** (or two-factor authentication, 2FA, and more generally **multi-factor authentication**, MFA), so a hacker needs not only my accounts (from my computer) but my phone as well (or vice versa if my phone is attacked). IT literacy means keeping up; two-step authentication is now getting old hat.[218]

sory ICSMA-18-037-02, dated March 2018, concerns GE Healthcare digital medical device vulnerabilities,[219] and lists 23 GE devices that are used worldwide and have a security problem. The problem can be exploited remotely with little technical skill. The NCCIC gives details, explains what GE has done, and has suggestions for managing the problems. Nevertheless, it all seems a bit hit and miss: these are bugs in medical devices that should never have occurred in the first place — and they should have been detected and remedied by GE rather than by independent researchers.

Indeed, in July 2019, GE reported cyber-vulnerabilities to some of their anesthetic machines, specifically their Aestiva and Aespire models 7100 and 7900. If these machines are connected to the internet, the bug allows a remote hacker to modify settings and, dangerously, also silence alarms. I was interviewed by the BBC about this problem, and I said my bit,[220] but I now know that the BBC learned of the problems before some hospitals had even heard there was any problem with their equipment — one hospital told me they first knew about the problem from reading "my" BBC news item!

GE Healthcare is reported to have said there was no "direct patient risk." In my opinion, this is a bit misleading; there is no patient risk so long as the anesthetist is alert to the problems. In law, the anesthetist is responsible, but in reality if their anesthetic machine is tampered with and has silenced alarms, isn't this a bug (which you can blame on GE or the hacker exploiting the bug) rather than an anesthetist's responsibility?

GE's disclosure of the problems followed a contorted pathway down to the key people who could do anything about it. This is unacceptable at many levels. Fortunately, most hospitals don't have anesthetic machines routinely connected to the internet — but this is no real protection, as it only takes a few seconds of internet connection for things to go wrong.

One anesthiologist was reported as saying:

> The likelihood of harm being caused to a patient through any hacking of the devices is "incredibly small" — patients should be reassured that their anæsthetist will be monitoring them constantly, and will have received many years of training to rectify immediately the situation of a device failure.[220]

It's understandable that they'd want to reassure the public like this, but this sort of public gloss on a serious, avoidable, problem won't help improve the quality of digital healthcare.

It's baffling that many well-published attacks like WannaCry and others seem to have changed so little. Old systems are still being used; new systems continue to have basic bugs that leave them vulnerable to hacking; regulations and IT management haven't tightened up.

In October 2020 — over three years after WannaCry — a Finnish psychotherapy center, Vastamo, was hacked. The hackers published sensitive information of at least 300 people online and sent emails to the center's patients to extort cash.[221] The center's patients include children, and its data includes transcripts of sessions.

Why wasn't all the center's sensitive data encrypted securely, so that even if it was stolen, it was useless to the hackers? Put in other words: why was the database design so buggy, why was such a bad system procured, and why wasn't it fixed?

In May 2021 — over fours years after WannaCry — another cyber attack affected *all* of Ireland's national and local Health Service systems. The attack meant that all computer systems had to be shut down.

Anne O'Connor of the Health Service Executive told the Irish broadcaster RTÉ:

> ... we will be in a very serious situation and we will be
> cancelling many services. At this moment we can't access lists
> of people who are scheduled for appointments on Monday, so
> we don't even know who to cancel.[222]

Clearly, and soon, if not yesterday, healthcare services will have to start training patients as well as staff about cybersecurity: once patient health data is hacked and, very likely, combined with other hacked data (such as hacked credit card or bank details) patients will *very easily* be persuaded to part with everything.

It's hard not to ask very basic, but probably quite harsh-sounding, questions about multistep security, backups and other protections, and proper organizational IT support, whether in Finland, Ireland, or — with WannaCry — everywhere. On the other hand, cyber attackers are nasty people, and we can't just blame the victims. Indeed, cyber attack methods are changing all the time, and it's hard, even for full time cyber professionals, to keep up. I've left further discussion of these sorts of problems to the book's further reading[a] — where I mention RIPPLE20 and other bugs that have compromised *billions*[5] of devices.

The scale of the problem — and the fact that things don't seem to be getting any better in digital healthcare — is utterly shocking.

———————————◆———————————

I wrote this book on my Apple MacBook Pro laptop. I've set it up so I have to log in with my name and password to use it — so if my laptop is stolen, the thieves can't log in and use it. But a determined thief could unscrew the back and take the laptop's disk out, and plug it into another computer they do have a password for. To stop that being a problem, I also encrypt the disk itself. That means to access any data on it, even if you take it out of the computer, you need the disk's own password as well.

I also back up my laptop several times a day, and I backup to four different locations, just in case any of them get into trouble. For instance, two of the backup locations are in my own house, so if somebody broke in and stole my raid disk systems or if the house burned down, I need to make sure I have independent backups. Two of my backups are not networked, so they cannot be hacked.

I don't just backup, I also use a version control system so that I can recover today's work, yesterday's, or recover work from any time in the past. That's in case I accidentally make a mess of my data and back up the mess — I'd then want to recover the previous day's work, not the messed up work.

I've also got firewalls and stuff to reduce the risk of any cyberattack getting to my laptop in the first place.

Since I'm writing a book about bugs, you can be sure that fate is determined to make an example of me by ensuring lots of things go wrong at

---

[a] See Chapter 33: Good reading, page 471 →

once! I have had disk drives fail in the past, and to be honest, although I have data that goes back to the 1970s, my current redundant backup system only works back to 2017.

At least that's what I do. I don't have any patient data on my laptop, so my approach is pretty relaxed compared to what professionals *should* do.

LifeLabs is a Canadian medical lab test company that handles data for 15 million patients, including their addresses, passwords, birth dates, health card numbers, and medical lab results. LifeLabs reported they were hacked in November 2019, and they lost patient data, some of it going back to 2016. Here's what we know:[223]

- LifeLabs paid the hackers a ransom. This implies that LifeLabs have no off-site backup that was not also compromised by the attack. In turn, if LifeLabs has recovered data (thanks to paying the ransom), this implies that they will have no way of checking if the "recovered" data has been compromised by the hackers. For example, it would be easy for the hackers to change lab results for all patients, possibly causing life-threatening consequences, and LifeLabs would have no idea that had happened.

- LifeLabs have no idea whether the hackers have distributed the patient data any further. The hackers could make a lot of money selling the patient data. This implies the data was not encrypted, although encrypted data is still worth selling (though they would get less for it) because somebody may be able to break the encryption.

- LifeLabs is now offering a free year of protection, including dark web monitoring (to see if the data resurfaces) and identity theft insurance. A year's protection seems little compensation for criminals getting access to information like your home address and using it next year.

- The chief executive of the company, Charles Brown, called the incident "a wake-up call for the industry." That suggests they've been asleep. He hasn't been paying attention to cybersecurity problems — WannaCry was worldwide news two years earlier — and he hasn't been thinking about how to make his company more secure. Furthermore, it has been reported that he doesn't know if the LifeLabs hacked medical test data was encrypted, which certainly suggests he has very little idea about cybersecurity or how his company runs its digital systems.

- The easiest way of cracking encryption is to use **social engineering** — for instance, tricking passwords out of LifeLabs employees. Given how ignorant the chief executive is about cybersecurity at his company, how many of his employees know about phishing and other social engineering tricks?

I think we can all agree with Charles Brown: the incident certainly was a wake-up call.

I must admit I was surprised that WannaCry didn't immediately result in worldwide legislation to force LifeLabs, Ireland's HSE, and Finland's Vastamo — and all the others — to wake up; clearly some people have carried on as if nothing has happened. For LifeLabs, "carrying on" resulted in an unnecessary loss and likely corruption of data for *millions* of patients.

Like the US National Cybersecurity and Communications Integration Center, the UK has its own National Cyber Security Centre (NCSC) too, and it lists plenty of problems, including US and UK hospital cyber incidents. Cybersecurity is a very serious global problem. Cybersecurity problems aren't healthcare's fault, although it's easy to make cybersecurity worse (like by not securely backing up data).[224]

Somehow, healthcare clearly needs to have much better awareness and much more effective procedures for dealing with digital problems. I am mystified that there is no legislation or regulation in place to make sure these sorts of things happen. How can a company managing millions of patients' data be surprised by cyberattacks? Nobody is listening. What we need is at least this:

- National systems need to sort out their procedures. In the UK, NHS Digital said it could not confirm the extent to which the Aestiva and Aespire machines were still in use across the NHS. Why don't they keep inventory? Basic stuff.

- Hospitals cannot procure digital systems without being fully aware of safety and cyber issues. Levels of acceptable performance must be specified in contracts. The entire burden of working out technical details of what's required needn't be on hospitals: manufacturers should be helpful and open about these issues, and hospitals can select what they want for given systems. But to be silent is not an option.

- Manufacturers must be more proactive in notifying hospitals of problems, and must provide effective solutions. Of course, manufacturers should follow best practice.

- Security updates must be handled systematically. In a national healthcare system, it is surprising that this is not centrally co-ordinated.

- Front-line staff — all staff with IT access — must be trained and be more aware of digital risks.

- All the above applies to cybersecurity problems and to all other forms of bugs and software upgrades.

Part II ◇ Treatment ◇ Finding solutions

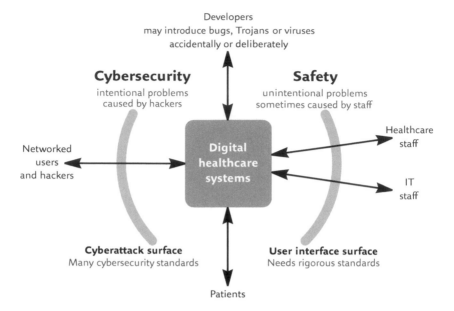

Figure 17.2. A digital device responds to the network and to users in essentially the same way. In addition, developers may introduce weaknesses, accidentally (e.g., bugs and viruses) or deliberately (e.g., Trojans and other malware). Poor design and programming on either side is dangerous.

Cybersecurity, rightly, has a very high profile, as it is obviously important to get right and to have the best defenses against malicious attack. It's obvious that there are bad people out there who want to hack systems, so we would be irresponsible to ignore the threat. But the opportunities these people have to hack are created by poor-quality software. Sure, the "evil hackers" get in and poor cybersecurity exacerbates the problems, but the root cause is that software bugs and weaknesses leave the front door open.

In contrast, virtually no clinician is trying to hack in or cause system problems: the problems happen unintentionally — and the clinicians are labeled as "blundering" or "bad."

We often overlook the fact that cybersecurity problems have the same causes as all other problems with risky digital healthcare: namely bugs and poor-quality software.

The picture (figure 17.2) illustrates the point. On the left, programming bugs are deliberately exploited by hackers, mainly via the internet and Wi-Fi software. On the right, bugs are mainly encountered unintentionally by users, doctors and nurses, operating the equipment. Don't just concentrate on cybersecurity, as there are bugs on both sides.

There is a complication my diagram doesn't show. Some cybersecurity problems happen when internal staff (including contractors) fall prey to phishing or other social engineering scams. One common phishing attack happens when one of your colleagues has already been attacked, and they then (unwittingly) send everyone on their address list an email, including sending you one. You then get phished, with some plausible-sounding email. It only takes one person to respond, and the chain of deceit expands its range by stealing another address list. Since the email apparently comes from a friend or a senior manager, eventually somebody falls for clicking on a dodgy link, typing in their password, or giving away some other information.

I was recently sent a phishing email, apparently from my Head of Department, saying he was in a meeting but needed an Amazon voucher to give to a student as a prize. I like to be helpful, but if I'd sent "him" a voucher, I'd have lost the money to the hackers who sent the email.

Hackers and criminals are devious, and they are not at all obliged to follow my diagram (figure 17.2)! They may, for instance, send phishing emails to the good staff on the right side of the diagram to trick them into breaching security or causing other problems *themselves*. Or they might even put bugs *inside* the digital healthcare system by planting devious software in it when it was originally programmed — such bugs (or Trojan Horses) then will stay hidden until the hacker wants to exploit them at a later date. This attack happens surprisingly often when disgruntled programmers try to get their own back on their employers.

We would be being incompetent if we did nothing to defend ourselves against hackers. Lots of money is therefore invested in cybersecurity, but mostly at national level, as, for instance, in the UK National Cyber Security Centre. We would still blame ourselves — or our staff — if we got attacked.

Thinking about security is completely different to thinking about safety. In security, the obvious culture is that we need to fix the root causes of the problems, namely we need to fix our software vulnerabilities quickly and effectively. In contrast, the usual safety culture is that, instead of fixing the problems, we rarely even notice them and then we blame the nurse or doctor. Therefore, unlike security, there is nothing else to do!

WannaCry basically stopped systems working, and it attacked only old versions of Microsoft Windows (such as ones running MRI scanners), so that many digital systems thankfully escaped its attack. In general, attacks can do much worse damage — and eventually they will. They can directly change the drug delivery rates on infusion pumps remotely, or even reprogram a heart pacemaker actually inside a patient.

A **cybervulnerability** in a St Jude pacemaker led the FDA (the US medical device regulator) to require 465,000 pacemakers to be reprogrammed to fix the bug. Nearly half a million patients therefore had to visit hospitals for the procedure. Meanwhile, hackers would have been aware of the pacemakers' bugs and the patients' vulnerability if they'd wanted to exploit them.

Part II ◇ Treatment ◇ Finding solutions

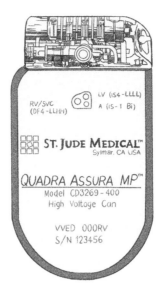

Figure 17.3. Drawing of a typical St Jude heart pacemaker implant, small enough to fit in your hand, or inside your chest if needed.

What's especially interesting, again, is the huge interest — and huge amounts of money — in a cybersecurity vulnerability that threatened patients, but the widespread lack of interest in risky healthcare more generally. We need to focus some of that technical energy into improving all of healthcare, not just cybersecurity.

It was a security company called MedSec Holdings who found the cyber-vulnerabilities in the St Jude pacemaker. However, instead of telling the FDA or St Jude, MedSec revealed the flaws to Muddy Waters Capital, who then sold St Jude shares short to profit from the anticipated fall in their share price when the public learned of the bugs.[225]

In the end, about $1 billion[5] was wiped off St Jude share values, which made it vulnerable to takeover. Abbott (another medical device company) then bought St Jude for a bargain $25 billion.

The short-selling activity, MedSec argued, was to fund their core business of finding security flaws. It's ingenious, dubious ethically, and certainly shows disregard for patient well-being.

On the other hand, MedSec claims that if they had done the conventional thing, which would have been to tell St Jude privately that they need to fix their problems, then St Jude would have just swept the problems under the carpet. That wouldn't have helped patients. In the end, St Jude wasn't able to sweep anything under the carpet.

MedSec made huge profit while risking St Jude going bust, which would have endangered at least 465,000 patients. MedSec also revealed there were bugs in the pacemaker, encouraging hackers to attack patients with St Jude implants.

Behind all that, of course, are the questions like these:

🡒 Why does a pacemaker have a bug, in this case, not "just a bug" but a serious cybervulnerability that makes the bug exploitable over the internet or in some other way remotely?

🡒 If a pacemaker does have a bug, why it isn't easy to fix? If the bug can be exploited over the internet, why can't St Jude patch it over the internet?

🡒 Why doesn't a pacemaker (at least for most problems) fail gracefully,[b] so it isn't an emergency to fix it?

🡒 Why didn't St Jude work with effective cybersecurity laboratories so bugs like this weren't a surprise?

🡒 Hindsight is a wonderful thing, of course. But the St Jude pacemaker wasn't the first pacemaker ever. Where is the learning — where are the open standards — so that pacemakers are improving? What other companies have learned from St Jude and improved their practices?

If you want to become an investigator, go to the FDA's reporting database. Their database is called MAUDE, the Manufacturer and User Facility Device Experience.[226] You'll find stuff like this:

> **Event Description**: It was reported that the patient expired. There is no known allegation from a health care professional that suggests the death was device related. The cause of death was unknown. No additional information was available at this time.

On the whole, these FDA incident reports aren't very helpful, and compared to, say, the detailed evidence around car and aviation crashes, the medical reports are scandalously vague.

Why didn't St Jude upload all the data from their device and know what was going on? In aviation it is routine to analyze black box data. For any medical device manufacturer to say to the FDA that "no additional information is available at this time" is a euphemism for saying they don't want to disclose data or bother to collect it in the first place. In contrast, publicly available, well-written, extensive reports are available for aviation accidents.[227] One wonders why aviation is getting safer and digital healthcare isn't — we'll look more closely at that story in another chapter.[c]

---

[b] See Chapter 21: Graceful degradation, page 292 →
[c] See Chapter 26: Planes are safer, page 347 →

In order to improve the risky digital systems, safety needs to be understood and treated as seriously as cybersecurity. This involves financing digital safety research and hands-on digital safety in healthcare adequately, and improving regulation to make it happen.

It's obvious to everyone that consumer digital technologies are amazing, so — the thinking goes — we just need to update healthcare to catch up. But, no, we must stop thinking about the latest digital as an automatic improvement, or even as an improvement over tired, obsolete, digital that's years behind the gadgets in our pockets.

Digital is only an improvement *when* it's resourced properly, with "resourced" meaning more than money to buy new stuff, or somebody on the Board, or even some supportive politicians. Again, no. We must learn the right lessons from WannaCry, Finland, Ireland, St Jude, and the too-many other such stories.

Reliable and safe digital healthcare needs teams of people at the center, who are properly qualified and professionally well-informed about how the latest digital works, including having thorough knowledge of cybersecurity, and all the other intricacies this book talks about.

Digital healthcare is not a job for enthusiasts.

It's no good having an IT Department who are run off their feet.

Digital healthcare must be done by professionals and resourced properly, just like any other sort of engineering that lives depend on. Until that happens, I think it'd be easier and quicker to set up formal two-way links between healthcare and every university department of Computer Science. After all, universities are *already* training the next generations of both hackers and professional software engineers.

Until some ideas like that, or better, are taken seriously, this chapter on cybersecurity disasters will just keep getting longer and longer.

Who is profiting from our data? Is Artificial Intelligence (AI) the solution to better healthcare?

18

Who profits?

Jack Singer faced a lawsuit. He had developed a new eye surgery technique for removing cataracts, without needing any stitches, so it the surgery healed faster. He had started teaching the method. And then the lawsuit came. It wanted him to pay royalties to someone who'd patented the idea already. Samuel Pallin was demanding $10,000 per year. Fighting the case cost Jack his job, and his clinic, and left him a bill of over $500,000.

Jack's case is not unique.[228] He died in 2011, and will be remembered as the doctor who, through his hard work (and the help of astonished colleagues), finally won the right for all doctors, particularly ophthalmologists like him, to perform surgery without fear of interference from patent holders.

Things have changed a lot since Singer's 1993 law suit.

Today, most of us willingly sign up to give away almost everything that defines us. Google know where we are and what we are doing — they know what we are interested in. Facebook and Twitter know all our friends and interests. Amazon knows what we buy. All these companies, to varying degrees, make a living out of advertising and propaganda, selling our data, and predicting what we'll do next. Facebook is now notorious for the huge business it has in forming people's opinions — and influencing the outcomes of national elections and referenda.

Contrary to privacy laws (such as Europe's GDPR, the General Data Protection Regulation) we also give a lot away *without* noticing, let alone signing it away. Many medical websites, like WebMD, Healthline, Babycentre, and Bupa, share our data when we browse them, generally with companies like Facebook and DoubleClick, Google's advertising subsidiary.[229] These companies argue that the amount of information we give away is "not sensitive" (who defines what's sensitive?) and that they don't sell it (though they must gain commercially from doing it, else why do it?). Yet even if our own personal information is tiny, by the time the website aggregates millions of users, the information has serious value.

Fix It: See and solve the problems of digital healthcare. Harold Thimbleby, Oxford University Press. © Harold Thimbleby 2021. DOI: 10.1093/oso/9780198861270.003.0018

The business these companies really have is different and hidden from the businesses we can see and think we're experiencing. We think we have a free and wonderful experience. After all, Facebook and WhatsApp and the others are free to use. However, in thinking it's free, we under-value what we are worth — where are we, what products are next to us, what targeted adverts will work best, who are we talking to (and where are they, what shops are they in ...)?[230] Indeed, Facebook is developing a new app, Preventive Health, to leverage users' health concerns, starting collecting data on — sorry, "helping" — users with, flu jabs, cancer screenings, and blood pressure tests.[231]

Such are the features, subtle side effects, and monetization that very few users expect to have. They create a privacy-destroying surveillance commercial world that, if nothing else, has no place in healthcare that otherwise respects confidentiality.

Of course, when we go to the doctors, a clinic or the hospital, our medical information, what drugs we use, our diseases, and mental health, and more, is recorded. That data, too, is widely shared. Of course, the healthcare system needs our medical records to treat us effectively, and it needs to review its data to see how it can improve.[232] Delays in adopting best practice or unusual increases in deaths, for instance, need investigating. The data is also used for medical research and developing drugs and other treatments. Who owns this data? Naturally the doctors, the hospitals, and larger health organizations, like the NHS, which has collected some of the largest medical datasets in the world, want to profit from the data they have collected — and they do. The NHS data alone is worth about £10 billion[5] a year.[233]

Industry is pushing hard into a Wild West of unregulated territory. The concepts are completely new, on an unimaginable scale, and years ahead of the traditional concerns of medical regulators. In 2019, Facebook had around 2.5 *billion* users,[5] and the other popular apps have similarly huge numbers, yet the regulations they work under were designed in a simple world where the snake oil salesman had a hundred customers and sold things you could see and take to a laboratory to test. The good news is we'll discover new cures and ways of having a healthier population; the bad news is that the motivation is to make money, and the global scale of the operations means that the medical interventions — for that is what they are — are going under the regulatory radars.

I've already mentioned the Practice Fusion scandal,[a] where a widely used digital healthcare system raised advertising revenue, with a business model more like a consumer product might have. But Practice Fusion crossed the line from consumer advertising with consent (however vague) into secret, manipulative advertising, nudging clinicians to prescribe opioid drugs that gave Practice Fusion a significant additional revenue. We've already got an opioid crisis, and Practice Fusion is making money promoting it.

---

[a] See Chapter 2: Practice Fusion's nudging, page 18 ←

We do want manufacturers to monitor how their products are working —
it's called **post-market surveillance**. It's an important part of detecting
bugs and improving the safety of medical systems. Yet if the manufacturers
are recording most of what you do, like where you are and each dose of ad-
dictive opioid or your blood glucose levels, this private medical data easily
gets into the hands of financial credit agencies, foreign states, and more. And
when a system has bugs (as they do) or a cyberattack (as they will), all their
assurances about private data are void. If only digital healthcare had fewer
bugs!

The clash is that we want the power of new digital technologies to solve
healthcare's various problems and inefficiencies, but we currently want it for
free to use, just like consumer products like WhatsApp that *seem* free at the
point of use.

Our medical data, which is what healthcare is based on, is — or should
be — worth more than our consumer data, which has driven Facebook into
world dominance in social media. Our data will lead to new treatments.
Those treatments, based on our data, including our genetic data, will be profitable for the companies that own them.

This is new territory. Central to making it work smoothly are "big data"
and the digital technologies of Artificial Intelligence (AI) and Machine Learning (ML — not to be confused with mL, for milliliter). ML is a trendy type
of AI, generally associated with processing tons of data.

Google's DeepMind Health is a cautionary tale.

An arrangement between Google DeepMind and Moorfields Eye Hospital gave DeepMind Health millions of patients' eye images, for which Moorfields was paid £110,000.[234] As a result of analyzing this data, DeepMind's
AI can now, in principle, cut down on the time and cost of diagnosing over
50 eye conditions. This sort of technical advance may save the sight of thousands of patients and may save the healthcare system a lot of money.

All diagnostic methods have **false positives** (you are diagnosed with the
disease, but you don't have it) and **false negatives** (you are diagnosed as
free from the disease, but you do have it). Without basic information on the
false positive rate and the false negative rate, from which no diagnostic system is immune, it is impossible to say anything specific other than that more
research is needed. Indeed, this AI for diagnosing eye conditions from data
is an unclassified medical device, though aspects might be a self-certified
device: yet its only purpose is to drive critical clinical decisions that need
more careful regulation. But it isn't something like a textbook for teaching
a clinician who later exercises their clinical judgment; it's a bespoke system
giving (apparently) precise patient-specific information that leads directly to
serious interventions.

There is a twist to all improved diagnosis, called **lead-time bias**. The
better we diagnose illnesses, the more treatment is demanded. Since treatments have side effects, it's possible that earlier diagnosis paradoxically in-

creases illness. Even more paradoxically, the earlier a condition is diagnosed, the longer people apparently live with the condition: improved diagnosis seems to make treatment more effective, yet the patient has to live with the anxiety of knowing they have the disease for longer. Without more research, we can only say this AI might cost healthcare a lot more money to perform the required treatments, or it might improve people's quality of life with better sight, or it might cause increased anxiety in patients who are diagnosed and have to wait for (or cannot afford) treatment. We don't know — yet.

Clearly a lot more research needs doing, and in my view the priority should be to do it scientifically. Science creates public knowledge, it creates testable, reproducible knowledge that others can build on and improve. Science — or, rather, the attitudes that underlie science — are why we have all these fantastic things in the first place. To turn what should be science at this stage into business, intellectual property, copyright, commercial confidence is a travesty. Business can do that later, when we've worked out how to get things to work. Indeed, isn't that the core problem? Business has rushed into digital healthcare when nobody really knows how to do it properly, but business knows how to make money out of it in the meantime.

Moorfields was allowed by DeepMind to use their system for free for five years. This seems like a short-sighted agreement, as it hands all the long-term rights of the data and AI to DeepMind. DeepMind are surely making similar agreements with other hospitals around the world, not least to avoid training their AI systems on unrepresentative samples of the population.

In another project, a DeepMind app used at the Royal Free Hospital in London is integrating 1.6 million patient medical records and test results. This system saves some nurses around two hours a day each and costs the hospital nothing.[235] That sounds very useful — but what is Google's business model that makes it worthwhile for it to do all this technical work "for free"? What will Google use the data for in the long term? How will the world benefit?

The UK information commissioner ruled that the Royal Free allowed DeepMind access to patient data without consent. It's the start of a controversy most people don't begin to understand. For example, if a patient decides they do not want their data to be given to DeepMind (why help a commercial business with no payback to yourself?), it's too late, as their data was anonymized and DeepMind has already lost track of it.

An independent review of DeepMind said:

> All companies that wish to operate in the area of healthcare data ought to be held to high standards, but the onus is even greater for a company such as DeepMind Health.[236]

That's hardly likely to happen, as DeepMind itself has now disappeared inside Google, and this critical report seems to have disappeared along with it.[237]

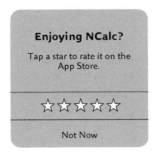

Enjoying NCalc?

Tap a star to rate it on the
App Store.

☆ ☆ ☆ ☆ ☆

Not Now

Figure 18.1. Rating dialogs like this pop up unexpectedly and obscure the screen while you are using many medical apps. The dialog obscures the app's screen and makes it impossible to use until it is rated or you tap "Not Now" and postpone the survey to interrupt you some time again in the future. The rating design here is based on the NCalc 2.0 app for calculating early warning scores for patients, which is not a task you can interrupt safely. In addition, using NCalc, adverts appear continually at the bottom of the screen. You have to pay to get rid of them.

In principle, the scientific value of this work is undoubted; in fact, it's amazing and could eventually help millions of people with sight problems worldwide (assuming we can reach them all with appropriate digital technologies). On the other hand, as Dr Singer found out, commercial interests take precedence, and when they do the scientific value is nil.

Apart from the big names, very few medical apps make money. If apps aren't charitable and don't have any other business model, they need subscriptions or must make money indirectly, typically by advertising or by monetizing user data (like the user's contact list), or by selling additional features, like getting the user to pay to block disruptive adverts.

NEWS is the NHS's National Early Warning Score, which helps identify patient deterioration; it's an important part of patient safety, particularly as deterioration (say from sepsis) is easy to miss. There are two versions of the NEWS score: the original NEWS (phased out in 2017) and the newer 2019 version, called NEWS2.

There is a "free" CE-marked app, NCalc 2.0, for NEWS scores, which runs both versions of NEWS (figure 18.1). It doesn't say which version it is running, and the app's Help menu option doesn't explain either. Users may be able to work it out by experimenting, because there is a menu to choose the version it isn't using, and if you select this menu option several times, you'll be able to work out that the menu showing NEWS or NEWS 2 means you are using NEWS2 or NEWS, respectively.

The point of using a NEWS app is to get a *reliable* early warning score quickly. So, why is it so hard to tell which NEWS score NCalc 2.0 is actually measuring? The need to make a good business out the app seems to take precedence. Indeed, the user is regularly blocked using the app while if collects marketing information (figure 18.1). In contrast to the eagerness for getting marketing data from users in the middle of trying to use it, the app provides no way to report bugs or to help make it more reliable.

The NHS National Early Warning Score is only one type of early warning score (EWS) to help anticipate patient deterioration. There are many other scoring systems. Interestingly, recent research shows that nurses can be more reliable than early warning scores like NEWS, and that some mix of nurse insight and algorithmic scoring may be better.[238] And of course there's no point using an app if the person using it either makes errors or misses the score or the significance of the score — it seems likely that nurse insight is going to be more effective in a busy clinical environment. There is a lot more work to do, in app development in what works best for patients, and in working out how to raise the funds to do the needed research, let alone in building a successful business out of it that doesn't compromise the value of the app. NCalc 2.0, typical of many medical apps, seems to have a way to go.

When I tried to track down the NCalc developers, I got a warning: "This website may be impersonating "www.lindummedical.co.uk" to steal your personal or financial information." Hmm. Their certificates aren't up-to-date.

A different app, the COVID Symptom Study by ZOE, like NCalc, took advantage of advertising to raise funds. Having access to users' personal details, ZOE sent an advertising email to users encouraging them to buy masks — raising questions on how the app manages user privacy. Prof Tim Spector, an epidemiologist leading the research behind the app, apologized in a follow-up email:

> We thought selling donated masks for charity would be a good opportunity to raise money for long Covid research, however, **we did not consider the implications of working with a commercial company**.[239]

My **bold** emphasis. Many users have said they will delete the app.

———————————◾———————————

AI can solve problems that humans struggle with, and it can solve problems faster, repeatedly without tiring, and more cheaply. That's very positive, but it may be a deal with the devil: to get the benefits, you (usually) sign away your rights to private data, so companies can make profits out of things you didn't even know about yourself, and — a key concern of this book — you lose scrutiny. When an AI system says a patient has a diagnosis, it generally can't explain why. If the AI has bugs, as it surely will, then, generally, you can't tell. Indeed, AI has at least two sorts of bugs: it can have conventional programming bugs in how it is implemented (so, under some circumstances, the AI will not work as intended); and AI can have bugs in its data

Box 18.1. Simpson's Paradox

Analyzing data reliably is very complex. In the diagrams below, four data points are used as a toy example to illustrate **Simpson's Paradox**.

On the left, four data points — perhaps obtained from measuring patients — obviously represent an increasing trend, which I've shown as a straight line. On the right, *exactly the same* data, but now split by gender, shows that male and female trends are in opposite directions.

For fun, I used a neural net to find the two regression lines below. Even though this is overkill AI for this job, evidently the AI doesn't help avoid the difficulties of reliable analysis.

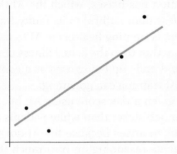

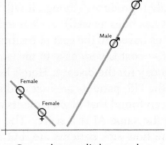

| All data, ignoring gender | Same data, split by gender |

Simpson's Paradox is relevant for both digital healthcare and medicine. It's been pointed out for a case where it affected the interpretation of a kidney stone experiment,[240] though in this case the problem was not the hidden variable of gender, but the hidden variable of kidney stone diameter. It's also resulted in confusion on pandemic severity.[241]

(meaning the AI has been trained inadequately or incorrectly). For example, an AI to recognize skin cancers from photographs may have a programming bug that ignores parts of the color spectrum; it may have data bugs because it was trained on white skin, so has not learned from samples of black skin cancers.[242] The final AI will have a mixture of both sorts of bugs, and it will be hard to eliminate them all, particularly as they interact, as my skin color example makes clear — moreover, the bugs may partly compensate for each other, which makes them even more obscure.

Now's a good time in this book to try to define **Artificial Intelligence (AI)**. AI is the deliberate approach to use data — patient data, financial data, X-rays, blood results, speech instructions, and more — in ways that we otherwise wouldn't know how to program. The computer "learns" or otherwise uses heuristics (a posh word for guesses) to solve problems in sophisticated ways that can't, or can't easily, be programmed directly by humans. It's pointless to define AI more precisely, as there are lots of vested interests trying to promote one exciting sort of AI over another.

AI got going sorting out the challenges of playing chess. Chess, although a hard game, is in principle easy for AI because everything is known about the game: where the pieces are, whose move it is. All the rules are well known and simple. However, healthcare applications of AI are much harder, because we don't know everything, and a lot of the data has errors in it, and we have little idea about the rules because we don't know the underlying science well-enough.

Training AI to learn "the truth" is very hard, so **proxies** are used. For instance: instead of training an AI how to recognize faces using data from everyone, a smaller, much more convenient sample of faces is used. Unfortunately, this proxy of the entire population has biases, which the AI then faithfully reproduces (though it will be *less* than faithful to its faulty training if it has bugs as well). A clear example is training healthcare AI to make decisions based on the cost of treatment, rather than the actual illness of the patient — cost is very easy to measure and ends up being used as a convenient proxy for the disease. Here's how AI training can go wrong:

In the US, patients are assessed and given a risk score using AI, but it's now been found that black patients are much sicker than white patients assigned the same AI risk score. The problem arises because the AI doesn't measure how sick patients are, but bases its reasoning on how much they pay — it's using cost as an easy, but as it happens unreliable, proxy for measuring disease. Since there is racially unequal access to healthcare in the US, data based on cost of care underestimates how sick the low-paying — predominantly black — patients are. This then leads to inequalities in program screening: the AI misleads the healthcare providers into thinking black people are less likely to require healthcare interventions.[243]

A further twist to this bias is that the AI system is a commercial system whose program and data is commercially confidential, so distentangling what it is really doing, and uncovering that what it is doing is incorrect — and leading to disproportionate harms to black patients — requires the suspicion and followed up by hard sleuthing.

There are four bits of good news:

① Although it is bad that any AI system is racist, at least we did notice that it *was* racist. The more digital systems systematize healthcare, and in so doing expose intrinsic problems such as racism (and healthcare's lack of interoperability, which we'll talk about in the next chapter[b]) the sooner these problems can be properly fixed. In the case here, the US healthcare system is racist, and the AI conformed to that culture, but at least its racism was exposed.

① Race is only one sort of bias; age and gender are others. The good news is that when a bias is recognized, we can automatically assess

---

[b] See Chapter 19: Interoperability, page 245 →

the system and decide how to manage the biases we find. For example, the Babylon app is gender-biased, which appears as bugs, and they could fix this bias automatically.[c]

🔹 Sometimes the biases are in the data, not just in the programs. Anemia is a serious health condition, but its definitions are gender-biased, so any app or digital system relying on standard definitions inherits the errors. For example, the World Health Organization's definitions of anemia are hemoglobin concentration less than 120 gram per liter for women and less than 130 gram per liter for men, values based on limited data from the 1950s and 1960s. These biases have recently been questioned.[244]

🔹 The scientists doing the research[243] are now collaborating with the AI supplier to improve its fairness. They are giving their time for free. They hope the idea will spread.

The biases of the AI training then reappear as subtle bugs when the AI systems are used.

Sexism is another huge problem, as a lot of AI training data has more male data — the data itself, then the AI using it, results in and perpetuates invisible women.[245]

Although we now recognize the importance of diversity in training AI systems, racism and sexism are only the simplest and most obvious of AI bugs — and ones I hope we all acknowledge when they're pointed out. Indeed, it is a worrying thought that racism and sexism are rather basic biases that we have names to describe and can recognize, which begs what other, perhaps unfamiliar, even unnamed, biases can — does — AI have?

Many of these problems with AI are not conventional bugs — "just mistakes" — but are more like biases. As such, they raise very interesting ethical issues, and ethics in AI has recently become a bit of a hot topic. Ultimately all bugs are about a failure of trust, and AI needs good ethical thinking behind it to ensure it's trustworthy.[246] The take-home insight is that if we have bugs in our ethics, the digital systems we build will amplify and blindly apply those faulty ethics. We'll then realize that debugging programs is trivially easy compared to sorting out their ethics — hence the interest: preventing bad ethics is better than curing it. Still, ethics should not be separated from bugs. If a system makes a gender-based mistake, that raises some ethical issues, certainly, but it's still a bug.

We have no idea what other latent bugs lie inside AI systems. Worse, AI has no notion of conscious ethics so that it can reason about what is right in the same sort of way humans share and have built into their humanity. The bugs in AI's ethics — the inability of it to reason humanely about its failings

---

[c] See Chapter 25: Gender bias in Babylon, page 342 →

— are going to be worse and have a bigger impact than AI's straightforward bugs.[247]

So if AI has bugs and learning bugs, why is everyone so excited about it, especially in a field where there should be little tolerance for error? Two reasons. First, the explicit reason is that AI can do complex things that cannot be done without it; this is a game-changer, especially in a complex system like healthcare. Secondly, the implicit reason is that as AI learns, what it has learned (which will include patient data and how healthcare staff operate) itself becomes exploitable and can make *more* money. The data and the inferences from it are valuable, and this drives the hype. I think there should be a **Cat Thinking Quotient** for the ratio between the excitement, expectations, and hype, and the risks of anything going wrong.

Unfortunately the excitement and rush for AI in healthcare has, in my view, overtaken sensible caution and proper scrutiny. Thanks to thalidomide, we would not approve unknown chemicals for the healthcare market, because they may have unknown problems. We now regulate drugs very carefully. Why, then, do we release AI onto the healthcare market when we have no idea what it's actually doing, and, generally, we even have no idea how any AI is really working. As I've shown, this lack of open scrutiny leads to unnecessary patient harm; indeed, it's often worse: racist, sexist, and other forms of unethical problems arise. We ought to be doing something about it. On the other hand, AI is causing lots of useful and deep questions to be asked — and it's increasing the awareness of how risky digital healthcare is. Indeed, AI has all the usual risks of bugs, plus new ones all of its own.

While AI gets going — wherever it is going — we are going to have problems with cultural and racial diversity, as well as economic diversity (perhaps the AI is mostly trained on patients who need the money for their time or samples). How will we get enough representative data into the training? If we don't solve this problem, healthcare AI will have biases we know nothing about until we start seeing problems. People may take years to develop skin cancer after a buggy negative diagnosis — so nobody will realize it's wrong. This is the well-known problem of **algorithmic bias** — and just like most normal human biases, the digital systems are oblivious to the problems.[248] And, of course, so are their users — if they were able to recognize the biases in the data, they probably wouldn't need to be using AI in the first place.

The sheer complexity of AI makes it unaccountable. Besides, the current state of the art in AI and AI regulation and scientific rigor is way behind the state of the art in chemistry and pharmaceuticals, even considering their state at the time that thalidomide was developed.[d]

That sounds like a strong statement; but the fact is that by the time of thalidomide, chemistry had been an increasingly mature science, at least

---

[d] See Chapter 8: The thalidomide story, page 81 ←

since Mendeleev's periodic table of the 1870s — so at least 80 years — and had developed many sophisticated techniques, like mass spectroscopy. It is public knowledge exactly what thalidomide is as a chemical, and any chemist can perform experiments on it, and so on. In contrast, we are still learning what AI is and developing new variants; almost all AIs used in healthcare are proprietary, and their characteristics are unknown to and untestable by the wider scientific community.

Ordinary digital systems do exactly what their developers tell them to do. The developers write programs, which are basically lists of hopefully carefully pre-planned instructions. We've seen there will be bugs when things go wrong, but on the whole the computers will obey the programs, including the bugs. In contrast, the basic idea of AI is that the computer works out its own programming. It can then do things that the programmers haven't fully worked out themselves. People get quite fussed over the exact definitions of AI and ML, but the point is, if something could be done by an ordinary computer program that we (or somebody) fully understood, that wouldn't be worth calling AI. Machine Learning (ML) is one way of getting this leverage.

For example, how would you diagnose skin cancer? Nobody knows how to write a program to do that. Instead, we do know how to write programs that *learn* to do that. The programs are shown hundreds of thousands of pictures of skin problems, along with what dermatologists think of them.[249] Gradually the program learns what features cancer has. After thousands of examples, it should be able to learn to do as good a job as the best dermatologists. If so, we've got ourselves an AI that could be put in an app on a mobile phone and could help anyone diagnose skin cancer from a photograph.

Unfortunately, we rarely know exactly what AI systems have actually learned. In the skin cancer example, some AI systems were trained on real images, and they learned that cancers often had rulers (to measure the size of the cancer) next to them because dermatologists like to measure cancers more often than they like to measure non-cancerous spots.[250] Recognizing a ruler in a photograph doesn't help diagnose any cancers that dermatologists haven't seen and haven't measured, but AI doesn't know that.

Inevitably, AI was rushed in to help with the horrendous pressures of the COVID-19 pandemic. Hundreds of AIs were specially developed. None of them made a difference, and some were potentially harmful — worse, many hospitals signed non-disclosure agreements with the AI developers, so we have no idea what was used and whether it was safe.[251]

Chest scans seem like a good thing to train AI on to recognize a respiratory disease like COVID-19. Unfortunately for AI, many scans also include the texts of radiographers' interpretations. The AI then naturally learns the obvious fact that a scan that a human says shows symptoms of COVID-19 is likely to be COVID-19. The AI hasn't learned how to diagnose COVID-19 as it's learned to cheat by reading the notes! This is called **incorporation bias**, because the AI's training data incorporates test results or human diagnoses as well — it isn't learning from the data alone, but from the errors and biases of the likely imperfect tests and diagnoses that are incorporated in the data. It's probably learning to pay more attention to the incorporated data than the raw data it's supposed to be learning from. In fact, AI generally has an easier job than actually understanding anything: clinicians tend to write more about interesting diagnoses, so the AI learns that longer annotations (and pictures of dermatologists' rulers for that matter) mean problems. The reality, of course, is the other way around: diagnoses don't cause disease.

We can train an AI system to recognize skin cancer because there are libraries of thousands of already-classified pictures. (Even then, real diagnosis won't rely just on images — there will be a biopsy and histopathological examination, among others.) In many other health application areas, there is very little existing data to go on, let alone data as well-organized as skin cancer images. For instance, driverless cars use AI to understand how to drive, but they have to be trained by many thousands of poorly paid workers who classify road images.[252] Where are the thousands of workers, poorly paid or not, that are medically qualified and willing to classify medical data or medical images reliably?

Understandably, the people who develop AI systems need to get them out into the market. Why wait for lots of classified training data, when you could start using the AI and let it train itself on the job? (This is how doctors train, after all.)

Unfortunately, we have no idea how to use as-yet unreliable AI. How can it be used safely when it hasn't finished learning? How will we (or it?) know when it "knows enough" and can be relied on to be safe? How will it justify its decisions?

For a few amenable problems, like diagnosing from pictures of skin cancer, AI is amazing, but for the vast majority of clinical problems, we have little idea how to make it effective. With humans, even a trainee doctor has had twenty years education before becoming an effective healthcare professional, and of course all human doctors start off with a deep understanding of what being human means; AI has no such luck. It will need to work out these hard problems before it can be trustworthy in healthcare.

Humans have had millennia to evolve and develop social norms. Each of us individually still takes a couple of decades to mature into adulthood. So why do we expect AI running on a digital computer, which is very definitely not human and shares none of our social and biological heritage, to understand human things in the space of days?

The more successful AI gets, the more intelligent it gets, the less obvious it is who — or what — should be accountable for it working correctly. On the other hand, AI by its nature will be full of huge amounts of valuable data and will have money-spinning applications. Hospitals will probably pay for AI with expensive subscriptions. AI will make a lot of money, so it's going to get better — if the regulation and accountability are worked out.

> **Box 18.2.** Problems with spelling correction
>
> Dr Rana Awdish (@RanaAwdish on Twitter) tweeted:
>
> > Worst autocorrect to date (sent to a patient): Your goat
> > would be best treated with asteroids ("fixed" both gout and
> > steroids).[253]
>
> Naturally, spelling correction has attracted a lot of research. A research paper by Kenneth Lai and colleagues[254] is a good place to start. It takes a programmers' AI approach to an abstract problem based on spelling correction: they have a neat algorithm for correcting spelling mistakes and it "achieves good performance on a variety of clinical documents."
>
> But they did not explore whether it *actually* helped anyone do a better or safer job — which, surely, is the whole point. It corrected spellings, but brought a risk of a misplaced certainty. They did no User Centered Design, so while it is an interesting algorithm, it's a very risky digital idea to rush into healthcare without more work.
>
> Worse, I think, is that the algorithm uses a Machine Learning approach. It does not use a simple list of words, so it's effectively impossible to check its spelling corrections for accuracy. It isn't as simple as checking a conventional dictionary, which is relatively easy; there is no "dictionary" as such.
>
> Imagine, a user starts to type **phenobarbital**, but in error it changes it to **pentobarbital** without the user noticing. This is a dangerous error — one drug is on the World Health Organization's List of Essential Medicines; the other is used in the US for executions.
>
> I haven't done the experiments, but I suspect a much better use of the Lai algorithm would be to compose a list of confusable words like phenobarbital/pentobarbital and warn everyone — including digital systems — to be extra vigilant when any of these words are used. (To add to the confusion, drugs have different names in different countries, part of the problem of **internationalization** discussed in box 25.1.)

Part II ◇ Treatment ◇ Finding solutions

AI magic works in a completely different way from human intelligence. That means that when it goes wrong — as everything does from time to time — it will go wrong in strange and unexpected ways.

A clear example of this is some experiments done with the AI used in driverless cars.[255] Driverless cars can read traffic signs — they have to be able to, so that they can obey them. So when they see a "Stop" sign, they should obey it. And indeed, driverless cars have been trained to be able to do this *apparently* very well.

Yet it can go wrong in unexpected ways. Graffiti on signs, which humans would ignore, can completely change the AI's interpretation of the signs. The experiments found very simple — apparently innocuous — graffiti that confused AI into recognizing Stop signs as speed signs (figure 18.2). This is a serious bug, and one wonders if the "driver" would be made responsible

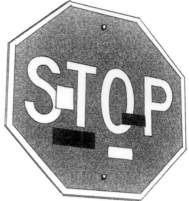

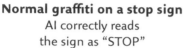

Normal graffiti on a stop sign	**Adversarial graffiti**
AI correctly reads	AI buggily reads
the sign as "STOP"	the sign as "45 mph"

Figure 18.2. Innocuous-looking graffiti on road signs shows how sensitive the AI in driverless cars is to small problems. If AI can make these serious mistakes, what mistakes does it make that are harder for us to notice?

for the problems that may follow.

An easier to understand, but no less serious, bug in AI was when a road sign showing a speed limit of 35 mph had black tape put on it (just to the left of the 3) so it looked a bit like 85 mph. A Tesla car then accelerated to that speed.[256] In other words, the car's AI was completely unaware of the context. To any human driver, the sign was obviously wrong, but to an AI system, the sign-recognition AI read 85, no other context was considered, and so that's the speed the Tesla then accelerated to.

AI in healthcare *will* go wrong from time to time, perhaps due to a deliberate adversarial cyberattack, as with the speed signs, or just by accident. When it goes wrong, the clinicians will be blamed for the errors that originate in the digital software.

Recent work has started to understand these problems with AI.[257] That's promising, of course, but it does rather highlight that the AI "solutions" promoted for healthcare are still having their problems sorted out.

AI isn't so much unproven technology, as technology that doesn't (yet) work reliably enough for healthcare. If we were thinking about promoting exciting drugs to cure a disease, we wouldn't want to use new drugs that were still being fixed to get rid of their side effects.

———————————■———————————

Eric Umansky has sleep apnea. He uses a CPAP (Continuous Positive Airway Pressure) machine to help him sleep. Without it, his airways might close, and he'd wake up repeatedly throughout the night and then fall asleep during the day. It's an essential device. His doctor prescribed him a new mask for it. But his insurance company, UnitedHealthcare (www.uhc.com), would not pay for the mask because of what they knew from the data they were collecting from it. Eric knew nothing about the data collection, but UnitedHealthcare thought he'd been using the machine for under three and a half hours a night. Actually, he hadn't been using the machine all night because he needed a new mask! Nevertheless, his insurance company wouldn't pay until he could prove he was using the machine all night.[258] It's a Catch 22. UnitedHealthcare's "reasoning" doesn't help Eric's health, which is the point of having the insurance. What it does help with is giving the insurance company excuses to reduce their costs — and of course, they can sell the data on to third parties to make more money.

Digital healthcare promises financially rewarding innovation. Certainly, if manufacturers don't make money, we won't have any technology. Without technology, healthcare will be stuck (an argument I've heard many times). Therefore, the argument goes, it is essential to relax regulation to free tech companies to innovate and provide new solutions. After all, they claim, current regulation is almost entirely based in a pre-digital world, and is unnecessarily restrictive for digital innovators. Those arguments wouldn't gain muster in, say, aviation.

The UK Government handed Amazon rights to NHS data. It's interesting reading these extracts:[259]

> Licensor hereby grants to Amazon and its Affiliates, a non-exclusive, worldwide, perpetual, irrevocable and royalty-free license to (a) access and use Licensor's application program interfaces, which will enable Amazon to obtain Licensor Content (the "Licensor API"), (b) access and use any systems, programs or software made available through Licensor APIs, and (c) use, copy, cache, store and make backup and archival copies of all tools and documentation related to the Licensor API ...

> Additionally, Licensor hereby grants Amazon and its Affiliates a non-exclusive, worldwide, perpetual, irrevocable and royalty-free license to make, have made, promote, market, advertise, publicize, distribute, offer for sale and sell Solutions and any products or services that use a Solution and the right to sublicense the foregoing rights to manufacturers of AVS Products and Amazon Associated Properties.

When Privacy International tested Amazon's Alexa with health queries, such as "Alexa, my period is late, what should I do?" Alexa would often give answers that did not come from NHS data. The Mayo Clinic was one of the alternative sources of information Alexa relied on, for example. This raises questions about the nature and relevance of an NHS contract when Amazon already has other health data.

The UK Secretary of State for Health, Matt Hancock, says the NHS must embrace technology and that the services Amazon provide could cut pressure on the NHS. Yet it has been reported that the deal gives Amazon free access to NHS data, as well as using the NHS logo, but the NHS gets no benefits if Amazon develops apps, and Amazon isn't paying anything for the benefits it's getting.[260] Whatever the Government's motivation, it's strange to give all the benefits to an international company and provide no help for the NHS. If the NHS set up a subsidiary, it could have done even better than Amazon — and the NHS data would stay in the UK inside the NHS. It seems to me that Amazon's much better understanding of AI and digital technologies has run circles around the NHS and the UK Government.

So much for today's problems. How are we going to have effective regulation that can handle new technologies like blockchain? Blockchain has been promoted widely — and wildly — for its uses in healthcare. It is, many argue, the solution for everything. I went to a medical workshop on blockchain, and heard from an excited doctor that it will solve the problem of having to log in lots of times. It won't.

Blockchain was originally developed for transferring money between parties who did not know each other and without using trusted institutions like banks.[261] It is therefore ideal for activities like exchanging money with people in foreign countries, particularly ones that have repressive governments (as their banks are unreliable or may be spying on their citizens). It's also ideal for illegal activities like extortion and drug dealing, for exactly the same reasons. Indeed, blockchain was used to support the Bitcoin payments demanded by the WannaCry malware.[e]

I may want to transfer money from my account to somebody I don't know so I can buy something over the internet; I do not want to get into an argument over whether I trust them or whether they trust the bank I use. I want it to work. Conventional trusted bank systems do this, and blockchain does it without banks.

On the other hand, none of healthcare is "untrusted." I never want to transfer my patient records to somebody I don't trust. I want to keep them, and I want doctors and nurses I know to have full access to them. If I transfer money, my bank account loses value accordingly by simple arithmetic. Blockchain handles that. If I transfer my neuropathy problems to a neurology consultant, I've still got my problems. My medical record works in a completely different way to a bank account. (An exception to trusted actors in healthcare is humanitarian work undertaken in oppressive states, where

---

[e] See Chapter 17: WannaCry warning screen, page 212 ←

> **Box 18.3.** Digital and pharmaceutical development costs
>
> Digital healthcare manufacturers complain that developing systems is costly, and they suffer from **regulatory burden** so asking them to do more to improve their systems is a step too far. Yet digital systems are cheap to develop in comparison to drug development. To research and develop a drug costs billions,[5] but a medical app can be developed in a few weeks by one person.
>
> Thinking more about how the pharmaceutical industry achieves quality will help improve digital healthcare. The business incentives are very different. If a drug causes patient harm, this is a disaster for the manufacturer and there's an incentive to improve it. If a digital system causes harm, it's likely to be blamed on the clinical staff. Patient harm is not as serious a business concern as it is in pharmaceuticals.
>
> Digital systems are continually updated after release, often charging customers for bug fixes. In other words, unfinished products are the way digital business works. Potentially some of the bugs that should have been fixed are never detected in the field, so the manufacturer saves the costs of fixing rare bugs. In contrast, a changed drug is a different drug, and needs new evidence of clinical effectiveness.
>
> Drugs are well understood and relatively easy to regulate. In contrast digital systems are complex and cover a huge variety of applications and uses. There are medical apps on handheld devices, many PC applications, they can be embedded inside medical devices like infusion pumps, anything with a Wi-Fi connection, and they are even inside rechargeable batteries. Digital systems are harder to regulate.
>
> There is a lot of competition in drugs. Several manufacturers can make drugs for the same diseases, and they compete with each other. They may be **biosimilars**: drugs that work in similar ways but do not infringe patents. In contrast, how digital systems work (apart from a few **open systems**) is proprietary knowledge, and competition is much harder.

it isn't possible to establish with certainty that relief workers are who they claim to be, or that even genuine healthcare workers and their data are not being monitored for political purposes.)

Of course blockchain can do more than this — it's certainly acting as a stimulus for new ideas in healthcare. But it's sobering that a recent survey of 43 blockchain developments showed that *none* of them worked.[262] The systems were originally described in glowing contracts like "operational costs ... reduced up to 90%," or "accurate and secure data capture and storage." The survey found no evidence that blockchain achieved any of these claims. Worryingly, the survey did not find any lessons learned or practical insights, something you'd expect for any technologies in development. Finally, not one manufacturer or developer was willing to share data on their results or processes. The industry is opaque.

We haven't yet worked out the technical or the business models to sustainably support the healthier digital future we dream about. While we fail to think through digital carefully, the legal precedents — like manufacturers requiring *us* to indemnify *them*[f] — build up and set precedents at our expense. They encourage a blind faith in digital that benefits the investors and not the patients. We buy into it because it's exciting, not because it makes sense.

Here's a typical problem. Until recently, the NHS shared patient data with the Government Home Office, which used the data to help trace people who had, perhaps, breached immigration rules. This has now been stopped after a lot of pressure from doctors,[263] but it's an example of the questionable way people just start using data and digital "because they can" in ways that would be completely unacceptable if we spent a moment thinking about it more carefully.

In other words, the regulations (and our thinking about them) are being out-paced by digital.

In the UK, general practice doctors are paid based on the number of patients registered with them. In a geographical world, this means that doctors are paid in a predictable way, proportional to the size of the local population who live near the doctors.[264] Along comes a digital innovator, such as Babylon, which provides a digital doctor's surgery and an app to access it. In a short space of time Babylon had registered 40,000 patients from across the whole country, most of whom, of course, must use it remotely. It achieved this phenomenal growth in just two years.

Most of Babylon's patients come from outside the region. Babylon's huge patient pool means that the local NHS funding body where Babylon is based, the London Hammersmith and Fulham Clinical Commissioning Group, now has a £26 million deficit.

Of course, Babylon has taken patients away from other areas, which you might have thought would save them money. However, the national funding system does not respond immediately, and the savings elsewhere are not used to subsidize Hammersmith and Fulham, since each area gets its funding set centrally.

There are more issues. Babylon is tending to register young technology adopters from across the country who like its service. This cherry-picking leaves behind the other patients who, being generally older, are less healthy. Because these left-behind patients tend to be sicker, this increases the healthcare costs per patient if you are a conventional doctor treating patients in person rather than virtually.

Cherry-picking also skews the funding in other directions.

Babylon's local, geographical, NHS funding body loses money paying Babylon for patients at the standard rate, because it assumes an average mix

---

[f] See Chapter 15: Mersey Burns app warranty, page 193 ←

of patient needs. But as Babylon's patients tend to be unusually healthy, Babylon gets relatively more money than it needs to treat its digital patients.

Funding models (as well as insurance models) will take time to respond to these rapid digitally-driven changes. By the time it's worked out a fairer solution, the digital innovators will be on to the next idea to make money out of the system.

Again and again, we see that digital health regulation is not fit for purpose, as the purpose is changing so fast. Old assumptions about healthcare are changing too rapidly for regulators. Digital start-ups can innovate to circumvent the intentions of the original regulation, and they can make huge returns on investment.

The standards and regulations we need are public goods, and — for the time being — our governments are so driven by the multi-national lobbying of Cat Thinking excitement[g] that we risk losing sight of what it's all about.

The traditional oath, "first do no harm," based, as it is, on Hippocratic wisdom dating back 2,500 years,[106] urgently needs updating to accommodate the new digital issues and challenges we face today and tomorrow. While we still think of harm primarily in terms of disease, we ignore the social determinants of health, such as wealth, education, politics, and religion,[265] as well as access to reliable digital healthcare information. In particular, we gloss over the serious harms caused by loss of privacy, loss of confidentiality, the loss of genetic data, financial exploitation, and more. These things form the whole basis of our own identity. Digital businesses are increasingly developing disruptive business models that are challenging the assumptions of healthcare. This is understandable, as there is much money to be made through innovation in these areas, but until there are clear cases made out that AI, blockchain, and other digital innovations, *actually* improve health (rather than, say, make apparently impressive diagnoses), it's more likely they will first be improving profit, which ultimately will be at our expense. Why fix bugs when it's more profitable not to bother?

The global scale of the digital healthcare market has disrupted centuries of thinking about healthcare. The scale and the technological innovations live in the loopholes of conventional regulation. There are astronomical financial incentives, so it's inevitable there will be new forms of criminal activity, as well as normal sharp practice in business exploiting the regulatory loopholes.

We need very careful national and international intervention to ensure proper safeguards for this very rapidly developing area. We need international collaboration, and we should start today with international think-tanks to work through these challenging issues — not least to find ways to for regulation to be sustainable — we don't need solutions that work for today but which will be obsolete after the next digital innovation.

---

[g] See Chapter 3: Cat Thinking, page 25 ←

Interoperability — or, rather, lack of interoperability — is a besetting problem in healthcare. We need digital to work seamlessly — to interoperate — across all specialties, disciplines, and healthcare institutions (taking due account of privacy, cybersecurity, and so on). It requires new thinking to get there.

19

Interoperability

Healthcare has developed over centuries, and most of it is not doing anything that's particularly easy to computerize. For example, one reason the singer Michael Jackson died is that he played off various doctors to feed his drug addictions, but none of them knew what the others were prescribing. So, if we just automate what doctors do, we don't solve another problem — doctors don't share patient records, and they don't share information effectively. Whether Jackson had a right to keep his full medical history secret from his doctors is one question, but if we digitize *exactly* what doctors do, we inevitably end up with what are called **interoperability** problems.[266]

Interoperability is of course a good thing. The opposite of interoperability is fragmentation, though it's a word that's rarely used. Whatever it's called, when systems don't work well together, it's a mess. Programmers, at least ones in the US, call them **stovepipe systems**, evoking the image of chimneystacks and stovepipes rising high above a town, each separately and independently belching its own plume of polluting smoke.

A typical example of a stovepipe system is a system that requires its own user names and passwords, instead of relying on a common user ID and password shared with all the other systems. It was easier for the programmers to build it like that when they developed it, but it makes it much harder for the users *every* time they use it.[7]

In contrast, a good example of interoperability would be email. You can use any type of email system to send email, and your email can be read by anyone else. You could send email with any old app that you just fancy using. It can be read on a website using a Firefox browser made by Mozilla, or read with Google mail, Microsoft Exchange, on a big PC or on a small iPhone, whatever. It all works. The reason is, email has standards, and all these systems work with those standards.

Once you've got something to interoperate, it's tempting to add extra features. We must all have received an email with an attachment that we

Fix It: See and solve the problems of digital healthcare. Harold Thimbleby,
Oxford University Press. © Harold Thimbleby 2021.
DOI: 10.1093/oso/9780198861270.003.0019

can't read at some point! The email works, but we haven't got interoperable standards for whatever the attachment is. Sometimes that's a problem; sometimes it's essential — as in getting encrypted emails about human rights issues out of oppressive states, where you really *don't* want some people to read them. The problem lies in getting the right balance.

I had a minor operation in hospital. I've never seen so much unnecessary paper that could have been easily digitized away!

I had a couple of inches of the radial nerve in my left hand removed for a biopsy. My local anesthetic had hardly worn off when the hospital gave me my discharge letter, a paper letter for me to take to my local doctor so he'd know what had happened to me.

Naturally, I opened the letter and read it. It was a photocopy of a paper form that the ward nurses had filled in by hand. No doubt the original was already on its way to be filed away in the basement of the hospital. For my own interest, I photographed the letter on my iPhone.

Once out of the hospital, I dropped off the paper letter at my GP surgery, as I had been told to.

When I later went to the surgery to have my wound checked. I'd been told to do this as it might have got infected, but the nurses knew nothing about it.

The surgery had lost the letter. Worse, until I asked, their systems didn't know they'd lost a letter. Maybe they lose letters all the time.

It took me a moment to realize I could solve the problem. As I had photographed it, the letter was available in paperless form on my iPhone, which I had with me.

Fortunately, my hand healed well, and I'm typing this without any problem. The NHS is amazing — it got the actual surgery done efficiently — but the digital side of the NHS is a mess. Ironically, by photographing it on my iPhone, not only did I hint at some future paperless healthcare world, but I actually solved a problem.

If the hospital and GP surgery shared their information, if their databases were shared and interoperated, the hospital nurses needn't have filled in and photocopied a paper form, and they need not have wasted any time finding my GP's address and writing it by hand on the envelope. The hospital needn't have relied on a patient carrying the paper letter to their GP. The letter would not have got lost (by the GP), and two surgery nurses (and the patient!) would not have wasted 15 minutes looking for it. The paper letter need never have existed in the first place. What a lot of wasted time and opportunities for errors.

How many of these unnecessary paper steps raise potential errors, and how much more efficient and cost-effective would a decent digital paperless approach be?[95]

We've already seen how Denise Melanson died from a calculation error.[a] The pharmacy's drug bag label could have been printed with the clear answer, or better still the pharmacy or even the bag could have programmed the infusion pump directly — that is, interoperably, perhaps with a barcode, an RFID tag in the bag, or a wireless connection to the pump[267] — then there would have been no calculation errors. Typically, nurses scribble down the doctor's instructions for the drug infusion from one computer screen or from the drug bag, do the calculations to find the right dose, and then walk to the infusion pump and enter the numbers into it. For high-risk drugs, like Denise's fluorouracil chemo, a second nurse must double-check that the pump is programmed correctly.

The cost? Johns Hopkins Hospital's Peter Pronovost worked out that, on a 12-bed intensive care unit, manual double-checks together add up to two full-time nursing positions.[268] It's not just time, though: having more staff time freed-up through interoperable systems would reduce errors — and when you reduce errors, you also reduce the staff time needed to sort them out and investigate them. Interoperability drives a virtuous circle.

Lack of interoperability is not just a problem within wards or within hospitals; it affects whole countries. Patients often attend two or more hospitals, typically to get specialized care; in the UK, patients often attend two or more hospital trusts (groups of hospitals). A study in England showed that most trusts that commonly share patients cannot share patient records.[269]

Here's a simple example of an interoperability problem. Consider some date written down, say 4/8/12. Unfortunately, this can mean at least six different dates (12 August 2004, 8 December 2004, 12 April 2008, 4 December 2008, 8 April 2012, or 4 August 2012) — assuming the date only refers to some date in the twenty-first century, an assumption which would repeat the mistake that led to the Millennium Bug. Indeed, there are more alternatives if we allow other centuries. A computer needs to know exactly what we mean; it'll just assume one of these meanings — and it may not assume the same date that was intended by the user, nor need it assume the same date as another computer would from the same input. That would be a serious interoperability problem.

The international standard, ISO 8601, requires a date like 4 August 2012 to be written as 2012-08-04 (when it is written without words). This makes sense, as it puts the biggest unit, the year, first, although few people do that (though many in China do). Indeed, date formats in the UK and in the US are different — internationalization and interoperability aren't just computer problems, but cultural problems.

The main solution is better programming, and improving healthcare so better programming is possible — programming, done properly, makes many problems in healthcare visible. The user interface should validate and dis-

[a] See Chapter 5: Denise Melanson's fatal overdose, page 49 ←

Part II ◇ Treatment ◇ Finding solutions

ambiguate dates before they even get into any computer, and then everything in the computer should be handled as a standard timestamp. There should never be any need for programmers to convert dates, nor for different systems to get into problems over interoperability. Unfortunately, solving the problem is not as easy as getting every manufacturer to agree, let alone fix, the old systems that have already been badly built.[23]

That's just date interoperability confusions!

Interoperability as a whole is a huge trans-national problem — patients don't stay in one country, and their medical records ought to follow them around the world. Until we sort things out, it's very likely all their dates (at least) will get mixed up.

Dr Marie Moe is a patient who travels the world. She has a heart pacemaker. (We've already met her before in this book.[b])

Her pacemaker malfunctioned when she was on an international flight. After the plane landed, she was rushed to hospital. They rolled in a trolley with four different pacemaker programming devices from four different manufacturers (figure 19.1): pacemaker programming devices are all different, thanks to interoperability problems. Luckily the hospital had the correct pacemaker programming device.

The problem with the pacemaker needed diagnosing, but the hospital technicians could not read its settings because it was an unfamiliar make of pacemaker. Indeed, they would not even have known what sort of pacemaker it was if Marie had been unconscious! There ought, surely, to be a set of international standards for interoperability of medical implants so that any hospital can access the relevant data? Indeed, if there were such standards, the safety of implants would be easier to check when manufacturers were seeking approval, and it'd be much easier for hospitals to check implants were safe.

Marie's pacemaker malfunctioned because of cosmic rays. (There are more cosmic rays high up where planes fly.) Although such a malfunction is strictly a bug,[270] at least the pacemaker detected the error and went into a safety mode.

The safety mode switched to an old type of pacing in case the leads used inside the patient were of the "old type." Often when they do pacemaker replacements, they keep the old leads in the patient if they are still working, to avoid disturbing them, to have a less risky surgical procedure. However, Marie did not have those types of leads.

Fortunately, the wiring configuration error made it obvious to her that the pacemaker was malfunctioning. She survived again, and even went on to successfully run in the New York Marathon.[c]

Why is interoperability such a problem? Surely fixing it should be a no-brainer, and something built into national strategies? Unfortunately, non-

---

[b] See Chapter 4: Marie Moe's pacemaker bug, page 46 ←

[c] See Chapter 30: Marie Moe runs New York Marathon, page 427 →

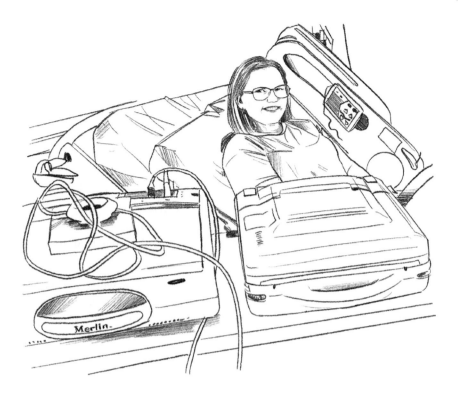

Figure 19.1. Dr Marie Moe getting checked up after her pacemaker problems. In front of her is a trolley of four different types of pacemaker programming device.

interoperability makes a strange sort of sense, for all the wrong reasons.
Let's explore some of these reasons for failing interoperability:

- Most computer systems are proprietary — that is, they are developed by companies which make money out of providing them and servicing them. No company wants to manage patient data and let *another* company benefit from all their hard work. So every company has proprietary "standards" which are their intellectual property that nobody else can use — at least not without paying licensing fees, if at all. These are new problems that computers have created, and at least in digital healthcare I don't think we have yet found the happy medium.

- Hospital procurement rarely requires interoperability as a contractual requirement — it'd be too tedious to spell out all the details of all the systems that must interoperate. So the hospital ends up acquiring non-interoperable systems and often signing away its rights to free and easy access to all patient data because the new systems don't fully interoperate with everything else. (It would cost more if a new system was interoperable — and as nobody has costed interoperability failure, why ask for it?)

⬙ Because computer systems are expensive, healthcare systems end up buying lots of smaller, cheaper, systems that don't do everything. This saves money, and also avoids reliance on one supplier (who might go bust, or suffer a cyberattack), but ends up with real interoperability issues. Again this is a new digital problem, unlike the sorts of supply problems that might affect other forms of healthcare.

⬙ There are lots of wonderful people in hospitals who want to fix problems. Most hospitals have hundreds of spreadsheets and other systems knocked up to solve real problems — unfortunately, quite independently.

⬙ The problem has been going on for years, and getting worse as each "solution" is brought in for *part* of the problem. Fixing or upgrading the digital healthcare in one area — say, radiography — doesn't improve interoperability; in fact, it almost certainly makes it worse.

⬙ There are international standards (called SNOMED-CT, HL7, ...) but they are still evolving. We need to acknowledge that digital healthcare is still a new idea, that healthcare is amazingly complex, and we are solving this amazing problem for the first time. We haven't finished yet. Worse, every week somebody announces a new healthcare intervention (say, genomics), and this changes everything that needs standards. We haven't even got standards for standards, and they will be continually evolving for the foreseeable future.

⬙ When things go wrong, the lack of interoperability makes investigations a nightmare, as nothing works reliably with anything else. It's rarely anybody's responsibility to make things interoperable.

⬙ Copyright, privacy, commercial confidentiality, software licensing, patents, digital rights management (DRM), and many other routine digital business ideas conspire to make interoperability harder. These ideas, and more, make sense in the commercial world, but they do not make as much sense in healthcare — mainly because some or all of a digital solution remains owned and controlled by a company rather than being able to be freely used and modified by the healthcare system. Consider that a non-digital medical device would not constrain how it is used, or require its use to share patient or other data. How much a digital device should share data needs debating; so far, the balance has fallen in the manufacturer's favor.

> **Box 19.1.** Adding value or managing risk?
>
> Organizations have two sorts of people. Some people — like doctors and nurses, cleaners and sterilizers — add **value** to the organization: in hospitals, these people work with patients. But some people — like financial directors — worry about **risk**. Since adding value sometimes runs risks and may create incidents, you need both types of people to run an organization.
>
> Managing risk tends to be done by managers, and their managers, all the way to the top. Hence strategic people, at the top of the management pyramid, tend to spend a lot of their time thinking about risk and damage limitation. John Seddon's insight[271] is that these risk-averse people at the top of an organization are the very people who authorize and buy the computer systems.
>
> Hence hospital computer systems tend to be designed and purchased in the first place for managing risks, such as asking to confirm that various procedural steps have been taken so that the organization cannot be sued. Helping patients or clinicians comes in second place.
>
> For example, having the wrong people access patient data is a risk that managerial thinking wants to avoid. The priority is to *stop* the risk of the wrong people using data, rather than to *help* anybody to use the data. Result: lots of logins and passwords to do anything, and interoperability fails.

All of these reasons for interoperability problems make sense. Together they create a *culture*. When you go to any experts on the issue — say, the manufacturers — they think within that culture. Change is going to be difficult. Unfortunately, digital healthcare will remain risky until the problem is addressed from the top, particularly by tighter regulations that require interoperability.

A more mature approach is to think about *how* to solve problems first, using **Computational Thinking**.[d] This of course relies on admitting and seeing *that* there is a problem to solve in the first place, and that of the many ways of solving problems some may be better or worse than others. Computational Thinking is very clear that different forms of thinking are required for different forms of problem.

Hill climbing is a popular way to solve simple problems: if you are climbing a hill, obviously, you need to go upwards. This is what mountain railways do — they have no choice but to climb hills! (Hill climbing is also called the **greedy method** — just choose what seems to be the biggest and best thing first. Climb the highest hill.)

Let's say, some years ago when everything was simpler, you wanted to digitalize healthcare. Hill climbing would decide what was easiest or cheapest to do first, do it — climb the closest or most visible hill — then see what to do next. Sometimes, this strategy works. Sometimes, though, you discover

---

[d] See Chapter 13: Computational Thinking, page 151 ←

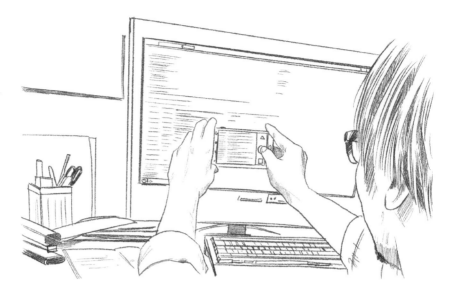

Figure 19.2. Lack of interoperability forces a doctor to photograph patient records with a mobile phone app. While this may help get things done, let's hope it doesn't cause problems. What if they take several photographs of different patient data and get them mixed up? What if they lose their phone or have it stolen? Bad guys could get patient details.

you've climbed the wrong hill, and then you need to climb the better hill you can see somewhere else. To get to your new goal, you first need to go downhill — your earlier decisions have turned out to be wrong. For example, you might decide the first thing to do, and indeed the easiest to do, is to get all the financial services computerized. You then look at pharmacy and physiotherapy, and see they need billing to work in different ways. You now have a conflict, and either way, the earlier financial system is a big system to change. It's hard to avoid an interoperability problem.

Mountain railways are a lot easier to visualize than healthcare problems. Given a hill, put a mountain railway (or a computer system, or …) on it, and you can get to the top of *that* mountain much more easily and quickly than climbing it yourself — just as digitalizing a problem makes it easier, all things being well. But what if you aren't climbing the right hill? What happens if you should have got rid of the hill instead? What happens if you are in the wrong area altogether and should be exploring a different mountain range where the mountains are higher? What happens if your passengers need to connect with other transport? Regardless, now that you've got a mountain railway, you're left with an investment that is now holding you back. Not only is it holding you back, but you've got all sorts of maintenance issues, staff, and consumables to sort out every day to make your wrong solution

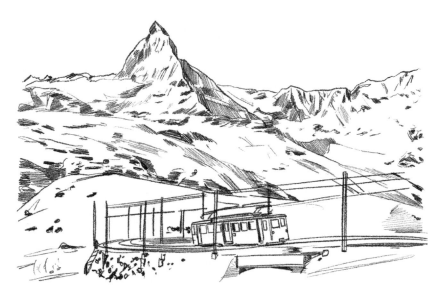

Figure 19.3. Hill climbing seems to solve problems but doesn't always find the best solution. The train here is climbing hard and will get to the top of the Gornergrat. It will finish nowhere near the Matterhorn, despite the Matterhorn being nearly 1,500 m higher: so hill climbing gets to the top of a hill, but never connects to the next hill even if it's higher.

work as best it can. You'll be tempted to advertise your mountain railway to attract more use, ignoring all its inconveniences. Basically you started off with an exciting, greedy, idea and now you've just got a white elephant that needs maintaining. The point is, you wanted to climb a hill, but now that achieved goal restricts what you can do. You can't so easily climb other hills.

Hill climbing is a very simple AI technique for solving simple problems, mainly ones that only have "one hill" to climb, so "up" solves the problem. Many problems can be solved by hill climbing, and many more problems can be quickly, but only approximately, solved by hill climbing. AI also offers lots of more sophisticated ways to solve more complex problems better. Viewed like this, what AI can offer healthcare are powerful ways of thinking about and solving problems that aren't as easy to solve as you might at first think. Indeed, AI is only one area of Computer Science; there are many others to choose from. Using Computer Science to help solve problems by thinking clearly is exactly what Computational Thinking is.[e] So if this sounds far-fetched, how, in more detail would AI help? First, any AI developer would ask about *exactly* what do you want to achieve and what data have you got? In contrast, many people just run into solving problems without planning —

[e] See Chapter 13: Computational Thinking, page 151 ←

> **Box 19.2.** Interoperability isn't just a digital problem
>
> Interoperability is usually thought of as a goal for digital systems, and interoperability, or, rather, the lack of interoperability is seen as a specifically *digital* problem. Not so. The hill climbing analogy makes it clear that lack of interoperability is a *symptom* of a particular, limited way of thinking applied to problems that need a more general approach.
>
> Take the naming of drugs.
>
> Drug names are often confusing. The drugs called clonidine and klonopin are typical examples. These two real drugs have very similar-sounding names, and they are too easily confused. You may want to find clonidine for your patient, but you misread and picked up klonopin. Or the other way around.
>
> How do these naming conflicts happen? Each manufacturer was climbing their own hill, determinedly following the path of their own drug-naming process. Managing drug names centrally would mean limiting the creativity of drug manufacturers and limit their freedom of expression. So, each manufacturer invents a drug name pretty much without reference to anyone else, as long as it doesn't conflict with patents or drug names already registered.
>
> Every so often, then, two or more different drugs will end up with very similar names. If those drugs ever end up in the same room, eventually somebody will pick up one, thinking it's the other; after all, the names are practically the same.

another example of the greedy approach. Often it works well-enough, but some times the landscape is too complicated, and you only find out that your quick approach doesn't work well enough when you're already committed to delivering it.

One of our repeated errors in thinking about digital is that we expect easy solutions to healthcare problems — we want to be greedy. Indeed, we see amazing digital solutions everywhere, like WhatsApp, so we think it should be easy to get healthcare to work if such amazing things were quickly brought in.

WhatsApp is very popular in healthcare. About a third of hospital clinicians use WhatsApp or a similar tool.[272]

The error is thinking that WhatsApp solved a problem; no, it created a "solution" to something that we now realize we were all missing, after the fact. It wasn't a defined problem beforehand. Nobody had specified what doctors want, and then set out to build it. WhatsApp did not so much climb a hill as build its own new hill.

If you want to solve an existing problem, such as anything in healthcare, you can't ignore history, **standard operating procedures**, regulations, and lots of other very tedious and complex constraints on your creativity. Instead, WhatsApp got lucky and happened to build a hill doctors wanted to climb —

a hill of exciting apps. The conventional alternative, trying to build the hill you think the doctors are on, is much harder.

In my view, WhatsApp should not be being used in healthcare. It doesn't even have a CE marking. Why do you think it's free? Its business model means that it collects data that healthcare should not be giving away without proper information governance. Their legal information includes these points:

> You provide us with the phone numbers in your address book on a regular basis ... we collect information about your activity how you interact with others ... we collect information when we you access our services ... we collect device location information ... we receive information about you from other services ... businesses you interact with provide us with information ... a business on WhatsApp may use another company to assist in storing your messages ... we help businesses who use WhatsApp measure their effectiveness and understand how people interact with them ... we share information with Facebook Companies ... we may transfer your information to any of our affiliates, successor entities, or new owner ...

None of that fits very well with information governance best practice. WhatsApp and many other apps let you use them to disclose all sorts of information inappropriately for healthcare (figure 19.2). Worse, WhatsApp has bugs that can be used to send you fake information and deceive you into revealing sensitive information to third parties: you've already agreed you're happy to lose your information, and your faith in the app can be further exploited by hackers.[273]

Now, back to interoperability. Interoperability problems are not all due to poor digital systems, bugs, and poor programming. Interoperability problems arise primarily because of independent development of "solutions" that seem fine on their own in isolation — in other words, they arise because of hill climbing being used, when hill climbing is not the right way to correctly solve the problem.

A core, critical reason for interoperability problems is that nurses, radiotherapists, psychiatrists, neurologists, general practitioners ... all work differently — they are all working on different hills. Connected digital systems then make these differences very visible, as a lack of interoperability. The lack of interoperability, the different cultures, different procedures, they were all there before digital, but nobody had noticed or, at least, nobody had worried about it too much.

In the old days, everyone exchanged paper (or faxes) and the human brain converted everything. In contrast, in the new digital age, specialties hit problems when they try to share patient or other data, since they separately developed their own digital systems to suit what *they* did, not to suit other specialties. Worse, what people do even in the same specialties varies from hospital to hospital.

Many hospitals had already started developing their own digital solutions as early as the 1970s. All these systems were polished in their own separate ways. Today, now networks connect everything, the fundamental lack of interoperability in healthcare has become visible. It's become an embarrassment — but it's as much to do with what clinicians wanted as with manufacturers never delivering total solutions for an entire country. It's a tough nettle to grasp, because interoperability means that some people have to give up the ways they have been working.

One lesson to learn from all these problems is that healthcare should not buy digital "solutions" as such. It should not bring in a solution and expect it to work. There should be a period of testing and polishing to get rid of the snags, and this has to be done across the country, not just in individual regions or hospitals. It also has to be done across specialities to make sure it interoperates within hospitals as well as between them.

Healthcare should procure systems, and pay for them only when or as they meet (or exceed) defined performance criteria. If something turns out not to be interoperable and impacts effective healthcare, then if nobody had paid for it fully in advance, the manufacturer would soon put the problems right.

If anyone could demonstrate that harm had decreased and staff across all disciplines were happier, that would be a landmark achievement, regardless of whether it was paperless, or used AI, precision data, Internet of Things, blockchain or anything else trendy.

Yet people *have* shown improving interoperability reduces harms and generates other improvements, such as working faster and more efficiently. The internationally agreed barcode standard, GS1, which is used for marking and tracking everyday products from cans of beans to drugs, is so useful because it is an interoperable standard. When hospitals adopt it, errors are reduced. The Royal Cornwall Hospitals reduced error rates in pharmacy dispensing by 76% thanks to using barcodes *which were already there.*[274] Somehow these sorts of achievement don't get built on, because people are so keen on piecemeal solutions.

We are going to have to wait for SNOMED-CT and the related clinical standards to settle down *and* be widely adopted, both by manufacturers and by healthcare professionals. There will then be a huge legacy of patient notes, on paper and digitized, that will need sorting out. This is a problem that will take mature thinking and will take years to achieve. Until we are more strategic, every day is postponing the ideal world of full interoperability.

Lack of interoperability is a symptom of poor systems thinking, a symptom of letting systems just grow regardless of standards. The cure isn't just "better" digital — it involves improving health systems and health system *thinking* too, so that we are clear what we want the digital to do.

Improving things also means reconsidering whether failing interoperability is, in some cases at least, a symptom that healthcare itself needs improving — it's far easier to make successful digital systems interoperate when the healthcare they are supporting itself is interoperable!

Part II ◇ Treatment ◇ Finding solutions

Understanding how humans make mistakes in predictable ways is the first step towards making fewer mistakes. This applies to clinicians, and most especially to programmers — whose mistakes end up as bugs affecting thousands of users.

20

Human Factors

We all like to think we are better than we actually are. We make mistakes from time to time, but often we don't notice them. In fact, if we noticed them, we either wouldn't make the mistake, or we'd correct them immediately. Furthermore, when we do make a mistake, our pride makes us diminish our role or deny the error, or even blame somebody else.

I'd certainly rather imagine that I am perfect. Like most people, I like to think I'm above average.[275] If I knock a glass off the table, my *immediate* reaction is to shout, "*Who* left the glass there?" I knocked it off only because somebody else left it there!

My wife and I make a good team. When I am driving, Prue sometimes shouts, "look out ..." and of course I immediately deny I've made a mistake or that I could possibly be *about to* make a mistake and hit somebody. Fortunately, our mature relationship takes priority a millisecond later, and I apologize. When I think about it, I'd much rather she shouted at me than that I run somebody over.

That's just my personal "culture of success." But in both healthcare and programming we are in understandable, but unhelpful, *social* cultures of success. Obviously we don't want to harm patients. To become professionals, we've had to pass exams, so we *know* we are good. We are surrounded by equally excellent colleagues ... and so on, and sometimes these things grow a culture of infallibility where we undervalue teamwork and even questioning whether we might be making mistakes. Why do we need teamwork when we know we are good?

There's another twist. In almost all jobs, people are working at their limits. Nurses are overrun with too much to do, and surgeons have to focus on complex procedures that, if they went even slightly wrong, could kill patients. Programmers, too, have to solve problems at their mental limits; if they didn't, their products would not be competitive in the business world. Everyone's work therefore requires full attention, which then in-

Fix It: See and solve the problems of digital healthcare. Harold Thimbleby,
Oxford University Press. © Harold Thimbleby 2021.
DOI: 10.1093/oso/9780198861270.003.0020

evitably leaves little or no head space for being aware of their own limitations and the errors they may be making.

Human Factors gives us an explicit toolkit to help make systems better fit in with our true human skills and limitations. It reminds us, for instance, that we naturally overlook things, but we do so in predictable ways. When I am fatigued, when I am cross, or when I am under pressure I will make predictable types of mistake.

Some organizations explain away incidents by blaming "the human factor," really meaning that some user or operator made a mistake and really they are to blame. This is totally inappropriate. Everybody makes slips and mistakes. If you ever hear somebody blaming "the human factor," tell them no, what failed was the system design that allowed a predictable problem to happen.

In healthcare, it has become popular to talk about Human Factors and patient safety in one breath; Human Factors failings led to some patient harm, and now this or that needs doing. This focuses the insights of Human Factors onto the clinicians most closely involved with the incident, those at the sharp-end. But *everyone* — even, and most especially those not in the room at the time — laid the context down for the harm to happen or, at all the other times, for the successes to happen.

Clinicians, managers, administrators, designers of **standard operating procedures** (SOPs), people who procure equipment, people who design and implement the digital systems, the politicians who get excited about certain sorts of "solutions" ... and so on: all these people and roles are, of course, human, and all of them, without exception, will fall into certain sorts of traps, traps of thinking, traps of doing, oversights, misplaced certainties, unknown ignorances, over-confidences, and more, that create the circumstances where over-worked, pressurized carers and patients have to work together. Things will, from time to time, go wrong, and what Human Factors teaches is that things go wrong (and things go right) in predictable ways.

We used to think that bad humans cause errors and problems. Human Factors is the study of how people work, and since we now know from Human Factors that humans do things in predictable ways, we now see error as a *symptom* of poor system design. Systems — especially digital systems — should be designed for human error, to block it where possible, to warn when it happens, and to help manage recovery from it when it has happened. Emphasizing the role of Human Factors in designing and creating systems is called **Human Factors Engineering**, or HFE for short.

What are some of these predictable Human Factors issues? We know that we have limited brain space — everything has to fit inside our skull. When we focus on a problem, we inevitably lose awareness of some other things that are going on, because our brains can only do so much. If we paid attention to everything, we would be utterly distracted. So, we get **tunnel vision**. Our attention tunnels into what we are doing, and it inevitably loses track of everything else. We are built like this, and often for important problems our hormones get involved too, and we end up with no choice but to be carried along by the excitement of the problem at hand. It's not a deliberate choice to become unaware of everything else, it's something predictable and happens to everyone.

Some people call tunnel vision **loss of situational awareness** or **inattentional blindness**, emphasizing how we blindly lose track of parts of the wider context of what we are doing. The important point is that you become *unaware* — you have lost awareness of parts of your situation. You are too busy doing something to take in any more information. When something happens in that situation that affects what you are doing, you very likely don't notice and then bad things can happen.

For me, there are problems with the term "situational awareness." It is never obvious at the time what the "situation" is that we're supposed to have lost track of. Criticizing somebody for losing situational awareness is easy, because after an incident, in hindsight, it's "obvious" what the full situation was supposed to be. In hindsight it therefore appears that it must be the nurse's or pilot's fault, as they lost track of the full situation. But it wasn't obvious at the time what the critical bits of the situation were — if it had been, they would have tried to avoid the incident! So, by definition, using the term situational awareness starts off implicitly blaming the person at the sharp-end, the person nearest the incident.

Tunnel vision and loss of situational awareness, whatever we call it, is something that happens to people. The point is, it happens *predictably* when too many things are going on and need to be dealt with at once. It is therefore much more productive to focus on the causes rather than the consequences. **Task saturation** is a better term; it emphasizes the role of asking people to do too much. Their work becomes too demanding, and they respond by focusing more on the main task that needs doing. They cut out of consciousness the distractions and the less important tasks. The problem is that sometimes some of these secondary tasks that are not being attended to turn out to be critical.

A familiar example of task saturation happens when people get glued to their mobile phones as they walk around town. They cross roads while still reading their phones and happily texting away. Lost in thought, they are most likely unaware that they have lost critical awareness of road safety. Fortunately, this task saturation usually doesn't matter: they cross roads safely most of the time, and so they are unaware of the risks they are running. But one day, they may become casualties because they didn't notice a danger.

Similarly, car drivers can get lost in using their phones: they don't realize how unaware they are of the road, and then they become a risk to themselves and other road users. This is why use of mobile phones (particularly by young or newly qualified drivers) while driving is banned in many countries: they *are distracting*. As you get sucked into the phone conversation (or

> **Box 20.1.** Magic makes digital healthcare safer
>
> The magician and computer scientist Prof Paul Curzon offered to show me a card trick. I picked a card at random from a pack he'd shuffled, and then — without looking at it — he knew what it was. I was amazed.
>
> He did it again. I was amazed again. He did it again and again. I had no idea how he was doing it. People started coming over and watching us. They started laughing. Paul was distracting me, but they could see how I was being tricked. I was feeling increasingly stupid, as I had no idea what Paul was doing.
>
> Tricks rely on **misdirection**, getting the audience's eyes to follow the wrong things. It's the magician saturating you with distracting tasks you don't notice, and your tunnel vision being misled into concentrating on the wrong thing and not seeing how the trick works.
>
> In the normal Human Factors of tunnel vision, errors are unintentional accidents, but with magic, the Human Factors are shamelessly exploited.[276]
>
> I can reveal one of Paul's techniques. He had several tricks up his sleeve (see the Good reading chapter for some of his ideas[a]). As soon as I thought I'd worked out how he was doing the trick, he would use *another* trick. So whatever I guessed — I think he's changing the pack of cards to one that is *all* Queen of Hearts??? — he'd do the trick again but in a different way and make my guess wrong! (I'd no idea he was so devious.) I was fooled even when he did it slowly so I could watch each step very carefully. Somehow I was missing something, but I had no idea what.
>
> The connection with digital healthcare is that digital systems *accidentally* trick us into making mistakes we don't notice. Understanding how magic *deliberately* tricks us into making mistakes can help us make safer digital systems!
>
> _____
>
> [a] See Chapter 13: Computational Thinking, page 151 ←

working out how to use your phone!) your tunnel vision helps concentrate better on what you think you are trying to do, and inevitably you lose track of everything else. You don't even realize that you are no longer aware of the rest of the world. You stop driving safely, and, worse, you aren't even aware that you aren't driving safely. Using the phone is demanding all your attention, and the road awareness you've lost is not noticed.

Many airplanes have crashed because of task saturation. Here are two key stories that helped aviation wake up to the importance of Human Factors issues:

- In 1969, Scandinavian Airlines System Flight 933 flying from Denmark to the US crashed into the sea near Los Angeles. The pilots were so preoccupied with the nose gear light not going green that they lost track of their altitude. Fifteen people died.

- In a similar story, in 1972, Eastern Airlines Flight 401 crashed, killing 101 people. When the pilot came in to land, the front wheel down light did not come on; was that because the light had failed, or the wheels weren't down? The pilot put the plane into a holding pattern while he sorted it out. Unfortunately, nobody noticed that the autopilot disengaged as they worked on solving the landing light problem. With no autopilot, the plane slowly descended, nobody noticed, and the plane crashed in the Everglades.

- In December 1978, the United Airlines Flight 173 crew was starting to land at Portland International Airport when it had a problem with the landing gear. The captain decided to fly in a holding pattern so they could sort out the problem. The captain worked on the problem for an hour, and ignored hints from the crew that they were running out of fuel. Only when the engines ran out of fuel did he notice this far more serious problem. The plane crashed on landing. Ten people died.

Although these are clear examples of task saturation, there are two remarkable things to point out here. These are *old* airplane crashes. Aviation has improved a lot since then. Secondly, the details of the crashes are easy to find out. Many are collated on Wikipedia and in lots of other places. Aviation is getting safer,[a] and it's open about its accidents and investigations. It wants to learn from them. It clearly has.

Here's the thing. When you have task saturation you don't know that you don't know what you are unaware of. If you were aware you didn't know something, you'd know it — and you'd need awareness to know that, something you don't have spare capacity to notice because you are focused on doing your job. This is why good teamwork helps: other people may notice what you don't notice, and if they point this out successfully, you may be rescued from your unawareness.

———————————————————

In March 2005, Elaine Bromiley, a 37-year-old wife and mother, went in for a routine, elective operation on her sinuses.[277] As soon as she was anesthetized, there were problems with her airway. Staff in the operating room tried hard to sort out the problem. The nurses watching, seeing the problems, brought equipment for a tracheostomy and cricothyrotomy[278] and booked a bed in the intensive care unit to help her recovery. But the doctors were too intent focussing on the technicalities of the airway problem, so they didn't notice that the situation was rapidly deteriorating into an emergency. Elaine was short of oxygen. They struggled for about 20 minutes. The nurses who did spot the problem did not speak up, because the doctors were "in charge."

---

[a] See Chapter 26: Planes are safer, page 347 →

Elaine died from brain damage caused by lack of oxygen.

Martin Bromiley, Elaine's husband, has turned this tragedy around. As an airline pilot, he is familiar with Human Factors and how teams in aircraft cockpits work safely together. Aviation has had its share of disasters, but it has learned from them, and aviation safety is continually improving. Central to this is a positive attitude to Human Factors, and a willingness to recognize and learn from mistakes and near mistakes — incidents that would have happened but for some successful defense stopping them.[279]

Martin's Human Factors insights — plus his amazing humanity — turned around the disaster of losing his wife into a powerful lesson. The very powerful story is available as a video, and it is already saving lives. Martin founded the Clinical Human Factors Group, CHFG, which makes the broader case for Human Factors in healthcare, and it is already transforming daily practice and saving lives. The CHFG has a great website — chfg.org — which has many useful pointers (including the video) and lots of resources. I strongly recommend it.

Martin saw Elaine's preventable death through the lens of his professional experience as a pilot, and this enabled him to turn it around. Later in this book, we'll discuss the successful way aviation has improved safety, primarily by having an open, non-blame, and inquisitive attitude to failure.[280] Indeed, Human Factors was brought into aviation as a response to inquiries into several major accidents. In contrast, healthcare seems to prefer to treat incidents as unfortunate, isolated events that do not have any systematic basis that would be worth exploring.[281] Human Factors belies that. People — whether pilots, clinicians, or programmers — all succeed and fail in the same ways.

———————————■———————————

Teamwork is a special case of **redundancy**: critical information may get lost or corrupted for all sorts of reasons, but humans are *more reliable* at handling the same thing when it is presented in multiple different ways, and that can be done by involving different people (and computers) in the team, even when the original task itself doesn't have much redundancy. However, designing systems to be redundant, which (if you didn't know Human Factors) might seem pointless, reduces the chances of error. For example, wrong patient errors are hard to avoid, but the more ways the patient's identity is presented (their name, their date of birth, their address, their clinical condition, their identifying number, their photograph), the easier it is to identify errors and correct them before harm happens. Hence computer systems, and indeed any systems, including paper systems, should be designed to increase redundancy.

There is always a trade-off, however. If you designed a system with a million items of information to redundantly double-check against the patient identity (what if they are a twin?), you might be very certain the patient in front of you is the right patient, but you'd run out of time to do anything else.

After an incident, such as operating on the wrong patient, the point of the investigators' job is to uncover what the people caught up in an incident were not aware of at the time. This is one of the logical problems for accident investigations, because the investigators themselves aren't doing the same job as the people were when the accident happened. They therefore have a very different point of view than the people had at the time of the incident. Maybe they are sitting back in their offices, relaxed and comfortable, with as much time as they want to do *their* job. Maybe they have all of the incident details laid out in front of them. It's then a short step to blame the pilots or clinicians for not having known what is now obvious.

Evolution gave us tunnel vision because it can be a very useful thing. All complex tasks require proper and full attention to be done well. You must ignore distractions, and tunnel vision does this for you automatically. Occasionally, though, for some random reason, something horrible happens outside your conscious attention and you ignore it because you are focusing on the "more important" job at hand. If the horrible thing then escalates into patient harm or an aircraft crashing, you may become aware of the problem too late to do much about it.

There are many solutions to task saturation.

- Train people to be calm, to have team colleagues who watch their backs.

- Have computer systems that help by spotting errors, patient deterioration or some other unusual behavior. Computers should be designed to be part of the team.

- Design better systems and procedures to reduce task saturation. Note that good system design also enables having better and safer procedures to use those systems.

- Stress, fatigue, uncomfortable working conditions, hunger, being late, and in a rush ... all of these reduce performance and increase error. Most of them create a vicious cycle: stress causes error, and errors increase stress. Deliberate techniques to manage stress help,[282] but the techniques are not just the responsibility of the sharp-end people — the design of the work, the management, the building design, the computer systems that have to be used, even the car parking, are all part of the parcel.

Of course, to design anything first requires doing experiments to find out what the real problems are, and to assess whether our planned interventions will really work. Ideas that seem obvious may not be as effective as expected in the reality of pressurized clinical work, for instance.

Having clear checklists (which mechanically make us go through things we may otherwise unintentionally miss out) is one of the simplest things

Part II ◇ Treatment ◇ Finding solutions

to do. For instance, the WHO Surgical Checklist[283] takes people through a list of essential checks, such as checking we have the right patient in front of us, before commencing surgery. The checklist significantly reduces task saturation, because the task is driven by a simple list rather than trying to remember things while performing a complex task.

As recently as 2019, Lourdes Hospital Transplant Center had two patients in the hospital with the same names and similar ages, and they performed a kidney transplant on the wrong patient.[284] Surely, every hospital's computer systems should be part of the team and *automatically* warn when treating any such patients: you've got some patients with confusable names — be doubly careful!

The executive vice president of the hospital, Reginald Blaber, said the incident was "unprecedented." No, no, no, the confusion *was not* unprecedented. The "unprecedented" confusion happened seventeen years after Sir Liam Donaldson, the UK's then Chief Medical Officer, highlighted that name confusions are *well known* causes of errors in his widely reported article, "An organisation with a memory."[285] Blaber evidently wasn't in charge of an organization with a memory.

Blaber also said that measures had been taken to ensure the problem would not happen again in his hospital. Why hadn't those measures been in place at least since the WHO checklist of 2008, or since Sir Liam's high-profile work? Why are we only improving safety after an incident in a hospital, rather than using general Human Factors knowledge *for all healthcare*? Why are we always improving safety case by case, one hospital at a time?

As using the WHO checklist is patchy, why not have all digital systems programmed to help with it in *every* hospital? If digital systems took some initiative to improve safety, executive vice presidents needn't worry about understanding the details.

Unfortunately, so far, computers have generally been the source of mushrooming workload.[286] The frustration and pressures on users exacerbate task saturation and tunnel vision, and contribute to stress and, in the long run, to mental health issues. Poor design and bugs create pressures that reduce people's effectiveness; essentially, bugs become contagious by making other systems harder to use.

A very common problem of this type is **alarm fatigue** (I mentioned Jenny Lucca and Pablo Garcia's story earlier[b]). It's interesting to see the different sides to the story:

> ① From the nurse's point of view, the device alarms when it notices something has gone wrong. Often so many alarms are going off, and often for trivial reasons, that the nurse ignores them. Then, one day, an alarm goes off that matters, and something bad happens. The nurse is blamed for ignoring the alarm.

---

[b] See Chapter 10: Alarm fatigue, page 126 ←

- When a developer builds a device, they focus on *that* device and what it needs to detect and alarm for. This is tunnel vision — the developer is (understandably) ignoring the wider situation. In fact, the developer has no real awareness of the rest of the ward where the device will eventually be used.

- The result is that devices alarm independently, and often overwhelmingly. It's then natural for nurses to ignore them, thanks to tunnel vision. Often nurses will just turn them off to reduce distraction.

- We know that busy nurses can only pay attention to so many alarms, and any more alarms is counter-productive. Blaming a nurse for missing an alarm does not improve the system or make it safer. Doing the research so we know how to design systems to avoid alarms that will get ignored because of tunnel vision would make systems safer; after the research, the results could then be turned into a standard or a regulation. Then there'd wide uptake of the better approach.

- Standards or regulation could dictate a maximum number of alarms, but the real art of regulation is to require the improvement in safety, and let manufacturers work out the best way to do it. This, in fact, is just good Computational Thinking, avoiding implementation bias and over-specificity on how to do it.

There is nothing special about bad programming creating bad design in digital healthcare — it's just poor HFE. Tunnel vision leading to error is what happens to everyone, especially when faced with complex problems under pressure. Human Factors applies to pilots, car drivers, patients, clinicians, and programmers alike, it isn't just an "end user," nurse, or doctor thing. Indeed, Human Factors applies upwards through management, building design, digital system design, and even into the design of standard operating procedures (institutionalized as SOPs) and regulations. Human Factors is everywhere. Equally, opportunities to make strategic improvements is everywhere. It isn't ever a matter of blaming the end user for "failing," when the system led them astray.

Here are some core Human Factors ideas and issues. As usual, I've put technical terms and the first use of standard phrases in **bold**.

Ignorance and **unawareness**. We don't know anything until we do an experiment to measure it. This is a more general observation than that we don't notice our own errors; we don't notice much at all. Careful experimentation is always required to figure out the true facts from our (usually over-simplified) imagination. The cure for ignorance, even deliberate ignorance, is evidence. **Unconscious incompetence**, a special case of ignorance, arises when we are ignorant of our lack of skill and competence in some area.

Box 20.2. Simplistic Human Factors backfires

It's possible for naïve Human Factors to backfire: there is a mistaken interpretation where the nurse or doctor is blamed for not using Human Factors properly. "They should have used their Human Factors knowhow to avoid the problems."

Hospitals have projects to "design out error" — even the name of which creates a false belief that errors aren't or shouldn't be possible because they've been designed out. So when errors happen, as they eventually do, the staff must be to blame again.

First it was that they just made mistakes; now they've had the Human Factors training, they're making mistakes because they aren't using their training properly. They're *still* to blame. If they moan, then it's because they aren't being resilient, something else they've been trained about and "should" be able to do.

While it is certainly helpful to be **resilient**,[287] these views of resilience and designing out error are often manipulated to reduce the system's responsibility.

It's important to be clear what Human Factors resilience really means. Sometimes it is worth calling it, more precisely, **risk resilience**, to emphasize its wider meaning.

We say risk resilience because it is a wider resilience than the everyday sense of staff being individually "resilient." That sort of resilience means things like not being stressed when things go wrong.

Risk resilience, more usefully, means providing a *system* that is resilient to errors: errors are often avoided, but if errors happen, they are rescued and recovered from. A team is better at risk resilience because it can detect, block, and manage errors in lots of ways — there are many pairs of eyes watching out. Risk resilience means learning and working out how to provide an increasingly resilient environment — and increasingly resilient digital systems.

Unconscious incompetence sounds critical, if not rude. But I myself am unconsciously incompetent about lots of things — the point is, I don't know what I am unconsciously incompetent about! So I have opinions about all sorts of things. Worse, because these are strong opinions of mine, and which make sense to me, why should I even think to check them? It's only when better-informed people around me challenge my ideas that I realize I am ignorant, despite previously having strong views. Unconscious incompetence is why people don't know they are not good at digital healthcare, despite, most likely, having a lot of experience of consumer digital innovations and strong views on what they like.

At the moment, then, any enthusiast can pass themselves off, to themselves and to other people, as a digital expert. Until we have training, qualifications, and regulations on who can practice digital healthcare development, we will continue with the problems of unconscious incompetence.

Biases, or cognitive biases, are ways in which unconscious processes in all of us affect our decisions and thinking — without us realizing. For example, the **fundamental attribution error** is our bias towards explaining people's behavior by their personality. Thus, if somebody does something bad, we are biased to think that they *are* bad. In reality, when bad things happen, there are usually lots of explanations — the Swiss Cheese Model again.[c]

In healthcare, an important bias is **hindsight bias** — after an incident happens, like a patient being harmed, we now know more than anyone did while the incident was happening. We therefore judge everyone involved in the incident harshly because, surely, they should have known what we now think is obvious. It's too easy to over-emphasize what we *now* think people should have known or should have been able to anticipate at the time: we let the insights we've learned knowing the outcome to rewrite how people should have behaved at the time.

In healthcare, almost everyone is wonderful, and bad things *rarely* happen because anyone is actually bad; rather, bad things happen because of complex system problems, bugs, task saturation, under-resourcing, and so on. But with hindsight bias, we think we can see reasons why the nurse or doctor failed: things went wrong, surely, because the nurse was inattentive? We prefer this simple human story of betrayal by a bad person. Next, having started to think about how bad somebody is thanks to hindsight bias and the fundamental attribution error, we then suffer from **confirmation bias**: we tend to seek out more reasons why we are right, and we discount other explanations for the problem, such as the system problems. We rarely seek out evidence that we are wrong! Soon we have collected so much evidence that the person is bad, that we are convinced there are no mitigating circumstances. We stop listening to the important role of other factors.

In healthcare in particular, the mass media exploit our weakness for confirmation bias. I've already mentioned the *Daily Mail* story of a "blundering nurse"[d] that goes on to tell us how the nurse blundered. The alternative explanations get no serious consideration; why should they, if we think the nurse is blundering? We are **primed** (to use the technical term) to think the nurse is a blundering nurse, and confirmation bias means we get stuck looking for reasons to support our growing suspicions, and we ignore any contradictory information. The reason confirmation bias is an important Human Factors issue is that we are unaware we are thinking so selectively.

It gets worse.

Confirmation bias is what we do to ourselves, why we must take special care not to jump to conclusions and then just seek reasons to justify ourselves. But we also start talking more to the people who have the same beliefs as we do. Naturally, they help us entrench our views. In other words,

---

[c] See Chapter 6: Swiss Cheese Model, page 61 ←
[d] See Chapter 7: "Blundering" nurse, page 71 ←

we start imposing and drawing on confirmation bias in the people around us. In turn, they do it too, and it creates an avalanche of what is really narrow-mindedness. This effect is well known in social media, where people tend to live in **echo chambers** with people who agree with them and who don't try to seek out contradictory views.[288]

The surprising disciplinary action against 73 nurses I described earlier[e] was (I think) the echo chamber effect in action: everybody inside the disciplinary process paid attention to people who agreed with the gist of the allegations. Moderating or dissenting voices were not sought out. (The expensive court case that followed pitted the prosecution and defense teams against each other: a formal process, indeed a very expensive formal process, that tries to manage the Human Factors limitations of jumping to conclusions.)

When a group of people or a company develops a new digital intervention, like a medical app, they too inevitably suffer from the echo chamber effect. Again, it's not their fault, but part of the human condition we all share. The developers believe their product is great (else they wouldn't be developing it!). They then naturally collect supportive people around them. They build their own echo chamber. Soon, they cannot believe there may be any problems to fix or any bits to improve. *This* is why we have to put real effort into User Centered Design[f] and Formal Methods[g] in digital healthcare: both techniques bring outside and objective perspectives into the process to compensate for our Human Factors weaknesses.

I mentioned **cognitive dissonance** earlier;[h] it's another of our cognitive biases.[14] The idea is: if we find several ideas about ourselves that are inconsistent — dissonant — we'll try to resolve the dissonance in favor of bolstering our self-image. There are many ways to do this, but an easy one is to dismiss any negative ideas. So if we have spent years learning and using a programming language — why did we spend all that time on it? — it's much more preferable to convince ourselves and everyone around us that, we being sensible, it must be a really good language. Other explanations, that it took us a long time because it's an over-complicated language or (an even worse thought) that we are bad programmers, are too dissonant to contemplate.

It cannot go without being mentioned, but there is an important **substitution rule**.[289] If somebody else under the same circumstances would have made the same mistake, then it is not their fault, but it's the system that let them down.

The substitution rule isn't conventional Human Factors (though it captures some Swiss Cheese thinking), it's more like an *axiom* underlying all Human Factors thinking. In important ways, people are the same. Human

---

[e] See Chapter 8: Disciplinary action against 73 nurses, page 92 ←
[f] See Chapter 22: User Centered Design, page 301 →
[g] See Chapter 27: Formal Methods, page 379 →
[h] See Chapter 3: Cognitive dissonance, page 28 ←

Factors literally factors out this "sameness" and sorts out how it's organized and applied. The substitution rule says that, to the extent that people are the same, we cannot blame *them* for what they do, for *anybody* would do it — and we should know that, and find out why.

Overcoming or **mitigating biases** is very difficult, because we all suffer from them and they are deeply embedded in how we think — they are very hard to acknowledge, let alone to see. Human Factors provides a range of solutions, from training to anticipate when biases influence us, to effective teamwork particularly to encourage other people to stand back and help critique our biased thinking. An important technique is to have somebody in the team as an observer who is critically watching what is happening without getting too involved in it; they are outside the stress and tunnel vision of the raw action, and therefore have more cognitive capacity to spot things going awry. Effective multi-disciplinary teamwork fixes many problems — especially if the team includes a Human Factors specialist who knows what to look out for.

"Effective" is the keyword here — it is so easy to have ineffective, even counter-productive teams, and nobody will notice or try to fix the dysfunctional problems because they don't see them and, even if they do, they are not empowered to intervene.

Finally, and perhaps the central Human Factors trade-off is, despite the fact that in many ways people are all the same, people have **individual differences**. We are all different, and we are different in different, subtle ways.

It's fairly obvious that we are all different when we think about it, but when we design and build digital healthcare systems it's easy to overlook.

The classic mistake is that people developing systems do not realize that their users are different from them: users have different skill sets, they think differently, and they are working under different conditions. It's easy to overlook when we design any systems, from digital systems to standard procedures to follow: our ideas look obvious to us, but we — thanks to individual differences — are not the same as other people. What's obvious to us, especially as we've spent a week on our pet project, is not going to be so obvious to other people, especially when they are working under pressure.

Gender is an important individual difference, but it's easy to overlook, as we are whatever gender we are; we take it for granted much of the time, especially when doing complex tasks like programming.

Female doctors are faster and more satisfied with hospital digital systems than their male colleagues.[290] The research suggested that developing a greater understanding of the differences could help reduce staff burnout and help improve performance more generally — because men and women burn out differently, and if this isn't taken into account, we jump to the wrong conclusions about it. Such understanding could surely help developers build more effective and pleasurable digital systems, which would then be more effective for everyone.

Part II ◇ Treatment ◇ Finding solutions

Most programmers are male; perhaps as high a proportion as 90% (depending on what you count as a "programmer"[291]). One of the things that's obvious to them is that they are men. I'm one too, and I can say we don't go around continually reminding ourselves we are men. Similarly, programmers don't go around reminding themselves they are programmers, or men, or young, or whatever; they just are — it doesn't need saying.

Gender has a high profile — but there are other individual differences issues, such as race and culture. Knowing, as we do, that gender matters should drive wider appreciation of these other differences.

What teams do is help individual differences to be balanced out, and — at least when the teams work effectively — for team members to complement each other.

Color vision is another example of individual differences that is easy to overlook. About 4.5% of the population is color blind — and people can be color blind in many different ways. So, although color coding might be obvious to you, never rely on color; always add monochromatic cues, lightness, texture, or symbols — and do large enough experiments with a representative range of people with different visual abilities to check your idea works.

In healthcare it's natural to think Human Factors is the concern of people at the sharp-end: the doctors and nurses and other healthcare professionals, so that they can learn how to have fewer accidents and harm fewer patients. That's a helpful point of view, of course, but *everyone* in the system is susceptible too. The line managers. The people in procurement who buy new systems. The people who write standard operating procedures. The programmers who design and develop the digital systems. The regulators who devise the final rules. Human Factors is a universal human concern.

How do we defend against our built-in (and usually overlooked) Human Factors weaknesses? Of course, we know about Human Factors, and we know the terminology, so that problems can be called out and recognized — and discussed constructively in a non-defensive, non-argumentative way.

But real life is complex and demanding, and, certainly in healthcare, requires reliable performance under pressure. Teamwork, at least when it works, breaks up the load, and each person has a role mitigating others' Human Factors weaknesses. If one person is task saturated, another has their eye open for issues that person overlooks.

Cultural issues are part of Human Factors. Another person will not point out a problem if they feel what they say will be taken as unwelcome criticism, especially if the person in charge of the problem has "authority."

The WHO Surgical Checklist starts off by getting people to say their names, as this reduces the power hierarchy: it's much easier to help someone when you know their name.

Diversity, too, can make teams far more effective because different types of people see different things and respond in different ways — of course, some diversity can reinforce power hierarchies that make co-operation hard.

Box 20.3. Risks of international code and poor code review

On 21 July 2020, a TUI Airways Boeing 737 flight from Birmingham International to Palma de Mallorca airport had a serious incident after underestimating the plane's weight before take-off.

> The incident occurred due to a simple flaw in the programming of the IT system, which was due to the meaning of the title 'Miss' being interpreted by the system as a child and not an adult female. This was because in the country where the system was programmed, Miss is a child and Ms is an adult female. This issue had not been identified as part of the initial risk analysis and did not manifest itself during the trial simulations.[292]

TUI assumes any passenger checking-in as "Miss" weighs 35 kg, whereas a "Ms," who they assume is an adult, weighs 69 kg. It's a very unreliable approach, out-of-sight, and hard to scrutinize — and unnecessary when TUI already keeps track of whether passengers are infants, children or adults.

Since an explicit change was made to some code, somebody must have *decided* to do it. In a development culture where there is code review, somebody else would have reviewed the code and documentation, and asked, "why?" In a mature international development culture, the code reviewer would be aware of cultural differences, and ask why changes were made based on local cultural assumptions. If it was a "simple flaw," as the extract from the formal report above says, it should have been simple enough for a code reviewer to spot — if effective code reviewers had been used.

Following the incident, TUI introduced a daily manual workaround to ensure adult female passengers were referred to as Ms on the documentation. Of course, a manual workaround — to be repeated for every passenger on every flight — to fix a bug is much less reliable than fixing the program.

Computers should be part of the team too — by double-checking, asking for confirmation, warning before potentially unsafe acts, and more.

Code review is a special case of organized teamwork for developers. It is a formalized process where programmers challenge each other — "Why did you do that? What are your assumptions?" Code review uses one person's questions to probe into the areas another has possibly overlooked. In particular, ensuring teams are more diverse and using techniques such as code review, are practical ways to spread Human Factors insights across development teams. Users would then benefit from using safer and more effective systems.

Some aspects of good teamwork have become formalized on a much larger scale, changing our culture, and the way we approach problems. Science is perhaps the best example.

The reason why science has been so successful is that it encourages a belief in evidence, searching for reasons we may be wrong, searching for clear reasons, and then spreading the best ideas as widely as possible. Science encourages a culture of criticism — there is a formal role of referee, a person whose job it is to find mistakes. Sometimes referees are destructive in their criticism, but at least they stop erroneous science being published (which would perpetuate errors in the community); better referees identify problems, and sometimes solutions, to help the science get better before it is published. "What would a scientist do?" is always a good question.[293] Science's goal has been described as reaching consensus,[294] which is exactly how we might describe successful teamwork.

At its best, science also cultivates humility. We don't know what we don't know, and we don't notice we don't know things, so we have a natural tendency to succumb to our Human Factors weaknesses. Humility means not just seeking new ideas, but actively worrying that our Human Factors means those ideas may be flawed. We then devise ways to check whether they work. We'll see later[i] that good programmers deliberately fill their programs with things to check their assumptions all the time, and they use powerful computer tools to help — they know computers "think differently" to them (doing type checking, analysis, theorem proving, and more — things people don't do well on their own), so the computer's insights complement their own. Bad programmers just expect their programs to work.

If you thought Human Factors was straightforward, there is a **theory of irony** to complicate things.[295] If I ask you not to think of a cat, ironically you can't do that without thinking of a cat. Similarly, if you try hard to avoid an error, especially under stress, you are slightly more likely to make it. If you are in a team, trying to avoid an error makes you especially resent anyone pointing out that you are about to make the very error you knew you wanted to avoid. The ironic effect is counter-productive. Fortunately, previous practice as a team, especially when the practice has been part of explicit Human Factors training, helps appreciate the positive goals of the person interrupting you.

Human Factors is not just about human "problems" (like tunnel vision) but also celebrates human powers.[j] Humans are remarkable at human things — intuition, recognition, caring, talking, listening — solving complex, ill-defined problems efficiently. Our skills complement what computers can do, particularly when we are well matched to the computers. In particular, as I've emphasized, we work better in teams — this chapter's opening example of how my wife helps me drive more safely is a nice example of this — especially when those teams know and follow Human Factors principles.

---

[i] See Chapter 21: Computer Factors, page 277 →
[j] See Chapter 12: Safety One & Safety Two, page 145 ←

Jacob Braude made a career out of collecting good quotes. He once said, though possibly quoting somebody else:

> Consider how hard it is to change yourself and you'll understand what little chance you have in trying to change others.[296]

Chip and Dan Heath have written a powerful book, *Switch*,[297] on how to achieve change. When we want to change things, whether in ourselves or, more often in other people, we are often torn between our rational, logical reasons, and our emotional, intuitive feelings. Now visualize the process of our rational, logical selves as like riding an elephant. When we want to go somewhere, we tell the elephant to go there. However, if the elephant — representing our feelings (including our hormone-driven feelings I called Cat Thinking[k]) — doesn't want to, it's actually so large and powerful it can do what it likes, regardless of what the intelligent rider wants it to do. The elephant is a good model of why change is unlikely when our feelings and habits overrule it. But the Heaths add a nice twist: whatever the elephant wants, it will still walk down the path in front of it. Therefore, changing the path is the best way of getting the elephant to do what you want.

Here's a concrete example of the elephant model in action. You may want to lose weight, but when there's a plate of food in front of you, literally your gut feelings take over. Why not replace your plates with smaller plates? You've changed the path, and you no longer have to fight your feelings every mealtime.

In other words, since it is so hard to change ourselves and other people, a better way of improving the effectiveness and safety of healthcare is instead to improve the systems, and today that means designing better digital healthcare systems. Every bit of technology imposes a way of doing work *regardless* of the knowledge, habits, feelings, and abilities of its users. Good digital technology grounded in Human Factors can improve healthcare faster than any other intervention.

That insight also applies to system developers: it's hard to program better and more safely just by wanting to, but changing the tools and languages we use will have an immediate effect. This idea may seem like a burden for programmers, but for every programmer who becomes safer, potentially millions of patients benefit, so it's worth taking the idea very seriously. I'll talk more about this later.[l]

Of course there's much more to Human Factors than this brief chapter can cover. I hope I've got you fascinated. There are some suggestions on what to read if you want to find out more in the Good reading chapter.[m]

---

[k] See Chapter 3: Cat Thinking, page 25 ←
[l] See Chapter 27: Stories for developers, page 367 →
[m] See Chapter 33: Human Factors reading, page 483 →

Understanding how computers can avoid bugs and mistakes is the first step toward programming safer and more dependable systems. This chapter introduces some important software engineering ideas that can help make safer digital systems.

21

Computer Factors

Since we have Human Factors as the common and predictable ways that humans work, I've invented the term **Computer Factors** for the features of digital systems that critically affect how reliable they are. Analogous to Human Factors, Computer Factors are the systematic, regular ways that computer bugs appear and influence reliable work. Bugs are to Computer Factors as preventable errors are to Human Factors.

When something goes wrong — when an incident is being analyzed — it's routine to ask what Human Factors "went wrong" and what Human Factors lessons should be learned. There's even a nice introductory book called *Brain Bugs: How the Brain's Flaws Shape Our Lives.*[298] Of course, it's even better to use Human Factors first, to improve design, to help avoid things going wrong in the first place.

Equally, we ought to be analyzing all the digital systems and asking what Computer Factors are relevant, what things can go wrong, what can be improved, what factors we should look out for when we get new systems, and so on. Like Human Factors, Computer Factors focus our minds on critical issues that are otherwise easy to overlook and often result in bugs and other problems.

Just as Human Factors are features of humans that lead to specific sorts of behavior, often causing problems, Computer Factors are features of programs that often lead to bugs or other unexpected behavior. Like Human Factors, there is an interesting mix of whether a Computer Factor is the computer's problem or some programmer's fault. Often bad Computer Factors cause problems because the developers made poor design decisions a long time ago, and it's now too difficult to disentangle the facts.

Here's an alphabetical list of a few illustrative Computer Factors. The interesting thing is to get the ideas, and then use the ideas to seek out and manage other problems that may arise during development. In particular, I'm sure you can think of some more ideas — give your Computer Factors

Fix It: See and solve the problems of digital healthcare. Harold Thimbleby,
Oxford University Press. © Harold Thimbleby 2021.
DOI: 10.1093/oso/9780198861270.003.0021

> **Box 21.1.** The etymology and entomology of bugs
>
> In everyday English the word *bug* means an insect, or to annoy or to irritate — perhaps drawing on what bedbugs and other pests do. In computing and engineering, more specifically, *bug* means an unwanted or preventable problem. The engineering usage may well be traced back to the old Welsh word *bwg*, meaning a ghost or goblin.
>
> Thomas Edison first used *bug* meaning a problem in an engineering design in 1876, and it was rapidly popularized. In 1878 he wrote what is now one of the classic quotes about the inventive process:[299]
>
> > The first step is an intuition — and comes with a burst, then difficulties arise. [...] "Bugs," as such little faults and difficulties are called, show themselves and months of anxious watching, study and labor are requisite before commercial success — or failure — is certainly reached.
>
> In 1945, Rear Admiral Grace Murray Hopper found a moth inside Harvard University's Mark II electromechanical computer. She taped the moth, probably the first victim of electrocution by computer, into her lab notebook. She famously wrote, "First actual case of bug being found."
>
>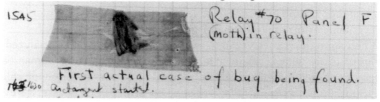
>
> This, the first bug you could actually *see*, has gone down in history.

names so that you can call them out and help others to understand and use them effectively.

- 🐞 **Antipattern**. I promised a list of factors that lead to specific sorts of unfortunate behavior, and thanks to choosing an alphabetical list of the factors, I have to start off with one that doesn't cause specific behavior!

  Antipatterns are the evil twin of **patterns**.[300] **Patterns** are good ideas for programming and building systems, whereas **antipatterns** are good ideas that are wrong and inappropriate in the current context. Every good pattern therefore has an antipattern — the temptation is to use an old solution as an easy fix because it had previously been a good idea in another place and time. Unfortunately, the antipattern gives the programmer unjustified confidence in the (wrong) solution, and they race ahead without proper checks. A specific example of an antipattern is given below, in its alphabetical place, at **premature optimization**; another example is the spreadsheet program Excel, which is amazing at doing many things, but this very power makes it a prime candidate to be an antipattern.[a]

- **Bad comment**. After a program has been written, people will have to come back to maintain it, modify it, or fix its bugs. **Comments** are essential human-readable explanations of what the program is supposed to do and how it does it. Often comments are inaccurate or just aspirational, and then the next programmer will misunderstand the program and make a mess of it.

  Bad comment is a good example of a Computer Factor. There is no bug-as-such in a program that corresponds to bad comments: after all, computers ignore comments, as comments are only intended for humans. Instead, bad comments mislead programmers, who *then* introduce bugs and other problems.

- **Buffer overflows**. Computers have a limited amount of memory, and the programmer has to allocate it wisely, trying to anticipate how everything will be used. If the programmer makes a mistake and the actual use of the program needs more memory, things will go wrong. Once a program has run out of memory, it is not obvious how to recover and do what the user wants.

- **Corruption**. Programs obviously use a lot of data, and sometimes bugs in the program (or cyber attacks) change the data. Then the program may do anything, and perhaps do anything under the control of some cyber attacker (or somebody accidentally behaving like a cyber attacker). Obviously programs should continually check data for integrity, so that any unwanted changes are blocked by **assertions** and **guards** immediately (I'll discuss these ideas more fully below), and thus not lead to problems.

- **Deadlocks**. Computers do many things concurrently, such as showing numbers on an infusion pump display, scanning for the user pressing buttons, and simultaneously pumping a drug into a patient at the same time. A simple deadlock happens when A is waiting for B and B is waiting for A, and then nothing happens! It's helpful to have a **watch-dog** that notices when nothing is happening, but the problem is that the watch-dog may not know what to do next, apart from barking to draw someone's attention to the problem.

- **Defensive programming — or failure to use defensive programming**. Programming involves human work, and therefore it is subject to error, and unfortunately some errors aren't noticed

---

[a] See Chapter 31: Using Excel in Test and Trace, page 440 →

without special effort. Therefore good programmers use **defensive programming** — using many techniques to help them (or help their programs) spot, and block or recover, from errors.

I think all programming should be defensive, so it shouldn't really need a special term — except it is useful when you ask a programmer how they're doing defensive programming, and you discover they don't have a good answer!

🄳 **Division by zero**. A computer can't divide by zero, so if a number is zero (perhaps because somebody set up a treatment forgetting to enter all the data) the computer crashes when it does what should have been a routine calculation (say, to work out how long the treatment will take).

🄳 **Infinite loops**. If a computer keeps on trying to do the same thing again and again, a so-called infinite loop happens. In the worst case, the computer won't pay attention to anything else, and it will appear to have frozen. (They aren't really infinite, just that there's nothing *in the software* to stop them.)

🄳 **Null pointers**. Rather than keeping lots of copies of data (and keeping track of changes) it is good practice to point to data — keeping track of its location. The pointer is then used as an efficient proxy for the actual data. Hours or days later, the program may try to use the pointer when it's wrong, perhaps even pointing nowhere. It's then a null pointer. Null pointers also happen when the programmer forgets to initialize a pointer to point to something in particular; again, it's then a null pointer. Many computer programs crash when they try to use a null pointer — note that the bug isn't the null pointer as such, but trying to use it is a bug. Modern programming languages make it very difficult or impossible to have null pointers.

🄳 **Out by one errors**. Often called **fencepost errors** (figure 21.1), out by one errors happen when the programmer has made a counting mistake in designing their program. Out by one errors usually result in corruption or crashing. Undetected out by one errors mean a program will carry on making more and more of a mess of things.

🄳 **Overloading**. In good programming, it is always clear what everything means. When anything is **overloaded** it is being used in more than one way, and sometimes — worryingly often — it may not be clear what it means. For example, the user is asked to enter a number that will be stored in the program variable n. A common, and problematic, overloading of n is that if it is zero, this is supposed to indicate that the user entered nothing, otherwise it's the value that the user entered. So what does it mean when the user enters zero?

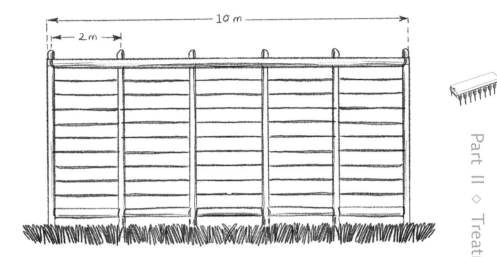

Figure 21.1. If you build a fence 10 meters long with posts 2 meters apart, how many posts will you need? Although it's obvious that 10 ÷ 2 = 5, the answer's not 5 posts, but 6 posts — you need one more post than there are panels.

A computer program may need to do several things, here represented by the fenceposts. But should it do as many things as there are panels or as many things as there are posts? Programming to solve problems without thinking carefully often leads to **out by one errors**, otherwise known as **fencepost errors**. (For short lengths of fencing, as shown here, the problem seems pretty easy because you can do it in your head. For fences you can't see — which is how programs work — it's much harder. Indeed, if you look closely at my simple diagram, even here you'll see I've got a different sort of error in the measurements: you can't give an exact answer without knowing how wide the posts are.)

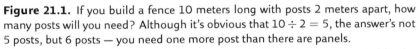 **Premature optimization**. Optimizing programs is a good idea — we want programs to run quickly and effectively. We certainly want to know where a program is "wasting time" so we can fix problems. But *premature* **optimization** is optimization's seductive antipattern. Here, we do the optimization too soon, before the program is finished and stable. Optimization always makes programs more obscure, as the programmers strain to squeeze seconds out of loops or calculations — but the original intent gets lost. Instead of doing it *right*, the emphasis has become doing it *faster*. The problem is, as a rule, speeded-up code is much harder to understand.

A much better way to do optimization is to get tools to do it — such as getting a better compiler — and then the programmers can program clearly, and leave the intricacies of optimization up to their automatic tools.

Timeouts. Many problems are "solved" by timeouts. If nothing happens for a while (like 30 seconds) the computer program assumes something else needs doing — perhaps a motor has got stuck, or the user has walked away. We can't do nothing forever, so the timeout triggers something else to happen. Sometimes, because actually the computer has no idea what's happening, what is automatically triggered is the wrong thing, and that's the timeout bug.

Type errors. Having types means you can't do some things — you can't do bad things by accident.

Types are the sorts of values used in programs. By naming the types, we can define what programs are allowed to do with those sorts of value because we named them. For example: "number" is a type of value you can add one to, or multiply by ten, and so on; or "string" is a type of value you can find characters in or make longer by joining with other strings. Types are usually related to each other, so they inherit properties; for example, an integer is a type of number, but it only allows whole numbers. It doesn't really make sense to add one to a string — this is almost always a bug you want to avoid: it's a type error. In typed programming languages you cannot freely mix up types, but in untyped languages you can make unnoticed errors (which a typed language would have caught) that then cause unexpected problems, perhaps only appearing years after the program was developed.[301]

Unpropagated updates. A programmer makes changes *here* but often forgets to make the corresponding updates *there*. Often, when there are many programmers involved in a project — possibly the programmers are spread out all over the world and work in different time zones — all the updates don't get made, because people lose track of everything that needs doing. Indeed, incompatible updates may be made simultaneously in different places.

Use error. The program gets a number or other data from the user and just assumes it is correct (see defensive programming, above). If the user makes an error that the computer ignores, then the bad data goes on to cause chaos, generally triggering an avalanche of further bugs.

Note: the correct terminology "use error" (not "user error") was explained in box 10.1.

Wrong operators. A very common problem in programs is that the programmer meant to write + but wrote *, or −, or = instead of == (all these examples just one keystroke wrong). Then wrong things will happen every time this bit of code is run. Unfortunately, it may be some time before this precise bit of code is run, and even longer before anybody notices anything going wrong. For example, x+0 and x−0 always have the same result, despite mixing up + and −. All bugs can hide themselves for a long time; they are then called **latent bugs** or **latent errors**.

There are very many more ways programs can go wrong — this brief list is by no means a complete list of Computer Factors and bugs.[302]

The key question is: how do you protect your programs from unhelpful Computer Factors? What, then, are examples of helpful Computer Factors? Here are some suggestions ...

The simplest idea is **redundancy** — which I also mentioned as a way to help in Human Factors.[b] Redundancy certainly helps humans, but redundancy is also a very good idea in digital systems.[303] Since our programming is unreliable, do everything in several different ways, preferably even by involving different programming teams. Then each way, although it seems redundant, can check the other ways. Different programming teams will have different assumptions and they'll make different mistakes. Redundancy works because the chances you all make exactly the same mistakes is very low, so when one part of a redundant system fails, other parts either recognize the problem and can stop things getting worse, or they can recover and keep the system working.

A special case of redundancy is **guards**. Guards explicitly confirm code will work and they make sure assumptions are met. Guards in computing are like the real-life guards that say "who goes there?" and if you haven't got the expected answer, you get stopped (or you're shot) before you can do anything you're not supposed to do.

Guards and **assertions** overlap; see box 21.2. Guards and assertions can be done in quite ordinary programming; they are basically just names we give to styles of programming so that we, as programmers, can think more clearly — in particular, so that we can *remember* to think more clearly, and talk to each other using shared ideas we all understand. Where are the assertions? Where are the guards? Are they clear? Do they **cover** everything that could happen?

Basically, guards protect specific code, and are a normal part of programming to handle different expected cases — though in much programming, the guards are often not laid out very clearly.

In contrast, assertions protect everything, and are there to detect and protect against bugs.

So, for example, a program might assert that a patient's BMI (body mass index) is defined and positive, since it doesn't make any sense for a program's variable BMI to be undefined, zero or negative. However, if we know the program doesn't have *that* bug, because it passed the assertion defined(BMI)

---

[b] See Chapter 20: Redundancy, page 264 ←

and BMI > 0, then — and only then — a BMI less than 18.5 would be an indication of anorexia — reporting that case could then be safely guarded by simply checking that BMI < 18.5. However, just guarding some code with the obvious if(BMI < 18.5) ... *without* any such assertion would cause chaos as the BMI variable might be, for some reason, undefined, zero, negative, or even somehow true or false.[304] If the BMI is bad, undefined or whatever, then there must be bugs of some sort, and the assertion will fail, so the programmer knows to fix the bugs, leaving the user to deal only with valid BMIs.

Interestingly, thinking as a programmer about assertions and guards immediately raises interesting clinical questions that may not have been addressed. First, if the variable BMI is undefined, is that actually an error: should it be trapped as an error with an assertion, or should it be handled as a problem for the user to fix with a guard? Has the program not made a clear enough distinction between the user not providing a BMI at all (yet), and the program not knowing what the BMI is? Obviously having a defined BMI ≤ 0 would be incorrect, and we have been told to guard for a BMI < 18.5 for possible anorexia, but this begs the question: what is the lowest a BMI can be and still be a legitimate value? So, asking these sorts of question, the programmer will be inspired to go to a clinician and ask: what sort of warnings do you need when the BMI is $<$ min, and what is min? A BMI < 13 can be fatal for males, and less than 11 for females,[305] so those cases need guards and a clear warning — and, to program *that*, we would also have uncovered that we need to ask whether the program should track gender as well. Programming problems with larger BMIs were discussed in box 13.3.

In a perfect world, neither might be necessary. It's too easy to forget we don't live in a perfect world, and things will go wrong for all sorts of reasons. Guards and assertions help stop the problems.

⚫ Good software has **guards** and **assertions**.

It's interesting to reflect *why* they are a such good idea for helping to make programs more reliable.

Most computer programming is **imperative** — we instruct the computer to make changes to things. Programming languages have **commands** — it's *imperative* the computer does what we command!

Imagine a program for handling the user entering a drug dose. Each time the user presses a digit key, the number the user is entering changes. Furthermore, it changes in quite a complicated way. If you want the details, it's like this: the number is multiplied by ten and the key is converted to a value which is then added to that number — *except* if the user has already pressed the decimal point; then the number is not multiplied by ten, but the value of the key is divided by a power of ten, depending on how many digits have been pressed since the decimal point. And if the user presses delete, then ... well, it becomes even more complicated.

As you can see, everything turns into an instruction to change something, and *hopefully* after all these changes the number is what the user wanted. Then there are the edge cases: What do you do if the decimal point is pressed more than once? What happens when the number is being entered into a window (such as the display on an infusion pump) which isn't big enough to display all its digits? What happens if the user presses lots of digits, so the number itself overflows? What if the user presses ▊0▊ when the number is already zero, should it display 0 or 00, as both choices make some sense? And so on.[55]

However it's programmed, almost everything the user does leads to some sort of change in the number's state. It isn't always obvious what to tell the computer to do, and often programmers accidentally overlook some of the tricky cases, so the computer may not end up in a well-defined, safe, intended state when it's finished. It's rarely totally clear what the cumulative effect, in every case, of all the changes is, especially when handling use error.

In contrast, assertions and guards are **declarative**. They declare something that must be true at all times. They say *what* is wanted, not *how* it has to be achieved. This makes them very much simpler than imperative instructions. They need not depend on previous instructions (like whether we have already handled the decimal point, and, if so, exactly how many digits ago) and *then* what do we *do*?

Declarative programming is simpler than imperative programming, but, more importantly, it is *different* — we express what we want the program to achieve in a very different way.

The point is: it'll be unlikely that the two contrasting styles of programming, when they are combined, will have exactly the same blindspots, so they won't have the same unnoticed bugs. Therefore, assertions or guards, which are declarative, will (very often) detect an imperative program's bugs.

For example, going back to reading numbers from a user's keystrokes, we can assert (that is, declare) the relationship between the keys the user has already pressed, KeysBefore, the latest key pressed, Key, and the outcome, KeysAfter, that must *always* be true as follows:

Key is a digit	KeysAfter is one key longer than KeysBefore
Key is delete	KeysAfter is one key shorter than KeysBefore
Key is decimal point	...?
Key is anything else	KeysAfter = KeysBefore
Key was not pressed	KeysAfter = KeysBefore

Already, as you can see, I'm asking questions about the decimal point case. It's trickier than it looks — it begs the question what should be done if the number already has a decimal point and this is another, if it's a new one, and whether we want to make the decimal point clearer by displaying a zero after it. If I'd been programming imperatively, these subcases would typically have been handled by getting on and just writing the code to do stuff. Trying to use assertions is getting me to be more thoughtful!

Even these *very simple and very clear* assertions will catch many bugs. We can already use these assertions, just as they stand, even before we've decided exactly what decimal points should do — the rest of the assertions are already helpful. This is a very remarkable fact: even partial and buggy assertions can reduce bugs in programs. Furthermore, we get these benefits without changing the rest of the program — which is a common source of unnecessary bugs.

When South Australia's hospitals using the Sunrise EMR upgraded their Microsoft Windows systems in 2021, they found that drug doses were being corrupted by duplicating the last digit.

Here are a couple of examples: a 15 mg drug dose became a 155 mg dose, and a 100 mg dose turned into a 1,000 mg dose. Yet if the Sunrise system had had simple assertions, these bugs would've been highlighted as soon as they happened. More to the point, the bugs would very likely have been highlighted during development and would have been fixed *before* the software was distributed. If the assertions had been written properly, standard bug logs would have been time-stamped and would have given a detailed breakdown of the scale and details of the problems. But, clearly, the system was not programmed very well.

The hospitals weren't even sure how many patients had been affected.

When asked how long the problem had gone unnoticed, South Australia Health's Chief Executive, Chris McGowan, said that it wasn't known.[306]

For hospitals, it's a no-win situation. It's worrying that updating an operating system breaks applications that patients depend on, but if you don't upgrade you may get cyberattacked because you haven't installed the latest security features. It's a no-win situation because digital healthcare is buggy.

The buggy Down syndrome program, which I talked about as an example of the Millennium Bug,[c] was written in the totally inappropriate, obsolete programming language Basic;[24] even so, its serious bug would have been detected and fixed *long before it had done any harm* if there'd been the simple and obvious assertion that a mother's ages must be a positive number.

If a human had been doing the Down risk calculations, instead of a computer, that simple assertion would have been totally obvious. Even if humans don't state all sensible assertions explicitly, it'd certainly have been obvious to anyone that a *negative* mother's age was an error! Why wasn't it obvious for the programmer to program the same basic check — especially after an earlier bug in the same program, which they'd fixed, involved not checking for a patient weight of zero?

---

[c] See Chapter 4: Millennium Bug (Y2K problem), page 33 ←

A Mr W updated the software in 1994,[22] which begs the question: why wasn't it already a *habit* to use assertions in any clinical program? Subsequently, 6,996 tests were carried out during the "reign" of the Millennium Bug. Why wasn't it obvious in the investigation of the Down bug that the program wasn't just wrong, which could have been an oversight, but wrong to the extent of incompetence because it had no assertions to detect its own serious bugs?

――――――――◾――――――――

Assertions can be used in any programming language.

In JavaScript, taking it as an example of a popular, more modern programming language, a simple assertion might be written like

if(...) alert("Assertion ... failed")

Then you'd do lots of testing to check that the assertion *never* fails with all the test cases you can think of. You'd then bring in users and let them do their worst, testing that no use error or bug slips unnoticed past your assertions. But if you programmed in a language like SPARK Ada, the compiler itself would check your assertions were correct, even before the program was ever run.

In other words, ordinary programming at its best can detect bugs, but Formal Methods can detect bugs before programs are run, before there is any possibility of patient harm. Even better, your program doesn't need to know what to do when an assertion fails — because in SPARK Ada it wouldn't even get as far as being allowed to run in the first place.

――――――――◾――――――――

Recall the Panama fiasco, where Olivia Saldaña González and her colleagues went to prison for manslaughter due to a radiotherapy machine's bugs:[d] the machine allowed the user to enter more than four blocks, but the program could only cope with at most four blocks. What Olivia did made no sense to the buggy program. It then failed, and overdosed the patients. Given the machine as it was, as we discussed earlier, the machine's programmer should have explicitly programmed some assertions and guards.

Here's how some very simple guards could have been used to check that what a user was doing in Panama made sense to the program:

Guards	What to do
if(number-of-blocks undefined)	intercepted a bug!
if(number-of-blocks < 0)	intercepted a bug!
if($0 \leq$ number-of-blocks ≤ 4)	treat the patient
if(number-of-blocks > 4)	this is an error; warn the user!

―――――――――――――――

[d] See Chapter 7: National Cancer Institute of Panama problems, page 73 ←

Part II ◇ Treatment ◇ Finding solutions

Notice that these guards make sense. They also make explicit that I think you treat the patient when there are zero blocks. To be honest, I'm not sure what to do with zero blocks — as I said above, thinking clearly with assertions and guards directly leads to asking important clinical questions that will need addressing.

Theses few guards are easy to understand regardless of how the rest of the program works. *How* the program worked out — or failed to work out — the number of blocks isn't mentioned, and doesn't distract us from thinking through what is correct. Clearly, the original programmers failed to think through the consequences of some possible bugs, perhaps because they focused on programming how to change the values, not on checking the values were within safe ranges.

As is good practice, these guards *explicitly* check all possible values that values, here number-of-blocks, can take, even ones that are apparently quite silly.[307] It's programs that *don't* handle "silly" and unexpected cases that go wrong and crash.

Here's an interesting question: why do the guards say 4 explicitly? As soon as you see the 4, you wonder why not 5 or 16, or some other number? Four seems a restrictively small guard to impose. Why is there any limit at all? Of course, it's possible that the radiotherapy machine only has four metal blocks (so that's where the 4 comes from), but clearly the programmer needs to have a chat with the engineer to find out. Possibly the end of that conversation will be that the machine is redesigned to have more blocks, or — the cheaper, hill climbing, solution — the programmer works out how to correctly handle the case if the user ever tries to use more blocks than there actually are. Either way: fewer bugs.

Instead, probably because they never wrote any guards and never noticed that their program had an issue with more than 4 blocks, the Multidata programmers didn't think (or think sufficiently) about the problem, and then the lawyers took over, arguing that it was the users' responsibility to check everything. This ensures the bugs "didn't matter," because the final responsibility was, or at least legally was, the radiotherapists' problem. Patients died because of bugs, but by this legal reasoning the clinicians had to go to prison — which doesn't fix bugs.

In a different world, the software would have been designed more carefully with assertions and guards in the first place. The radiotherapists would not be blamed, and they'd carry on treating patients, because the errors they made would have been blocked (or, better, correctly interpreted). With better software, the radiotherapists would have been even more successful in treating patients — there would have been no story for this book, and some people would have lived to tell different stories with happy endings.

In another world, following the problem, the manufacturer would admit that their programming made a critical contribution to the incident, and that they would fix the bugs as quickly and as safely as they could. Then, with better software, the radiotherapists would be even more successful treating patients in the future.

It's regrettable there was a bug, but surely we want to live in a world where we can learn from our mistakes and improve software? Even if we make mistakes, we want future patients to be better off — and we needn't lose good staff to prison. Sending staff to prison rarely solves any of the causes of the problems, and always increases workload pressures on the hospital, which itself will increase errors.

While guards help make programs more dependable, they are a waste of time if the programming language itself is not safe.

To illustrate this critical point about the need to use safe programming languages, here's a simple bit of JavaScript that you could imagine being somewhere inside some digital health system, like the Panama radiotherapy machine's program:

```
// user has asked for one more block ...
// check there aren't too many blocks already, then add the new block
if( blocks < 4 ) {
              newblocks = blocks + 1;
              if( newblocks > 4 ) ERROR! – surely can't happen?
        }
```

Imagine that this piece of program is run when the user has asked for one more block. The idea is that after confirming that the current number of blocks is less than four, which we do with the line "if(blocks < 4) ...," we then would want to add one more block, as the user requested, and set the variable **newblocks** to be **blocks+1**, which will be the new number of blocks the machine is to use. Seems easy enough.

Surely, **blocks+1** can never be more than 4 if we've already checked that **blocks** is less than 4? Well, you haven't take account of the very strange ways that some programming languages work.

Perhaps you are assuming the number of blocks is a whole number, as there can only be 0, 1, 2, 3, or 4 blocks in use in these radiotherapy sessions. Many programming languages could force that to be so, by using types, and thus they'd enforce that **blocks** and **newblocks** are integers (or even small non-negative integers in programming languages with better type systems). However, JavaScript doesn't care. It could be, due to a bug somewhere else in the program, that **blocks** has been set to 3.5, say. Unfortunately, while 3.5 is less than 4, unfortunately 3.5 plus 1 is 4.5, which is more blocks than the machine has. This would be an error.

You may now be thinking that the guard should be stricter: it should require that **blocks** is a whole number between 0 and 3. Unfortunately, in JavaScript (or any other unsafe programming languages) this still won't be sufficient.

Part II ◇ Treatment ◇ Finding solutions

If for some reason blocks has been set to "3" (which is less than 4, as the first guard will confirm), then newblocks will be made 31 and the second guard will fail. The problem here is that JavaScript is designed to make "3" and for 3 to be the same *sometimes* but not *always* — sometimes ignoring types is a deceptively convenient feature that makes programming easier, but other times it's a trap for the unwary. A mix-up could happen miles away, say in code written by a different person somewhere else in the world. The confusion may never be noticed until patients start being harmed, perhaps years later.

The result of these problems and the many other curious features of JavaScript is that JavaScript isn't suitable for use in healthcare — or in any other safety-critical area for that matter. Writing a guard that checks all the necessary conditions properly becomes so complicated that the guard itself becomes a source of bugs. The underlying problem is that JavaScript was designed to be easy to program in; it was not designed to be safe to program in. This serious criticism of JavaScript can be leveled at a lot of other popular programming languages used in healthcare.

———————————■———————————

Tools are special programs that check or help build more reliable programs. Fortunately JavaScript, being so popular, has lots of useful tools available, like Closure, DeepScan, ESLint, Flow, and PureScript. These tools are programs that read programs and look for common errors, and hence enormously improve the quality of projects. By the time you read this book, there will be other, no doubt even better, tools. Good programmers always build and use tools for their projects, as the tools encapsulate best practice in one place, and they can be reused time and time again with no further work.

I must add a warning: many apparently attractive tools do not help developers make safer or more secure systems. For example, NHS Digital has started using Nunjucks,[309] which makes rapid JavaScript and HTML development "a doddle," but it introduces new risks — the easier you make programming, generally the easier it is to overlook problems.

In addition, Nunjucks is itself rapidly developing (Nunjucks version 1 was released in October 2013; as of 2020 it's got to version 3.2.2), so, very likely, programs using Nunjucks will frequently change their meaning or stop working altogether as Nunjucks is updated. So far as I can see, there is nothing in Nunjucks to help check, let alone maintain, backwards compatibility to preserve things working as intended. Indeed, there are no tools to help ensure safe Nunjucks use — it's so recent. I've found no formal definition of Nunjucks, so I can't see how reliable tools for it could possibly be built.

The largest combined collections of research in Computer Science in existence, the ACM Digital Library and the IEEE Xplore Library,[310] have *nothing* on Nunjucks as of 2019. It would be easy to conclude that there is no research behind Nunjucks, or at least that there is no research behind it that has had the benefit of being peer-reviewed (that is, assessed by experts in

> **Box 21.2.** Good programs have assertions
>
> Guards — when used in good programming languages — aren't the only good programming idea for improving safety. Good software also has **assertions**. Assertions let the programmer check the right things are happening. The computer should use assertions to double-check its own calculations; ideally a different programmer will write the assertions, so they are as good as an independent check. It seems that Multidata used neither guards nor assertions.
>
> Assertions stop your program making mistakes, but what if there are more profound problems? If your program is confused, the assertions might be confused too. The solution is to do some of the assertions in a completely different place, with a different programming team whose only job is to make your system safer.
>
> Assertions have been around a very long time, and should therefore be standard practice. Alan Turing was already using them back in 1947:[308]
>
> > The programming should be done in such a way that the ACE [Automatic Computing Engine, a 1945 computer] is frequently investigating identities which should be satisfied if all is as it should be.
>
> In modern programming, using Formal Methods, both assertions and guards can be found and checked by the tools, by the computer itself both before and while a program is being run. Formal Methods makes the computer part of the safe programming team when the systems are designed. Formal Methods thinks faster and differently to slow, error-prone humans: in other words, Formal Methods are essential to help avoid bugs. Using Formal Methods can also find problems with assertions *before* a program is ever run; this is, of course, a huge advantage over having an assertion fail while running a live program!

the field). By way of comparison, SPARK Ada has over 100,000 entries in the ACM digital library alone — it is a programming language with a lot of worldwide expertise behind it.

It's always hard to get the right balance between rigor and safety, and power and wide appeal, but using the latest will always carry new risks. For example, whatever benefits Nunjucks is thought to bring, it introduces a *new* **cross site scripting vulnerability** (XSS) — XSS are bugs that allow hackers to bypass security checks, and hence compromise patient safety or confidentiality.

Programming languages such as SPARK Ada are intrinsically much safer than popular languages and environments like JavaScript and Nunjucks, and hence their tools are able to be much more powerful — and much more helpful to developers. Interestingly, none of the JavaScript tools listed above detect the guard problems we discussed, but SPARK Ada would not even allow a programmer to write code with those problems in the first place.

SPARK Ada is a *much* safer language to use, albeit somewhat harder to work with. But a very beneficial side effect of using SPARK Ada, or similar rigorous programming languages, is that, because they're harder to use, you have to employ better trained and more skillful programmers — which improves everything.

In safety-critical programming — which includes digital healthcare, but also aviation software, driverless cars, nuclear power stations — the program can't just stop when there's a bug. The program has to recover sufficiently from the error to continue; specifically, it has to **fail gracefully**. For example, in radiation treatment, you cannot just ignore an error or just say, hey, there's an error — the program *must* also stay sufficiently in control to switch off the radiation so the system is left in a safe state. That means the computer — preferably another computer that is at no risk of being corrupted by the error — has to take over control to shut down or otherwise manage the failure conditions.

Unfortunately, even with the best programming with the best programming languages and best tools, problems can still arise. Perhaps the device has been dropped and a wire has come loose, or a sensor has got clogged up. Under these circumstances even a correct program will struggle to do the right thing. One solution to fail gracefully is to have a **failsafe**.

It's important that systems fail safely rather than cause more problems when things go wrong (it's called **graceful degradation**). Failsafes are systems that are built to intervene when things go awry. Often failsafes are completely independent computers, so they don't get affected by the bugs that have brought down the main systems. In particular, failsafes should be *simple* computers.

———————————◾———————————

Traffic lights control traffic at a road junction or crossing, and they're complicated, so it's convenient and cost-effective to control them with a computer. It's then very easy to configure the same computer hardware to work for any junction, or to change it for new needs like adding pedestrian phases, to add special overrides, like when a fire engine wants to rush across the junction. (Set all traffic lights to red, so the junction is clear of traffic.)

An obvious assertion for a traffic light system is that there should never be conflicting green lights, yet if that assertion fails, things must have gone so wrong that you probably can't rely on anything *including* the assertion. Therefore traffic light systems — and all safe computer systems — use a *different* piece of hardware to do the safety checks. It's called a failsafe.

Here's a traffic light control box (figure 21.2), photographed in downtown Minneapolis, USA. The big box with a screen on it is a full-blown PC, running Linux. The small box next to it is a very simple thing, the failsafe,

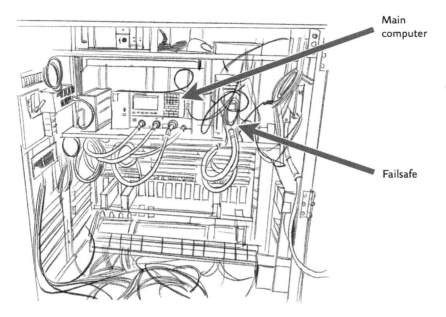

Main
computer

Failsafe

Figure 21.2. A roadside traffic light control box, with its door open showing its main computer and failsafe device. The failsafe is physically separate from the main computer, and of a completely different design; it also has a different job — to ensure any failure is made safe. The key thing is if the main computer fails you do not want the failsafe to fail for any of the same reasons.

whose only job is to stop the traffic lights going all green. If that ever happens, it takes over and makes the lights flash red in every direction.

If having a failsafe is routine for traffic lights, do your medical devices and systems have failsafes in them (do you know)?

Since we know medical systems have a pretty rough life, if they don't have failsafes, you can be pretty sure they are *not* safe to use. If things go wrong (say, the battery briefly comes loose), without failsafes the device won't know, and it won't take appropriate steps to recover gracefully or warn you that it's got a problem.

———————■———————

Failsafes are a good way to introduce **invariants**.

An assertion checks an assumption is true, a guard blocks something happening if an assertion fails, and an invariant checks something is true *all the time*. Failsafes are like guards that always keep checking the questions, and therefore failsafes check invariants. Moreover, failsafes don't just check invariants, but they are run in some separate hardware — if an invariant fails, there's generally something badly wrong, and you therefore really can't rely on any checks that aren't independent of the failing software.

In the Mersey Burns app there is a guard. The guard checks that no pre-scription calculation is made if the patient's weight is more than 30% out from a standard weight for that age of patient, unless the user confirms the unusual values. This is a guard because the app allows the unusual weights and ages until the step just before calculating the prescription when it checks them. The app's design assumes a discrepancy of up to 30% is more likely to be a use error, but as it could also be a real patient, the guards force the program to prompt the user to reconsider.

If it was an invariant — an explicit invariant that's checked — then Mersey Burns would *always* be checking it. Currently, you can enter an outlandish age and you have no idea until you try to get a prescription; that is, you have no idea until the guard warns you. If it was an invariant, you'd know straight away. It isn't obvious which is the right design. If an invariant calls out a strange weight, it might be that the use error is in the strange age, not the weight — for instance, the user is entering an age for a new patient, but the age has been left over from the last patient. The guard might first report the problem with the weight, but the problem is actually with the age.

You could do experiments to decide which design is better, but there is a third choice: the app should know when it doesn't know the age or weight. Indeed, a problem with the app is that the last patient's weight and age are automatically carried over to the next patient; it would be better if they reset to "don't know" and then you couldn't have a weight out by 30% if the age was "don't know."

This diversion into details of Mersey Burns makes a nice example of how thinking carefully through guards, assertions, and invariants helps make dig-ital healthcare safer and easier to use reliably. Indeed, as I keep emphasizing, thinking through guards, assertions and invariants helps make *any* program safer and better.

———————————— ∎ ————————————

A powerful way to reduce bugs is to use a **domain-specific language**. "Domain" means some intended application area — for instance, you could have a domain-specific language designed specifically to make it easier to program radiation machines. And, unlike a general purpose language, a domain-specific language is aimed at solving problems in a specific area or domain — it's limited in what it can do, but what it does, it does really well. As domain-specific languages are used so frequently, the idea is abbreviated **DSL**.[e]

Normal programming uses a general purpose language (such as C, Java, or JavaScript), and general purpose languages are designed to do anything. That is their power and their curse. A general purpose language allows the programmer to do exactly what they want to do, but, equally, it allows the programmer to accidentally do things they *didn't* intend to do! General pur-

---

[e] See Chapter 33: If you are a developer, page 484 →

pose languages therefore *encourage* bugs. In contrast, DSLs only do the sorts of things the domain needs. Even if a programmer using a DSL introduces bugs, the DSL, by design, can only do what makes sense in the domain for that DSL. (In contrast, a bug accidentally programmed in a general purpose language can do *anything*, even things that make no sense in the domain.)

The spreadsheet system Microsoft Excel provides a familiar example of a simple DSL. Excel has a simple language that allows the user to program spreadsheets to do useful things. To add a column of numbers, you might write =SUM(A1:A10). This conveniently adds the cells A1, A2 ... to A10. The colon notation makes it very easy to specify rectangular areas (usually rows or columns) and very difficult to specify what are almost certainly buggy areas that are not rectangular.

If you used a general purpose language, taking the sum of random cells in the spreadsheet would be easy — and usually wrong. Instead, the DSL makes it easier to do what you want, and much harder to do things that are buggy. In particular, the Excel DSL makes it impossible to refer to data that is not in the spreadsheet at all — this eliminates at a stroke one of the common causes of corrupt data we talked about above.

Let's say we develop a DSL for infusion pumps. We can now allow people to program their infusion pumps, confident in the knowledge they cannot cause basic bugs in the pump's operation. The "infusion DSL" doesn't allow anything to happen that an infusion pump cannot do — but of course the computer program that provides the DSL is running on a computer chip that can do anything. The DSL ensures the programmers can't do anything now except sensible infusion pump type things.

The standard example of using a DSL is to make it easier to **internationalize** systems correctly — to help get them to work appropriately in any country. The main software development is done in one country, but the product is shipped around the world. Programmers in other countries can customize the device (or app, etc) to work in their countries, using their own language and idioms, but the basic operation of the device cannot be changed — so new bugs are unlikely to be introduced — as the DSL doesn't allow the international programmers to change the basics.

An important example of DSLs in healthcare is **dose error reduction software** (DERS). Here the DSL is very simple: it only allows people to program about drugs and dose limits — a good DSL would structure and simplify the task so much it'd barely be recognized as *programming*. The idea is that a hospital buying a system, like an infusion pump, can program *anything* allowed in the DERS DSL, and it will (probably) be safe. If a general purpose programming language had been used instead, then programming "anything" could *really* do anything at all, including completely unsafe things, like maybe crashing the system so nothing works. The DERS DSL allows only plausible drug dose limits to be specified, so it automatically avoids a lot of bugs that could happen without it.

Part II ◇ Treatment ◇ Finding solutions

The point is, a DERS DSL "knows" about drug dosing, whereas the underlying general purpose languages have no idea, and would allow anything to happen. A very simple example a DERS DSL can enforce is that all drug doses must (obviously) be at least zero; the DSL knows this and can enforce it, but the general purpose programming language it was programmed in has no idea about drugs or doses — it would happily allow negative drug doses to be programmed! The DSL (*if* it's well designed) simply doesn't allow such silly bugs.

Before the invention of DERS, nobody would have countenanced a mere hospital reprogramming infusion pumps, because it would have opened a can of worms. DERS also nicely show a common advantage of DSLs: that is, DSLs are generally much simpler than general purpose languages. You do not need to be trained as a programmer to use DERS safely (of course, some DSLs are very sophisticated and do require specialist expertise to use safely).

It is critical that programming languages used in healthcare are safe and dependable, otherwise programs written in them won't be safe and suitable for use in healthcare. For example, SPARK Ada is (and it's used in defense, aviation, air traffic management, and so on), but JavaScript isn't. Here's a curious thing: a safe language such as SPARK Ada can be used to implement a DSL that isn't safe. Ada could, for example, be used to implement JavaScript — JavaScript is much more popular and widely known than SPARK Ada, so this might seem to make sense. It opens your "safe" SPARK Ada world up to all the advantages of JavaScript, like being able to run web applications, but *also* to all its unsafe pitfalls.

The problem is, however safe you might think SPARK Ada is, now the JavaScript DSL means it is implementing JavaScript. Therefore SPARK Ada is potentially as unsafe as JavaScript. SPARK Ada might correctly implement JavaScript, but JavaScript isn't a sensible thing to implement. More generally, just because Ada (or some other safe language) is used to implement a DSL does not mean the DSL is safe. The DSL has to be designed to be safe.

Most software is proprietary (it belongs to the person or company that wrote it), confidential, and secret, so nobody can run off with the ideas it embodies — at least, not without paying first.

Open source software is very different: everybody can see it, use it, look for problems, and improve it. Open source therefore brings potentially worldwide teamwork to everything it does. As a result, open source software is generally much more reliable than proprietary software — and if things go wrong (as they always eventually do!) — then open source communities will fix the problem. Often, bugs in open source systems are being fixed somewhere in the world while you are still fast asleep. With conventional proprietary systems, the manufacturers and their few programmers are often far too busy to help you.

Open source is a Computer Factor, so ...

- Ask to see the program code of any product you want to buy or use. Very likely, the manufacturer will refuse. You ought to ask, what are they frightened of you discovering?

- On the other hand, if a manufacturer uses open source software, their answer might well be, "thousands of the world's best programmers have already had a look ... here it is if *you* want to fix it."

- Open source programs are developed over the internet so that many programmers can scrutinize the code and contribute to it. Quality, security, and speed all improve enormously.

- One downside of open source is that making a financial return on programming costs is harder for the manufacturer. Instead, open source manufacturers provide other useful services, such as training and support.

- A worry lots of people have with open source is that, in principle, it allows hackers to inspect code for weaknesses, which they can then exploit — or, worse, they could insert their own bugs, Trojans, Easter Eggs and other problems directly into the code. Actually, these are risks of any software development — how do you know a company's employees are all good people? On the other hand, open source exposes the software to far more good people, and bugs and problems are found faster. Furthermore, code, if necessary, can be corrected very quickly after a hack if there is an international community of open source developers to help.

We can combine the best of Human Factors insights with the best of Computer Factors insights: programmers should work in teams — which is exactly what open source achieves. The idea is that other programmers in the team review what is being programmed, and spot errors and inefficiencies that one programmer would miss had they been working alone.

I visited one infusion pump manufacturer who did their programming in-house. They had just one programmer. I asked him how he did code review,[f] and he didn't know what it was. If the company's programmer does not know how to program safely, as he's "the expert," nobody else is going to realize the risks the company is running. Just one programmer is certainly asking for trouble, and programmers working in isolation without a formal process for code review is a disaster waiting to happen. If the manufacturer had been using open source, they'd have had lots of people helping them. Instead, working alone, they have no idea how risky their approach is.

---

[f] See Chapter 20: Code review, page 273 ←

Part II ◇ Treatment ◇ Finding solutions

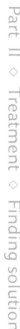

Box 21.3. Newer Computer Factors

There is a lot more to Computer Factors than what is widely known. For example, **digital cryptography** has transformed every area of IT, though much of it is invisible, hidden behind websites, streaming videos, bank transactions, and much more. Cryptography might be invisible, but it's foundational to everything in healthcare, from patient confidentiality to managing log-in passwords and providing cybersecurity.

Newer ideas like **public key encryption** (PKE), and **zero knowledge** are completely counter-intuitive. For example, you'd expect you'd want your passwords to be kept secret, but in a public key system, the passwords are made public — you can then do some *very* interesting and useful things. All the — partly justified — excitement behind **blockchain** and **bitcoin** is based on these ideas.

It's beyond the scope of this book, unfortunately, to explore how digital cryptography could help transform many aspects of healthcare. However, it *is* in scope to point out that many of the conceptual bugs we have at present, for instance with slow log-ins and multiple passwords,[7] arise because these newer Computer Factors are not being explored and fully exploited.

There are many more useful Computer Factors in modern programming, including:

🔹 **Version control**. Many computer tools are available to manage program development, including testing, documentation, and quality control. Version control tools like Git[311] also support open source development.

If you program and you don't know what Git is, it isn't the only version control software out there, but it is the best known system. It's time you found out and started using it or something that better fits your development processes — or, better, change your development processes to rely on Git.

🔹 **Iterative design**. Computer programs are hard to get right, but they are very easy to change. Iterative design[g] makes this official — acknowledging it's not possible to be right first time, test designs, see how well they work, and improve. The international standard ISO 9241-210 provides an official process for this (as well as having a lot of helpful ideas and good reading advice).

🔹 **Automated development**. Why do something when you can get a computer to do it?

---

[g] See Chapter 23: Iterative design, page 313 →

For example, why do all the hard work of testing when a computer can do it faster? I'll briefly discuss **fuzzing** later,[h] which is a fast, repeatable, and effective form of computerized testing.

- 🚹 **Formal Methods**. Formal Methods sounds sophisticated,[312] but really it's doing no more than using math to help program more rigorously. I think that using Formal Methods in programming should be no more unusual than using math to check that bridges, planes, or power stations are safely engineered. I'll talk more about this fundamental programming topic later.[i]

- 🚹 **Conceptual Design**. Overarching everything are the **concepts**, the deep ideas behind all the software and programming. If the concepts aren't right, really nothing matters. Not even the bugs, because the bugs may be relative to inadequate concepts, and then the foundations of the whole design need fixing not just the bugs — many of which will be just symptoms of the conceptual mismatch.[313]

Edsger Dijkstra wrote powerful essays about computing and programming.[314] They are required reading for all programmers. Fortunately, his essays are now really quite easy to read because he wrote them mostly back in the 1970s, an age where all programming was a lot simpler than what we are used to now.

Dijkstra made some very nice links between Human Factors and Computer Factors:

> If I start to analyze the thinking habits of myself and of my fellow human beings, I come, whether I like it or not, to a completely different conclusion, viz. [...] the recognition that, by now, brainpower is by far our scarcest resource [...] The competent programmer is fully aware of the strictly limited size of his own skull; therefore he approaches the programming task in full humility [...][315]

> As a slow-witted human being I have a very small head, and I had better learn to live with it and to respect my limitations and give them full credit, rather than try to ignore them, for the latter vain effort will be punished by failure.[316]

Of course there's much more to Computer Factors than this brief chapter can cover. I hope I've got you fascinated, now you've got the idea, and started off on thinking up your own Computers Factors, perhaps more relevant to your needs.

---

[h] See Chapter 28: Testing and fuzzing, page 389 →
[i] See Chapter 27: Stories for developers, page 367 →

Part II ◇ Treatment ◇ Finding solutions

However good a computer system is, it still needs to do what's needed — not what we think is needed. **User Centered Design** finds out how people really use systems, and how to improve their experience and reliability.

22

User Centered Design

Healthcare is a complex and messy place, but when we design a digital system, we must have a clear and precise idea of what we want, so that a computer can be programmed. Here are just a few of the inevitable problems that follow from this clash of precision with reality:

- Any "clear and precise" ideas will over-simplify lots of things.

- What the designers (developers, managers, politicians, ...) want may not be what the people (nurses, doctors, lab technicians, patients, ...) who'll use the system will want or find helpful.

- The developers, who program the systems, may not really understand the implications of their decisions, because they don't have the experience and expertise of the users.

- When people start working with a digital system, its "clear and precise" ideas will expose differences between what the computer makes them do with what they want to do. Indeed, especially when inspired by struggling with computers, what people want to do frequently changes — digital systems *become* wrong, merely by being used. People want to improve patient care, not answer to computers.

- Users may not know or they may misunderstand how a system is supposed to work — so features the developers thought were obvious may not be used, or may be used inefficiently or incorrectly.

- In an attempt to avoid these problems, systems are often designed so that they can be configured or customized by users themselves. Unfortunately, customizations may introduce new problems. Excel, mentioned several times in this book,[a] is a classic example: it allows

---

[a] See Chapter 31: Using Excel in Test and Trace, page 440 →

Fix It: See and solve the problems of digital healthcare. Harold Thimbleby,
Oxford University Press. © Harold Thimbleby 2021.
DOI: 10.1093/oso/9780198861270.003.0022

users to do anything, which may seem helpful, until you notice that being able to do *anything* necessarily includes the possibility of doing wrong things — bugs. Worse, bugs are all the more likely because most users don't know how to program safely.

Fortunately, there are powerful ways to help improve systems.

User Centered Design (UCD) is the part of developing digital healthcare systems to ensure that what you want to do is the right thing *for your users*.

UCD is usually thought of as an important process to help make a design easy and safe to use. Unfortunately, most manufacturers and developers are so familiar with their own ideas that they cannot imagine their ideas would be hard for other people to use. Indeed, manufacturers and developers are a very particular sort of people who have a unique view of digital systems, as they are the people who plan and develop them, and they think it's obvious their systems are easy to use. Conversely, politicians, managers and leaders in organizations that buy digital systems usually expect them to be effective — which is why they want them! — yet they can't possibly know until they check. There's a sort of inevitable conspiracy that UCD isn't necessary. Yet UCD is a powerful method to put diversity into digital system development, purchasing, and use, getting everyone to learn about the real lives of the other stakeholders. In short, you should always do UCD to find out how effective your systems *really* are and how to improve them for the people who use them in real life — whether you are a developer, vendor, or a purchaser, such as a hospital.

An important reason for using UCD is that many medical products fail in the market. Something like only a percent of medical ideas make it to regular use. UCD can help: it provides a way to test your idea with real users in real situations.[317] If nothing else, UCD quickly and efficiently helps you find out design problems that could make your product unsuccessful.

Another good reason for UCD is that it finds problems early. It is expensive to fix problems after a product is in production or is in use — it has to be recalled and fixed, and it's a loss of brand image. It's even worse to end up fighting legal battles caused by design errors — to say nothing of causing patient harm. UCD means you make better things that better suit what people need.

Arguing the case for UCD is made easier with these two very useful terms:[318]

- 🜋 **Work as done** — abbreviated **WAD**. This is what people actually do.
   ▷ Users stick post-it notes on equipment to remember essential things, like their passwords.[319]

- 🜋 **Work as imagined** — abbreviated **WAI**. This is what managers and others *imagine* is being done. Often, for all sorts of reasons, people don't quite tell the whole truth to their managers. Unfortunately, computer systems are often specified on what managers imagine is being done, often some "perfected" story passed up to them, and it may not be at all what the actual work as done, the WAD, is.

▷ Users fill in computer forms, and can only provide the details asked for. Often, things are made up just so that the forms can be completed. So management thinks things are happening as the forms say, but the forms aren't truthful.

The underlying concept behind these ideas is the user's **task**. What is the user's task? What task are they actually doing? What task do they want to do? What tasks does the digital system support? What's the difference between what the user thinks their task is and what the management thinks their task is? Has a **task analysis** been done,[320] so we *really* know the answers?

The WAD–WAI gap creates a vicious cycle of divergence. A computer system is brought in, which of course matches WAI, because that's why it was bought. Soon users start experiencing hindrances in getting their job done with the computer, so they start creating **workarounds**. They need to get their job done — generally helping patients — and the WAI system obstructs them. The simplest workaround will be that they lie to the computer. Then the management starts getting data that confirms their incorrect WAI view of the world! WAI and WAD diverge, so the next computer system will be even worse.

In contrast, UCD researchers go to the workplace (or sometimes a simulated workplace) and carefully find out what is really going on, the WAD, and hence how to design the computer systems to narrow the gap between WAI and WAD — to help make the computers work better in reality. Note that it isn't just that WAD is "right" and the WAI that is "wrong," it's also that the people doing the WAD do not understand the WAI point of view. It's a two-way understanding problem.

One example of the WAD–WAI divergence I've already mentioned is Seddon's ideas of value adding and risk-averse work:[b] value adding is work as done, but the work as imagined is worrying primarily about risk management. This different view twists the WAI perspective and takes it further away from the coal face WAD.

For a developer or manufacturer building systems that impact how people work, it's very important to be clear where on the WAD–WAI spectrum every idea lies. Given these very different cultures influencing the perspectives, it's even more vital to take UCD seriously. You need scientific evidence-based facts about what is actually done.

WAD–WAI is a very productive idea. Of course, there's lots more to it than we can cover here if you'd like to follow it up.[321]

---

[b] See Chapter 19: Managing value or risk?, page 251 ←

Box 22.1. How many users is enough for safe design?

If you happen to pick on a user who is color blind, then that one user will give you very useful insights — about color blindness. Even one user is then a useful input into an iterative design process: fix the color schemes, but you then have to test the next version on more users. The question is raised: how many users are required for an effective UCD study?

Widely quoted research suggests five is a good number of participants for user studies.[322] There are many flaws with this, including:

- Finding out what people prefer is easy and doesn't need many users; finding out what makes a system unsafe or safer requires systematic studies that you cannot achieve with five users.

- Most digital healthcare systems and patient care pathways are very complex, and five test users won't begin to explore enough of the system or how it is really going to be used.

- The number of users isn't a useful factor to measure; it's coverage multiplied by representativeness. Have you studied all of the system, do the users statistically represent the target population of users, and do your studies represent real use?

- Unless the studies are **ecologically valid**, you learn nothing about how the system will actually work under real clinical pressure.

Note that UCD studies don't much help in early design, since you need some sort of concrete design before UCD can get going. Once you have a concrete design, you've already made a lot of assumptions that users then take for granted, which then limits how constructive UCD can be. Instead, use expert designers to **sketch** the design, then use UCD to improve it.[323]

There's an interesting twist.

Before there were computers, there was paper, and lots of it. Just like digital systems, paper creates and imposes processes and procedures: instead of having to fill in things on a screen, you have to fill in things on paper forms. Paper forms were developed *before* UCD had been invented, and therefore — and this is the twist — the paper forms, although very familiar and seemingly central to everything, are *very unlikely* to be a good way of doing anything. So, if we go into an organization and do the WAD–WAI analysis, ask people what they want, unfortunately everyone is living in a culture steeped in paper rituals, and their ideas and wishes are almost certainly about improving the paper models, not about finding the best way for a new digital culture.

Computers can do things paper hasn't dreamed of. Obvious examples include digital signatures, passwords, email, default values, data validation, ... and lots more. Digital is different.

This is one reason why UCD emphasizes building digital prototypes to

evaluate, so that users can give feedback based on the new system ideas —
and the new ideas will need improving! — rather than just focused on improving the old systems.

The same problem happens when UCD is done to help replace some obsolete digital system with a great new system: many of the UCD ideas will
tend to focus on fixing the old digital system's problems.

Given WAD and WAI are well-known terms that make a useful — and
thought-provoking — distinction: the twist might be called **WAT — work
as twisted**. Work twisted by some obsolete, paper or digital, system. In
other words, WAT emphasizes that WAD is often WAT, and we need to work
out the **WAG — the work to achieve the real goals**. The goals of work are
not using computers or filling in forms, and not even doing that better, the
real goal — the WAG — is about improving patient outcomes. It's too easy
for UCD to focus on what user are doing now, rather than on where users are
trying to get to.

The goal of digitization is never to "go paperless" but to remove the
twisted WAI and WAD that led to wanting all that paper in the first place.

If the first question is, "are you using UCD?" the second question is,
"who *are* the users?"[324] Not being clear who the users are (and how they
actually work, Work As Done) is the quickest way of making a mess of any
digital system.

Virginia Mason, Seattle, is a hospital that asked itself what it was doing. It
had adopted the Toyota Production System (TPS, a type of quality management), which says if you want to improve quality, the first question to ask,
obviously, is what are you trying to do? They realized that their hospital was
not doing what they really wanted it to do. If they had computerized what
they were doing then, they would therefore have computerized the wrong
things, and just done the wrong things faster, and maybe more cheaply.

But, instead, they realized they were there to make patients healthy, and
to provide as pleasant an experience as possible for patients, families, and
carers.

Therefore, the patients (and family) are the users.

Not the clinicians. Not the finance department. Not the government and
its performance targets. Not the insurers. Not the digital system vendors.

Design systems to make healthcare systems better at what they are *really*
for: making patients healthier (including not getting unhealthy in the first
place), faster, more effectively, and, as often as possible, more enjoyably.

Happy and active ten-year-old Maisha Najeeb had an arteriovenous mal-
formation (an AVM), which for her meant a red mark on her cheek. She
had had the AVM treated successfully several times before at Great Ormond
Street Hospital for Children in London.

In June 2010, Maisha Najeeb ended up with brain damage when polymer was mistakenly injected by a radiologist during surgery.[325]

The operating room had two identical-looking 10 mL syringes; one for the X-ray contrast, which is used for guiding the injection of the polymer, and one for the polymer itself. Neither was labeled.

The syringes were mixed up, unfortunately leading to the polymer being injected and getting into her brain. Maisha is now in a wheelchair and needs full-time care. The NHS faces a £24 million payment over her lifetime. At the time, it was the largest compensation in a UK case of medical negligence.

Typically, clinicians make up drugs, fill syringes, label them, then put them into syringe drivers or give a bolus by hand. There are lots of steps in this sequence where errors can occur — and drug errors are among the most frequently reported incidents. Maybe computers, so often badly designed, just make the need for UCD very obvious, but note that UCD helps with *all* design, not just digital design.

Instead, manufacturers can and do pre-fill syringes (in quality-controlled processes at the factory) and barcode the filled syringes automatically. Then, when a syringe is used with a patient, a syringe driver can check and record that the right drug is being administered,[326] perhaps using a "dose error reduction system" or DERS.

If there isn't a suitable pre-filled syringe available in the operating room, as happens from time to time, the clinician will have to fill an empty syringe and barcode it themselves. The computer system, reading the barcode, will still think everything is working perfectly fine: scanning the barcode will confirm the right drug preparation is being used for the right patient. Unfortunately, if the clinician makes an error in the syringe preparation, say using the wrong drug but sticking the "right" label on it, the computer will still think it's correct, because it doesn't know any better.

The computer's assumption that the barcode is correct now positively conceals errors it was supposed to detect and block.

Clearly, there's a huge gap between work as imagined (what the computer is reporting) and work as done (what the clinician is doing). Some basic UCD work in the operating room is needed, and it will uncover the very reasonable everyday practice that shows that the computer system is not working.

In fact, the digital system has created a false sense of certainty. If a patient safety incident happens following a wrong drug error, the wrong lessons will be learned, and things will just get worse. UCD has huge benefits, especially in uncovering what we don't know we don't know.

The processes need improving, but you wouldn't have known that without the UCD step that took the trouble to carefully model real clinical practice.

———————— ■ ————————

But what is real clinical practice?

It's tempting to think that the problems with digital systems arise because developers just don't spend enough time listening to clinicians and getting to understand the complexities of healthcare.

That's partly true, and may well be completely true in some cases, but the fact is, healthcare is actually about patients. Patients are the real users.

Even when patients are unconscious, they are still a proper part of the system that UCD has to address.

Any work in healthcare systems UCD *must* include some patient representatives and carers, selected to be representative of the areas the systems are being designed for. Digital systems designed for supporting patients with infectious diseases are going to be different from computer systems for supporting palliative care, and central records must be able to cope with everything. If you don't ask the questions about users, you won't design systems that properly support patients for all conditions.

Computers tend to treat patients as either male or female, often down to just a choice of M or F labels, but in reality people are on a spectrum.

Thinking in terms of only M or F is bad enough, but when the computers get in the way and refuse to handle the reality of human experience, unavoidable bugs, errors, and potential harms get built into healthcare. For instance, in the UK, when a patient has transitioned to male, their medical records are updated as male. Yet their body may still be partly female. They may still have a cervix, but the computer systems, believing them to be male, will never call them in for a cervical smear. Then their blood levels make them anemic, because "the right" levels for a male body are higher than for a female body. Converse problems happen for transfemales.

Trans patients have reported that they have been refused tests because their recorded gender didn't match the test requested, despite blood samples being sent.

One transmale had their referral to gynecology for a hysterectomy refused on the basis they were male, so it was assumed to be a mistake. In another alarming case, labor was missed as a cause for abdominal pain in a pregnant transmale who was assumed to be obese. The baby died.[327]

It is a complex issue (with complex legal constraints too), but the root of the problem is that computer systems were originally designed for patients fitting a simplistic binary gender model. The problems highlight how UCD was not done adequately: designers just assumed patients had binary gender and they did not explore design issues with a representative group of patients. There is a now a serious legacy problem, catching up increasing numbers of patients in the simplistic binary gender categories. Given that healthcare IT systems should be designed to support all patients, it's a horrendous oversight.

Facebook allows users to choose from 71 gender options, including asexual, polygender, and two-spirit person, as well as "custom."[328] A user can also choose their preferred pronoun, so that Facebook can automatically generate appropriate text.

There's no reason why healthcare systems couldn't do something similar — but, and it's a big but, however obvious it sounds, it still needs very carefully checking out. There are two obvious problems, for instance: there may be some people for whom these choices don't work, or may cause clinical problems; secondly, the more complex the choices become, the more likely people — whether patients or clinicians — will choose or misread "the wrong one" and cause harms.

So here's what I think is a good idea (with the proviso that I have not tested it with anyone): instead of just the usual (and unfortunately dangerous[c]) binary F and M options, computers should show an additional text field where the patient can say what they like. This text should be visible whenever gender identity is relevant. UCD needs to be done to find the right balance.

However, there is a core idea here that could be really useful in addition to helping with the gender issues. It's now standard practice to teach clinicians: instead of asking "what's the matter with you?" you should ask "what matters to you?"

So why don't we ensure all digital systems, where it's relevant, have a field that allows patients to show what matters to them, including covering their gender identity and any other issues? It could be a tab on the screen so that it doesn't take up much space when other things need to be displayed, and it could provide not just text but audio or pictures that the patient supplies. Indeed, experiments have shown that patients pre-recording text saves time for the doctors and benefits the patients.[329]

It's nice that solving one problem could solve another problem at the same time. This binary gender mess gets solved, but the too-frequent dehumanizing effect that computers have on healthcare gets addressed too.

Thinking further ahead, asking "what matters to you?" could also help systems get future-proofed too (a bit) — say, for when patients start getting enhanced with implants and bits of robots and AI, or want to be able to say things about using their mobile phones — soon, patients will have interesting digital needs that are new to everyone. So a "what matters to me" box would help future-proof healthcare for when it becomes a whole different game (perhaps); it makes healthcare more human, and it gives patients a voice to say what matters to them. Every computer should know — and tell all healthcare professionals — what matters to their patients.

———————————————■———————————————

There is a very common design problem that UCD can sort out, which I'll illustrate with a user interface design issue with the Babylon app.

The Babylon app requires personal details from the patient: it needs the patient's date of birth, height, and weight. The screenshots show the form where this data is entered (figure 22.1).

---

[c] See Chapter 29: M/F abbreviation for mother/father or male/female?, page 413 →

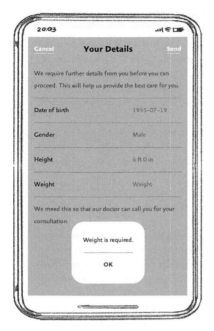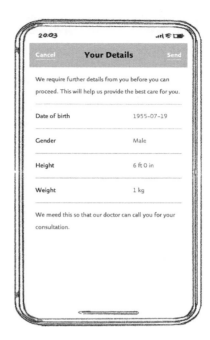

Figure 22.1. A common user interface design problem, here redrawn from the Babylon app (version 4.3.0). If you try tapping <u>Send</u> on the left-hand screen without providing all the data — perhaps because you don't know your weight and need to go off and weigh yourself — you get a warning, as well as a hard-to-read screen. You may lose everything you've done. As a workaround to avoid losing all the valid data you've already entered, a fake weight can be entered to keep the app happy (in the right-hand screen, I entered 1 kg). The app accepts the error of a nonsense weight (given my age and height!) but, so far, I haven't found any way the workaround weight can be corrected.

Without UCD, the personal details form will always *seem* to work: the patient always either fills in the form or cancels. It seems to work — so long as you never go and find out how it is *actually* used.

With UCD, though, finding out what users actually do, you discover a problem (provided you test enough users in enough scenarios). Shown on the left in figure 22.1, the patient has started to fill in their details, but apparently they weren't sure of their weight. But now Babylon's design stops them leaving the form partly filled in, which means they can't go and find out their weight without likely losing the other data they've already entered. (On many user interfaces, it's very common for forms to time out and delete all the user's work done to date.) So, as shown on the right in the figure, the user decides to do a workaround: they enter a "placeholder" weight of 1 kg,

> **Box 22.2.** Cloned documentation
>
> With digital, instead of typing something, you can just copy what you want and save all the bother, and the longer and more complex the text you want, the greater the benefits of cutting and pasting. Patients with chronic diseases who turn up time and time again with the same problems create the perfect case for cutting and pasting old notes. You get fewer transcription errors as text does not have to be typed again.
>
> Except, of course, when the original text has errors or is no longer relevant, or was written by a trainee or has other problems. Possibly the wrong text, perhaps from the wrong patient, is copied and pasted. The problem is called **cloned documentation**.
>
> There's a story of how one patient turned up to a consultation with 4,000 pages of notes.[330] Critical information would be well buried in all that cloning.
>
> Ross Koppel reports on another patient who had the same blood pressure for a month. When this unbelievable consistency was investigated, it turned out that the patient had a foot amputated a month before. The nurses had been copying and pasting blood pressure in the notes, rather than entering the patient's actual blood pressure. Another of Ross's cloned documentation examples regards a patient who entered the hospital unconscious after a car crash, recovered, and thankfully walked out three weeks later. His patient notes show he was comatose until just a few minutes before he was discharged.[331]
>
> Failure to handle cloning safely is an example of failing to do proper UCD and finding out how people really use systems. Once developers discover cloning happens, it is easy to manage it better.

which the app happily accepts — despite the age and weight being inconsistent. The plan is that the user will come back later and sort it out.

UCD would discover this sort of workaround — here, fibbing on a form — and it would probably suggest modifying the user interface to allow a patient to save a partially completed form. In fact, the computer could continually save the incomplete form automatically (perhaps keeping it separate from a fully-completed form), and, therefore, the app warning the patient the form is incomplete would be unnecessary. There is rarely any good reason not to save partial information to help a user.

Similar problems happen in hospitals. A nurse has to get the computer system to work, but they may not know some detail the computer insists on but which they think is unimportant. Either the nurse enters the correct data, or they make up something that keeps the computer happy — after all, the nurse wants to get the job done. They plan to come back immediately and sort out the problem, but life is complicated and they may get distracted. Sometime later, the incorrect placeholder data causes a problem for the patient.

> **Box 22.3.** Externalizing User Centered Design
>
> Businesses want to reduce their costs, and a standard way of doing this is **externalization**, displacing activities and costs onto other people, outside of the business. The highly-successful Swedish furniture store IKEA does this by getting customers to assemble their own furniture. Externalization means IKEA saves all the final construction costs. They are then more profitable.
>
> UCD is a cost for manufacturers, so what better than to externalize it?
>
> When a hospital buys a new electronic record system, this is usually installed over a couple of years and the hospital configures it and helps debug the system — at their own expense. This is externalized UCD. The hospital ends up with its own programmers and engineers and specialists, whole teams devoted to installing and maintaining the system. That is taken for granted in digital healthcare. It helps to call it by its name: **externalization**.
>
> Yet if you bought an ambulance, you'd expect all the development work to have been done before it was delivered. This certainly makes the ambulance a bit more expensive than it might have been (because development had not been externalized), but the ambulance works properly on the day it is delivered. The entire engineering project was done and completed by the manufacturers. In particular, safety and usability were not externalized.
>
> The topic of this chapter, UCD, is essential, but that does not mean *you*, the customer, has to do it. It should be done by the developers.

Without UCD — going and finding out what users actually do and want — this sort of problem is invisible. In the specific example here, if the patient comes to harm, the nurse will be blamed, yet the nurse was trying to do their job and the design of the system made it too hard to do it the official way.

———————◼———————

Henry Ford didn't invent factory assembly lines, nor did he invent cars, but he did build cars very efficiently: the Ford Model T was the result. He made the Model T — and sold it — in such huge numbers that its place in history was assured. Henry Ford is often quoted as saying that if he'd asked people what they wanted, they'd have said that they wanted faster horses.

It's a shame that Ford never said that,[332] but the pithy saying highlights dangers of UCD: if you ask clinicians or patients what they want, they probably don't want what will be best for them. Instead, we have to find out what people are actually doing (WAD), which probably isn't what they think they are doing or even what we thought they were doing (WAI).

This chapter's brief introduction to UCD hasn't covered everything. The next chapter is a short personal story to illustrate some of the points and the importance of iterating UCD to keep on improving. The Good reading chapter provides more on the wider subjects of UCD, UX, and HCI.[d]

---

[d] See Chapter 33: User Centered Design reading recommendations, page 482 →

User Centered Design means finding out how systems are used with their real users doing real tasks. The insights from working with users leads to design insights and ways to improve the systems. These ideas are formalized in the important idea of **iterative design**.

23

Iterative Design

I was posted a paper letter from my hospital with details of my next hospital appointment. I duly turned up at the Morriston Hospital a little before my appointed time.

On entering the main foyer of the hospital, I was asked to check in using the self check-in kiosks. There are volunteers on hand to help do this. The kiosks scan your appointment letter or the helpers can manually take your details. I had a letter, and scanning it was easy.

The kiosks then tell you to sit down and wait.

There are two sorts of computer screens in the waiting area; one for blood tests and one for everything else. The screens bing every time a name comes up, and when yours does you're supposed to follow the instructions on it. You then walk to the specified waiting area, tell another kiosk you've arrived (why?), and wait again for your name to come up on one of the screens there. When your name comes up, you are told which room to go to for your appointment. (The Morriston Hospital has around 100 appointment rooms in this part of it.)

This all sounds perfectly reasonable, and is no doubt much more efficient than the previous, pre-digital system, which might have involved a lot of staff time to manage different patients. I can imagine the new digital system being demonstrated: and it would all have seemed to work well.

Now look at it from my point of view. I don't think I'm a very unusual patient; thought I was stressed being in hospital as a patient for the first time.

While I sat and waited, I worried whether the system had actually registered me and put me on the waiting list.

There is no feedback that you are going to be seen at all until your name bings up — which might be thirty or more minutes of not knowing later. Maybe my name had already popped up and I'd missed it? I don't know how long I am going to have to wait, and the longer I wait, the more I think it's likely I've missed my name binging earlier.

Fix It: See and solve the problems of digital healthcare. Harold Thimbleby, Oxford University Press. © Harold Thimbleby 2021.
DOI: 10.1093/oso/9780198861270.003.0023

Box 23.1. How do you know when nothing happens?

I've been back to the hospital for several appointments. As an "experienced" patient, I've learned what to do, so I confidently walked up to one of the check-in kiosks.

On the front of the kiosk is a slot with large, apparently helpful, instructions:

→▊▊▊▊▊▊←

SCAN HERE

I popped my appointment letter in the slot for the computer to read the barcode at the top.

But nothing happened!

You need to first press lots of buttons on the kiosk to help it realize you are there and let it know what sort of appointment you are going to.

Why doesn't the barcode reader — which clearly knows when there is a barcode there to read — do something useful and help the patient?

Here's the UCD (User Centered Design) moral: when nothing happens, the computer won't know, and nobody is going to find out there is a usability problem just by looking at computer logs and what the computer knows. You have to go and see.

If a healthcare UCD case study isn't quite persuasive enough for you, here's a famous story: UCD identified a previously unnoticed problem that was losing a company $300 million a year. UCD made a surprising and enormous return on the trivial investment in doing it.[333]

There are lots of people here who got here before me. My anxiety rises.

Every time somethings bings, you have to look to see if your name is up there on one of the screens. I daren't read my book in case I miss my name.

Then I noticed there are two sorts of screens, and, clearly, my name might come up on the other sort — one I haven't been looking at. I got up and walked over to look more closely at one of the other screens to see if my name was there. Then I noticed the waiting area has *five* screens. Which is my name going to be on? I've no idea. Has my name already appeared on another screen and now disappeared? I've no idea.

Finally, my name did pop up on a screen I was watching, and I was told to go to another waiting area, Waiting Area 2. Where's Waiting Area 2? I got up and started to look around. It turns out they put small signposts up to help you on columns, but the signposts are at head-height. So you can't see them if anybody is standing in front of a column.

I then discovered I needed to check in again! I don't know why, though, worryingly, maybe I have missed my appointment, and I need to start again?

In hindsight — now I've been through the process successfully — I now know they have two checkins for everyone: the first one means you register to wait near the entrance to the hospital, and the second one is for checking in to a more specialized part of the hospital you've been sent to.

I sat down and waited in the new area.

There are 7 screens in this new room (it's a big room), and I walked around to see whether the screens were all the same, or different from each other, as they had been in Waiting Area 1. One was certainly different, and seemed to be only for patients having their plaster casts checked. It was a good job I hadn't sat down to wait there, as plaster wasn't my problem — but I did notice none of the other screens had told any plaster patients they would be watching the wrong screens.

I started looking around. Around the edge of this big waiting room I could see numbered doors, and, as the doors have windows, I could see that behind each door there are numbered rooms. I think it'd be clearer if the doors were called, say, A, B, C, so there is no confusion with the waiting room's own number or the numbered rooms beyond — it'd be tempting to run to Door 2 when my name comes up because I've already been told to go to Waiting Area 2, and maybe I'll go to the wrong room once I'm through the door. I think designing the system so it says "Please go through Door B to Room 5" would be less likely to get patients confused.

As always, UCD is needed. To anyone — you, for instance — sitting comfortably reading this book, saying "Go to Door 1, Room 3" seems perfectly clear. To the developers building the system, too, it would very likely have seemed perfectly clear too. But what happens with real patients, feeling stressed with lots to worry about, and in a noisy environment? Or people like me on their first ever visit to this part of the hospital, where everything is strange? Probably, the information has to be repeated at least twice, maybe more times, for real patients.

Anyway, after about half an hour in this waiting area, a screen bings. I look up, and, yes, my name is there. But everything vanished before I'd finished reading all the details — I think it said something about going to door something, room something. What? What? What do I do now?

I waited for my name to come up again, but it didn't.

I found a volunteer to ask what to do, and they walked off — I hope to help me! A few minutes later they came back and told me that my appointment has been taken by somebody else, presumably a pro patient. I'm told I'll have to wait again for another appointment.

Does that mean I need another appointment altogether, or do I just wait in the waiting area, or do I have to go back to first waiting area? Do I have to check in again? How long have I got to wait? Will I be next — so it'll be half an hour or so — or will I be put back to the end of the queue? The TV screens now say my consultant is running 45 minutes late, so what does that mean for me?

The old paper-based system gave patients a numbered slip of paper, and all the patient had to do was wait until a big number display counted down to their appointment number on their slip of paper. Crucially, this very simple system gave the patient two reassuring details the new Electronic Patient Flow Solution does not. The slip of paper was a tangible reminder that the system "knew about you," and the number display gave you a clear sense of progress. The number increased by one for each patient as they were seen, and you could see how the display was getting closer and closer to your number. When it got close to your number, you started to get ready to jump up. If you missed your slot, that was obvious too, as the displayed number would be larger than the number on your slip of paper — then you could go and try to sort it out.

With the old system, if a patient found it hard to understand, there were lots of other patients happy to help. The new computer system is much more complex and introduces interesting new problems: it knows people's names, so if you try and help somebody, you start intruding on their privacy. With the old paper system, the only thing you needed to know to help someone was their number. Everything else stayed private, so it was easy to help.

There were no surprises in the old system, and many reassurances to the patient that they were "in" the system. Like, you've got that bit of paper.

Clearly, the new Electronic Patient Flow Solution could be further developed to improve the patient experience and recover some of the safety features of the old system. Some patients already come with their own mobile phones, and they could easily start simulating the old paper system to restore the sense of progress. That would improve the system for some patients, and give the volunteers more time to help the patients with more serious problems.

Although describing my story sounds complicated, the story is a nice example of the tensions of digital system development from several different perspectives ...

The hospital staff now have less work to do, so that's good. The developers have made a high-tech digital system that obviously works, so that's good. Thirdly, the developers probably never seriously studied how patients use the system, for there are simple changes that would make the experience so much nicer. Or possibly, the advantages to the hospital make it seem obvious that the system is better, so why try to improve it?

In many hospitals, a digital system like this will be procured and installed by a manager. Does the manager really understand what staff and patients do? Have they bought a system that seems fantastic, but isn't quite aligned to what really goes on? Indeed, any new system like this hospital's self check-in kiosks will *change* how everyone behaves. So you can guarantee nobody really knows how this or any new system *will* be used. More to the point, even if anyone knows what patients do, they, too, will probably do something else after a new system is installed.

The developers have problems too. If they did do user studies, which is best practice, the users they are most likely to recruit into their studies would

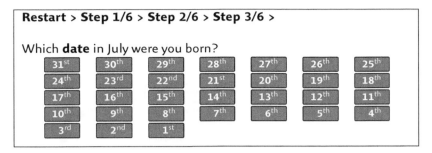

Restart > Step 1/6 > Step 2/6 > Step 3/6 >

Which **date** in July were you born?

31st	30th	29th	28th	27th	26th	25th
24th	23rd	22nd	21st	20th	19th	18th
17th	16th	15th	14th	13th	12th	11th
10th	9th	8th	7th	6th	5th	4th
3rd	2nd	1st				

Figure 23.1. The touch screen to choose your birth date when registering as a patient. Curiously, the dates are listed in reverse order, as shown in this schematic. This design choice is likely to increase errors. To recover from any errors, the user will need to press the not-very-clearly-named **Step 4/6** on the *next* screen correctly, because (although it doesn't say it), this screen is the fourth out of a series of six screens they have to deal with.

be frequent or regular patients — therefore they'll tend to be patients who are familiar with how the hospital works and where the waiting areas are, and so on. These patients are unlikely to be as stressed as I was on my first few experiences.

For obvious reasons, developers probably never or rarely recruit patients with mobility problems, with cognitive problems, with hearing problems (who can't hear the bings), or with sight problems (who can't read the screens). What about parents with children, whose lives are even more complex than mine?

Inevitably, the first system that is built is built largely on hope and fantasy, so it's important to evaluate it and find out how it works. Even if it works well, it will change how people work, so once it is in use, it may no longer be the ideal solution it was promised as. It is important, then, to have continual **iterative design**: after a system or device is installed and "working," there should be regular assessment of how it is working and how to improve it. For example, volunteer users can be interviewed every week, and then they can move on to using something like a suggestion box once they are trained to report their insights about how the system is working — or issues that are arising.

For example, when your birth date is entered, to help confirm who you are in the Morriston Hospital waiting room, the "calendar" of dates is, curiously, backwards, and upside down (figure 23.1). Why not put it the right way up to make it conventional and easier to understand? Or was it done this way to make patients more careful?

And, finally, what is the objective improvement?

The old system with its slips of paper was simple, easy to understand, cheap, and reliable. The new system is much more complex, slightly or a lot

Part II ◇ Treatment ◇ Finding solutions

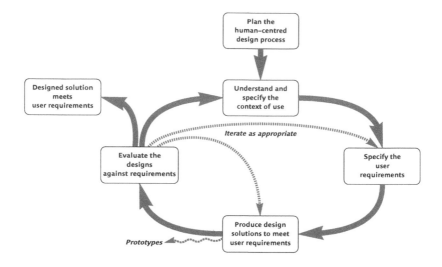

Figure 23.2. The recommended ISO 9241-210 design cycle. The oversight of the 9241 process is that "evaluate the design requirements" emphasizes empirical UCD methods, glossing Formal Methods and other software engineering methods (version control, etc) that should also be used to rigorously prove requirements are met *and stay met* as the design is iterated.

more efficient (I don't know), but it is certainly much more expensive than paper — and it's subject to cyberattacks and the costs of keeping obsolete technology working.

Reality is a lot more complicated, and if they go about installing it the wrong way, once patients start experiencing problems it will be too late — certainly expensive — to do much to improve it. It should have been designed so that it could be improved, so that there were ways for the system developers to learn, to get feedback, and to try improvements. Indeed, there's an international standard explaining how to do this (ISO standard 9241, especially part 9241-210) and if that standard hasn't been followed, then the system is, literally, sub-standard.

User Centered Design is the main way to help.

Last time I had an appointment at the Morriston Hospital, I bumped into my friend Mandy in Waiting Area 2. We had a bit of a chat. She'd been waiting a while. I asked if she'd checked in *again*. No, she didn't know she had to. So, she checked in again, and she was immediately called off to her appointment.

She could have been sitting there for hours longer if we hadn't met and chatted.

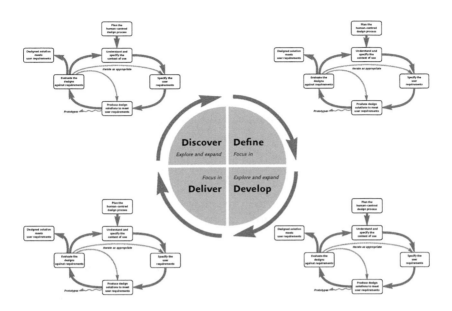

Figure 23.3. The recommended ISO 9241-210 design cycle (figure 23.2) should not be done on only a single product concept, and certainly not by doing only one cycle. A more mature process is to start with an open discovery process, developing personas, scenarios, and sketching[323] — typically involving product concepts in paper or wood — leading to a **minimal viable product** (MVPs, or the first nearly working design), then refining that to a defined product, which is then developed and delivered, through many ISO 9241 cycles until you *have evidence* that the delivered product is acceptable. The central organizing cycle in this figure is inspired by the UK Design Council's "double diamond" high-level approach to design.[334]

It's interesting to note that finding out Mandy had similar problems to me increases my sample of data from one user (me) to two (us). It's reassuring to know that I am not a totally idiosyncratic user![335] More data turns personal stories into systematic evidence.

Why don't some designers come round and interview patients and find out how their systems don't work for patients like Mandy?

A very simple thing to do (without fixing the rest of the weird system) would be for the many displays in Waiting Area 2 to remind people to check in again. In fact, in principle, the computer system knows who is there who hasn't checked in again, so why doesn't it say things like "beep beep Harold Thimbleby we know you haven't checked in again, please do so at the check in kiosks outside Waiting Area 2. We know you can't see them, but we're sure you can find them somehow."

I'm not joking.

Spelling out exactly what a helpful system ought to say would help the designers work out how to make a more helpful system.

There's one more point to make: it's a really good job that Mandy can hear the beeps, can see and can read the displays, and she can walk perfectly well! In other words, if you are going to do UCD, you do UCD for a representative sample of users, not just the unstressed and able-bodied — especially in healthcare, where, by definition, nobody is totally able-bodied.

My dentist works for a company that has just bought Clinipad[336] to replace paperwork. My experience, as a patient, is that the simple paper form I used to sign has been turned into an iPad nightmare. There are now two forms. Neither of the forms are fully visible without scrolling; some parts of the form are pre-filled; some parts you have to bring up a keyboard to edit; some parts you just scribble in using a special pen. It is very inconsistent and awkward.

It took me, with the receptionist helping, fifteen minutes to fill the electronic forms in, using two iPads and, for some reason, having to go back and forth between the two. I don't know how long people who aren't professors of Computer Science and totally familiar with iPads would take. I wonder how many new errors get through? For instance, I never saw any data confidentiality declarations, which are required by law. Somehow, Clinipad has turned a digital opportunity into something that is much worse than the original paper, and, at least for the patient, provides no benefits — like reminding you your medication list might need updating.[337]

Then when I got to see the dentist, her computer screen was wrong because the iPad's links hadn't updated properly. The dentist then spent a few minutes talking about resigning because of the new digital pressures and problems. But the paperwork has been automated, so the business managers will be happy — they don't see the struggles undermining the user experience.

It's not hard to think of lots of improvements to this system, just from my one-off experience, but it'd be much more useful to get some representative data. (Perhaps I am an unusual patient; perhaps my dental practice has pre-existing morale problems — who knows?) It wouldn't be difficult to get permission to sit in on a few dental surgeries, and find out what is really going on on the ground. Of course, this would need to be a long-term study, to balance out effects like initial excitement masking problems, or receptionists being able to use a system well immediately after training but, maybe, not six months later.

I was once working on the iterative design of a new system to be used in doctors' surgeries. We wanted to cover a range of conditions, one of which was dementia.

Unfortunately, you can't easily do UCD work with patients with dementia (or lots of other conditions, for that matter), so we used **patient actors**. The patient actor "with" dementia got lost coming to our session. This brilliant acting was very valuable in designing so our system could work well-enough to be trialled in a *real* doctor's surgery. Iterative design would then continue from a good starting point.

How do you brief patient actors? We spent weeks developing a representative collection of characters for the actors to play. We worked with doctors and real patients to make our characters cover the critical issues in as balanced a way as possible, as well as giving the actors a good background story for each of their roles. These briefs are called **personas**. We checked out our personas with consultants to make sure our descriptions were clinically correct. The right level of clinical detail depends on your project.

Personas can be used throughout design and development. The personas can be printed onto posters and put up in the developers' offices. The idea is that the personas have names, and the developers get to know them as real people. How would Donna use the system? Would Donna have the patience to do that? And so on.

Our persona for Donna is at the end of this chapter. Note that the persona doesn't say it's a persona: we treat Donna exactly as we would a real person.

Do be inspired by the headlines in the persona, and don't copy my Donna persona — it's to inspire you to think about *your* users. Doing the work yourself of developing personas is a very important part of the process, and helps the development team learn a lot about the users and their needs. As you do it, you talk to representative users and get all sorts of insights.

———————————◼———————————

Human Factors[a] tells us that other people are different, and they are different in different ways. It follows that when digital healthcare systems are designed, we have to test them out on real users doing realistic work — otherwise we have no idea what little we really know about the users' real work as done (WAD).

It's very hard to see problems in design, because when we design we know too much; we have privileged inside information about our systems that no user is party to. We don't know the half of the complexity of the users' work. We find our designs natural and easy, and we don't anticipate the errors users will make with them. The work as imagined (WAI) concept captures this: unless we try really hard, we live in a world that unintentionally just imagines what users do, and this is never what they really do, the WAD. Unless we do UCD, we have no idea. As soon as we start doing UCD, we see it is a process: we get evidence that we have to improve our designs to make them safer, more effective, more pleasurable to use. In turn, those improved designs raise new unknown problems that we have to go and seek out. We

---

[a] See Chapter 20: Human Factors, page 259 ←

need iterative design, and we carry on iterating until the design performs well for its intended purpose.

For conventional products, like cars and planes, iterative design comes to a point of diminishing returns, and a polished product is put on the market. Digital products, however, can always be improved even after they have been "finished" — just by downloading a software upgrade. It follows that digital products should be designed so that iterative design can continue, for instance through an ongoing process of collecting data about how they are used. For medical devices, it is, in most countries, a regulatory requirement to monitor patient safety by doing post-market surveillance, but iterative design says we can go much further.

We already expect continual digital upgrades as the manufacturers fix bugs and think of new features. So manufacturers are already half way there. Iterative design says, more strongly, that you should upgrade *for the users and their tasks*, not for the uninformed imaginary excitement of new features.

People choosing new digital systems to use need to be aware at least of the issues in this and the previous chapter. If you don't know about the essential role of iterative design (quote ISO 9241 to your suppliers), you will buy a *product*. Instead, you need to buy a *relationship* with the manufacturer, a relationship of continual support and improvement.

Box 23.2. Donna Meyer's persona

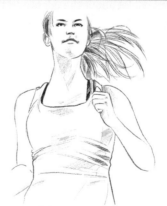

Donna Meyer, age 31

Donna's key phrase: **"I'm responsible!"**

Quick take
Conditions: Recovering from a leg injury. • Key technology: Very into technology; Fully geared for active lifestyle; Good at using social networks as fo-

rum to share fitness tips. • Housing: 2-bed apartment. • Situation: Spouse Frank Meyer, 32; Parents living 1.5 hours' drive away; No children; One 3-year-old golden retriever (Frank's dog). • Background: Associate technical manager in an international co-operation; Graduated in Electronic Engineering; Regular runner, has run 4 marathons; Food fads & Weight Watcher. • Changes: Recently broken leg in a rather serious incident; Just been promoted; Busy preparing to buy a house.

Donna's background unfolds

Donna has been married to Frank for 2 years. They are considering buying a house, and having a baby. Donna has just been promoted, and the new post requires a large amount of traveling around the globe.

Frank is also a very enthusiastic runner. The couple uses the same GPS apps and occasionally they enjoy a running match.

They have a dog, a very energetic dog, which enjoys being loved and stroked as much as it enjoys its toys and its daily walk. So that keeps Donna busy outdoors.

Donna's key goals

Donna has always been very good at multi-tasking and managing her own life. She looks forward to her new responsibility at work as well as getting herself physically prepared for being pregnant.

Though there is a lot on her plate, Donna believes she can manage this. However, her broken leg has been a problem: she's been in and out of the operation room a number of times, before finally — she hopes — being discharged a week ago. Donna is determined to have a fast recovery, and get back on track with her life.

Key symptoms

Her leg was broken. One of her wounds was infected, which has left a scar. She uses moisturizers a lot to ease the dryness and itchiness. She's still using a crutch, but has started to manage without it recently.

A day in the life of Donna

Donna gets up at 7am to allow herself enough time to have a healthy breakfast before Frank drives her to work. Sometimes she goes swimming in the morning for 40 minutes to an hour, as it's good for her recovery. She's very busy during the day, and sometimes has to work overtime.

She uses her iPhone app combined with other accessories to track her activities. She uses online forums at weekends.

Influences

Donna is very self-driven. She studies various rehabilitation treatments, and consults with her friends and clinicians on a regular basis. She's also taking extra care to comply with the prescriptions she's on.

Donna is different

Donna has a lot on her plate.

She's keen on getting back on track with her life.

Donna has discovered the advantage of using devices to manage not just her condition but her lifestyle in general. She's thinking she will continue using them after she recovers.

Developers and programmers need no qualifications to develop digital healthcare systems. We need to develop a qualification structure for digital healthcare, and do much more research on digital safety. Both will have a huge impact on frontline safety.

24

Wedge Thinking

My friend Dave Williams was flying back to the UK on an international flight from the US. There was an urgent call for a doctor on the plane to help a passenger. As he is a UK consultant anæsthetist, he immediately responded, but the US air hostess, misunderstanding the UK term, refused his offer of help, as she wanted a "proper" doctor.

In the UK, Australia, New Zealand, and South Africa, an **anæsthetist** is a specialist doctor with significant training in anesthetics and patient care. In the US, the **anesthesiologist** is similar to the UK anæsthetist, a doctor who specializes in anesthesiology and is qualified to make all anesthesia-related decisions, but an **anesthetist** is a non-physician who provides care before and after anesthetic procedures.

The hostess instead chose a medical student who'd also volunteered to help. The student would've had negligible training and experience compared to Dave's.

This is a small example of the problems of **internationalization** (that is, words and concepts varying across countries and cultures), and its potentially harmful and fatal consequences.

The relevance of internationalization to digital healthcare is discussed in box 25.1, but the point of this story is that even an air hostess recognized that a doctor needs proper qualifications to provide reliable care, even though, in this case, she didn't realize there are differences between the US and UK.

If something goes wrong when an anesthesiologist is looking after a patient on a plane, or more usually during surgery in a hospital, they have minutes, perhaps only seconds, to do the right thing. They work in a very pressurized environment.

If you want to be an anæsthetist in the UK, you must first be accepted to train as a doctor. It then takes a minimum of *fourteen* years in the UK before you'll complete your training (figure 24.1). Furthermore, you have to undertake regular updates and training to stay certified to continue working as an

Fix It: See and solve the problems of digital healthcare. Harold Thimbleby, Oxford University Press. © Harold Thimbleby 2021.
DOI: 10.1093/oso/9780198861270.003.0024

Airway management; Anesthesia for neurosurgery; Anatomy; Basic sciences to underpin anesthetic practice; Cardiothoracic anesthesia and cardiothoracic critical care; Core anesthesia; Critical incidents; Day surgery; ENT, maxillo-facial and dental surgery; General duties; General, urological, and gynecological surgery; Induction of general anesthesia; Infection control; Intensive care medicine; Intraoperative care; Management of cardiac arrest in adults and children; Management of respiratory and cardiac arrest; Neuroradiology and neurocritical care; Non-operating room obstetrics; Non-operating room orthopedic surgery; Obstetrics; Orthopedic perioperative medicine; Orthopedic surgery; Pediatrics, including child protection; Pain medicine; Perioperative management of emergency patients; Perioperative medicine; Pharmacology; Physics and clinical measurement; Physiology and biochemistry; Postoperative and recovery room care; Premedication; Preoperative assessment; Regional sedation; Statistical methods; Transfer medicine; Trauma and stabilization; Vascular surgery.

Figure 24.1. A selection of the many essential topics a UK anæsthetist must be examined on and pass to qualify so that they can use anesthetic machines built by unqualified developers — compare with figure 24.2.

anæsthetist. If anything goes wrong for an anæsthetist (or anesthesiologist), they might harm or perhaps kill one or two patients.

In complete contrast, if you want to build or program a device that delivers drugs into a patient, you can start making and programming an infusion pump or any other machine *immediately*. No qualifications whatsoever are needed (figure 24.2), whether you are a programmer or other engineer, and there are no requirements to undertake professional development, and no requirements to be certified in any way. You can program badly and have no risk of disqualification.

It's worth pointing out that while programmers may make mistakes, they do have lots of time, like months, to detect and correct bugs before their products are sold and used. In contrast, doctors and nurses need to get things right or sort out critical problems, often under urgent time pressures — so they have to be better trained and have to be more skilled.

If a device sells well, bugs in it have the potential to cause widespread harm. It could affect thousands or even millions of people. This is a huge contrast to the limited harms that anesthesiologists and other medical professionals can achieve, even over the course of their entire careers.

Modern digital devices are potentially far more complex and have far more scope for harming patients than the trivial Graseby MS 26 and MS 16As that were at the center of the Gosport tragedy.[a] The Graseby devices were

---

[a] See Chapter 8: Gosport War Memorial Hospital tragedy, page 84 ←

Figure 24.2. All of the topics a programmer must be examined on and must pass to qualify so that they can design and program healthcare systems, such as anesthetic machines — compare with figure 24.1.

so simple they weren't even connected to the internet, but then think of the scale of what Robin Seggelmann's Heartbleed bug did to more modern digital systems — it affected 4.5 million patient records.[b] Probably the true scale of the Heartbleed problem was much worse than this, as many hospitals wouldn't want to admit to the problems it caused, even if they noticed them. How many anesthesiologists can impact 4.5 million patients?

In almost all areas that society recognizes as being risky, you legally must have proper training and qualifications. You must have accreditation to certify that you've been trained to an appropriate professional standard.

Take installing gas boilers, like in your home. To install a boiler in the UK, you are *legally* required to be on the Gas Safe Register, and specifically approved for working on boilers. As a registered gas engineer, you are issued a card with your photograph, your registration number, and an expiry date and details of the different categories of work that you are qualified to undertake, like working on cookers, boilers, or gas fires. Furthermore, carrying out work without a current registration is illegal; doing so can result in fines and a prison sentence.[213]

None of this regulation is surprising; after all, people's lives depend on gas boilers not exploding or killing people with carbon monoxide.

In contrast, it seems strange to me that to build a digital device that injects potentially lethal drugs or delivers radiotherapy, you need no qualifica-

---

[b] See Chapter 27: Heartbleed bug, page 369 →

tions whatsoever. There is no requirement for you to stay up-to-date in your field. You don't need a photo card specifying your competencies. Yet digital health is a far more complex job, with more opportunities for life-threatening consequences than installing a pre-made gas boiler. There's also a lot more innovation in digital health, making it hard for programmers to keep up.

In healthcare you wouldn't trust a doctor or nurse who wasn't certified, so why would you trust an uncertified programmer? Indeed, the qualifications doctors and nurses have include legal issues like respecting patient confidentiality; you wouldn't trust a doctor who did not keep your information confidential — but no programmer or digital device manufacturer is required to respect confidentiality so rigorously. As Jesse Ehrenfeld, chair of the American Medical Association Board of Trustees put it,

> Physicians swear an oath to keep an individual's data confidential, [but] there's currently no such obligation for technology companies and data aggregators or the data brokers to whom they might sell information.[231]

Clearly, digital healthcare needs proper qualifications, accreditation, and regulations for all developers of digital healthcare systems and apps. There should be a legal requirement that digital healthcare programming must be done by appropriately certified professional programmers *and nobody else.* Some people won't like me saying this, but that also means that doctors should not program their own apps, and administrators and clinical technicians should not program spreadsheets. Potential fines and prison sentences would also motivate, and reduce cowboy work, and cybersecurity leaks. Ultimately, proper regulation would reduce patient harms.

There are sensible ways to transition to this ideal. For example, in the UK, years ago anyone used to be able to wire up their own house. Since electrical wiring shares many properties of digital healthcare — it may look like it works, it may be usable and pass tests that it works, but it may still pose very serious risks[338] — it is now legally regulated. However, as an unqualified electrician, I can still do my own wiring, but I am legally required to have the quality of my wiring certified by a registered person. When I sell my house, I also have to have appropriate safety certificates signed off by a certified electrician.

Not just qualifications and certificates, though — we also need a culture of **professionalism**. In other areas, a professional engineer is not just qualified and certified, but follows a regulated code of practice and has professional indemnity insurance. There is no need for a professional to have warranties, like we've discussed,[c] that deny all liability. Sorting out the qualifications digital health programmers need is not so hard — the Good reading[d] chapter provides a basis for a syllabus for developers.

---

[c] See Chapter 15: Who's accountable?, page 193 ←

[d] See Chapter 33: Good reading, page 471 →

> **Box 24.1.** Parallels with the German Enigma
>
> The World War II German Enigma secret code machine predates modern computer programming, but its design shows all the Human Factors failings in programming that we are familiar with in digital healthcare. Despite the overwhelming need to win the war, preventable design mistakes were made and perpetuated in the Enigma which significantly contributed to the Axis failure. Indeed, the very need to win a war created the tunnel vision that meant the Enigma designers overlooked many ways of making it more reliable to use. In turn, the design failings put pressure on its operators — often working under fire — exacerbating the chaos. In other words, the poor design at the blunt end created problems for users at the sharp-end.
>
> I did some research on the Enigma, and I showed it was an unnecessarily flawed machine.[339]
>
> Enigma operators were often executed as scapegoats when messages went wrong. In an environment like that, it'd be wise to keep quiet and just go along with pretending everything was OK! The stakes were higher, but the Human Factors problems, and the reasons they occurred, were the same as in modern healthcare.
>
> The designers having tunnel vision is one reason why digital systems have bugs and design problems. It's so hard programming that developers aren't able to pay enough attention to all the many critical details and complexities of healthcare, which then come back to haunt the users. Worse, because designers are deeply involved in their systems and know them thoroughly, they can easily kid themselves their designs are much easier to understand than they actually are. They know some of the "secret" tricks but don't even realize they are secret.[340] The only way out of these problems is to use UCD.[a]
>
> ─────────────
> [a] See Chapter 22: User Centered Design, page 301 ←

Part II ◇ Treatment ◇ Finding solutions

Doctors and nurses work at the **sharp-end**, where things happen quickly. We tend to focus on the sharp-end, as it's where harm is seen to happen. The **Wedge Model** (which I invented) emphasizes that the sharp-end is only part of a larger whole, and it should not be looked at in isolation.

There are all sorts of wedges. I imagine the sort of strong steel wedge used for hammering into logs to split them up for firewood. You push the sharp-end of the wedge into a block of wood and hit it hard with a sledgehammer, and the sharp-end is thwacked into the wood, splitting it apart. This familiar sort of wedge reminds us that the sharp-end of a wedge is useless without the thick end; without the thick end, you can't do much with the thin end.

Nurses work at the sharp-end, whereas developers and manufacturers work at the **blunt end**. Note that in the analogy, the thickness of the steel represents how much time is available at each end to do the job.

Because we tend to focus on what doctors and nurses do — it's usually they who end up in the news when things go wrong — we tend to think about and seek solutions at the sharp-end.

It is critical that people doing safety-critical work know Human Factors. The nurses might have had more confidence to speak up in the operating room when they were worried, and the surgeons would have welcomed their intervention rather than seeing it as criticism.

Yet there's another side to the story. The sharp-end of the wedge is used for splitting the log, and you hit the blunt end with a sledgehammer.

Could the manufacturers of tracheal tubes (the pipes that go down your throat and windpipe) put them in sterilized bags with "SPEAK UP IF WORRIED" labels on them? What could have been Human Factors training (perhaps last year and now forgotten) would now be prominently built into the system: it would give people permission to say something *and* it reminds other people not to be surprised or cross when somebody points out a problem.

Peter Pronovost, who was until recently an intensive care specialist physician at Johns Hopkins Hospital in Baltimore, tried an idea like this.[341] Very sick patients often need lots of drugs, so they need lots of intravenous injections and infusions. Inserting needles into people repeatedly has its risks, so these patients have a central line, a gadget that allows tubes to be connected and disconnected repeatedly without making more holes (inserting cannulas) in the patient's skin. Central lines also allow drugs to be easily put directly into a patient's heart, which can save seconds in an emergency.

Central lines are a good idea, but eventually they get dirty and harbor bacteria, then there will be a risk of an infection going straight into the patient down the central line. Obviously, therefore, central lines should be replaced every month or so with new, sterile ones. The trouble is that people forget to do this. Every year in the US, 80,000 patients get infected and about 30,000–60,000 die; that equates to about 16,000 infected and 6,000–12,000 dying in the UK (if we just assume the numbers are proportional to the populations of the countries — the health systems are pretty similar).

I am always astonished at how cavalier healthcare is about knowing what causes disease and death. What other industry would accept an *estimate* of fatalities somewhere between 30,000 and 60,000 from a common cause? If we faced the embarrassment of this avoidable death rate, we'd take central lines more seriously. Which is exactly what Peter Pronovost did.

Peter's solution was to develop a checklist of what needed to be done and when. He ensured patients had labels on their central lines, like "Replace before 1 July 2018."

Anybody who sees that label after June will ask why the central line has not been replaced. They might be nurses. They might be relatives. Blunt end thinking has sorted out a sharp-end problem. Peter Pronovost managed to get central line infections down to zero at Johns Hopkins Hospital. The checklist simply — but very effectively — turns the invisible and easy to overlook into something everyone can see and that is hard to miss.

Peter's book *Safe Patients, Smart Hospitals*, which I recommend reading (see the recommended reading list at the end of this book),[e] asks this question,

> ... an estimated 750,000 people [perhaps 150,000 in the UK] each year suffer a cardiac arrest in the hospital. Cardiac arrest is almost always treated with a defibrillator. Yet roughly 30% of the time, physicians operate these machines incorrectly. So why not redesign them so they are easier to use, or print clear instructions on the machine?

This is great blunt end thinking — improving the system improves the sharp-end for free. All we need to do is put the thinking into action. I'd add that if instructions aren't clear, then you must redesign the system so the thing is easier to explain clearly.[342]

The blunt end and sharp-end are metaphors, but we can use the wedge to visualize time and show all of the stages at once to make the stages of design and use clearer (figure 24.3).

When people save time, effort, and money at the blunt end, they cause preventable problems for people using their products at the sharp-end. Essentially, the money developers save loses money for the users at the sharp-end. A useful way to remember this is the term **technical debt**[343] — the developers are borrowing from users, and becoming indebted to them. When the cost of error at the sharp-end is so high, death and harm for patients and imprisonment, depression and suicide for clinicians, we really do not want technical debt.

It isn't really the developers' fault. Unlike the lawyers writing warranties who clearly don't want to be responsible, I believe that developers sink into "not thinking" by accident. They have a complex enough job just getting the stuff to work, let alone thinking of all the ways users may have trouble with it.

Student programmers on degree courses are usually taught about the *user's* Human Factors issues, in courses called User Centered Design (UCD) or Human Computer Interaction (HCI),[344] but they are very rarely taught about Human Factors as it applies to them and the programming process itself. Programming is really difficult, and it's hard to program and to keep track of all the details of the user's needs. When the user's needs are clinical, it's likely the programmer doesn't even understand the details anyway. The programmer suffers from task saturation and loss of situational awareness — having too much to do — and they rightly focus on getting their program

[e] See Chapter 33: Good reading, page 471 →

Part II ◇ Treatment ◇ Finding solutions

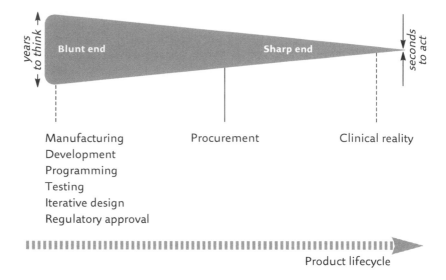

Figure 24.3. The wedge's blunt end and sharp-end show when activities happen and how long they typically take. The height of the wedge at each point schematically indicates the time available for each task. At the blunt end, designers have years; at the sharp-end, clinicians have maybe minutes or seconds.

to work, but they then inevitably start to lose sight of other issues, such as correctness, safety, and error handling.

These programmer Human Factors problems are almost exactly the same Human Factors problems as clinicians face at the sharp-end: task saturation, and loss of situational awareness.

An unfortunate consequence of being at the blunt end is that many errors are never noticed, so design errors get missed. At the sharp-end, things may deteriorate, and usually it is very soon obvious when something bad has happened. At the blunt end, the errors may have no consequences for years — and by then the programmers have moved on to other projects. So nobody is really aware of error when developing systems. Developers can live in the false bubble of thinking that "errors don't happen here."

The main solution at the blunt end is the same as at the sharp-end: effective teamwork. By working in a team, others can help spot oversights and errors. Other people should go over your code and query why you are (and aren't) doing things using code review.[f] Another pair of eyes spots errors you overlooked.

Pair programming is a very effective form of code review: two (or more) programmers work together, one using the computer, and the other

---

[f] See Chapter 20: Code review, page 273 ←

asking questions, critiquing the programming, and making suggestions — it's been likened to a pilot and navigator working together. By focusing on different aspects of the task, they free up their minds to be more effective. The Computer Factors chapter has many more ideas like this.[g]

Almost the opposite of pair programming in **N version programming** (NVP). Here, independent programmers build *different* programs from the same specification: these are the *N* versions. All the *N* versions are then run with the same test suite, and if they don't get the same results, then some of them must have bugs that need fixing.[345] NVP isn't perfect, as it's sometimes difficult to compare the results of *N* programs (if so, then the specification of what the programs are supposed to do needs improving), and programmers tend to make the same mistakes — but *N* programming will pick up lots of accidental mistakes, as they tend to be random. As always, reliance on one method is not sufficient, but the more methods that are used to improve the quality of programs the better.

Once you realize your own programmers are a risk — as they are — then there are lots of obvious ideas to manage this risk. Manufacturers could send their programmers off to universities to update their knowledge. External experts could come in and do reviews.

An interesting and very important teamwork idea is that the team need not all be in the room with you. There are international standards, for instance, developed by expert teams somewhere else. Their standards can help you think more clearly, and most have checklists and bibliographies of important things to consider. They are like somebody watching what you are doing, asking whether you have done the iterative design (or whatever). Even better, if you follow the standards, you can write it down in your promotional material: "Our products conform to international standards, ISO 14971, ISO 62366, ISO 9241, ..." They'll sell better.

- 🌓 This book isn't really the place to explain International Organization for Standardization (ISO) standards and all the others (IEC, ANSI, ...) — but they aren't all the very dull documents you might expect them to be. Most of them, especially ISO 9241-210, have lots of useful background information in them in addition to the raw standard.

- 🌓 If you buy stuff (say, in hospital procurement), then you *should* pay attention to standards, and make sure you buy products and systems that conform to the latest safety standards. Ask for documentation from the salespeople — they should be happy to provide it.

- 🌓 If you are a patient in a hospital, you might like to make sure (or get a friend to make sure) the devices — monitors, infusion pumps, ventilators — connected to you conform to all relevant standards. The

---

[g] See Chapter 21: Computer Factors, page 277 ←

Part II ◇ Treatment ◇ Finding solutions

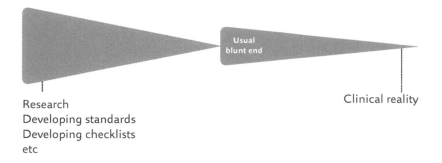

Research
Developing standards
Developing checklists
etc

Clinical reality

Figure 24.4. The Two-Wedge Model shows there's a longer process of research and development (represented by the thicker wedge) going on before any particular system's blunt end even begins.

> few days I've been in hospital, I've looked up the devices used on me; it seemed like a good use of my nerdiness and otherwise spare time in a hospital bed.
>
> This sounds like a lot of work. Instead, we need a change in the way devices are made and labeled, so that it's easy to find out how safe they are just by looking at them.[h]

International standards are examples of experts doing work long before the blunt end in the Wedge Model: standards bodies are teams of people working out how teams of people can better build and design digital systems (well, except when Human Factors and other pressures undermine them). In fact, since a wedge is a good analogy, two wedges must be even better ...

Prior to and supporting everything going on at the blunt end of the single wedge (development, testing, regulatory approval, manufacturing) is research, creating standards, and developing checklists that are then used at the blunt end.[346] The timescales of "Wedge Two" (the wedge on the left) are in decades and longer, but the impact is huge, as the research and standards eventually feed into regulation and every product at the blunt end of Wedge One (the wedge on the right). Increasing funding for research in digital healthcare safety could be the most effective form of long-term investment in healthcare.

Look back at the bar chart on causes of death.[i] More than £500 million per year goes into cancer research in the UK alone.[347] It's needed, but think what a fraction of that amount could do for research in preventable harm, and in particular for improving the safety of digital systems. It would have an immediate effect.

---

[h] See Chapter 29: Safety ratings will improve healthcare, page 401 →
[i] See Chapter 9: Preventable error bar chart, page 113 ←

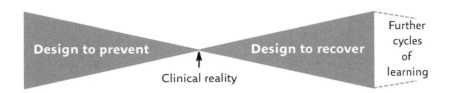

Figure 24.5. Wedges can inspire all sorts of helpful models. Here, a **Bowtie Model** shows two sides to the story: all the factors leading up to clinical activities, and the analysis and learning that follows clinical work. Ideally, in turn, this leads to learning that feeds into the next wedge — as sketched on the far right of the diagram.

Unlike cancer or any other disease, digital systems are involved with every patient regardless of their disease. Digital also impacts "hidden" areas of healthcare like sterilization, blood transfusions, and pathology labs, as well as hospital finance, patient appointments, and lots more. Investment in the safety and reliability of computers would certainly compare very well with cancer research in terms of improvements in health per pound — and, unlike cancer, the field is pretty much wide open for research. There're lots of avenues to explore and opportunities to find real improvements.

Part II ◇ Treatment ◇ Finding solutions

Why is poor-quality software so widespread? Simple bugs might seem trivial, but they are very common and don't help patient safety — they make everyone inefficient and error-prone, if nothing else. Health would improve if we paid attention to digital details.

25

Attention to detail

When I went to see my GP (my local doctor), he filled in a form to ask for some blood tests. In the picture of the form (figure 25.1), what I want you to notice is that my long name, Harold Thimbleby, is printed in full, but the doctor's name has been cut short; he isn't Richard Jon, but Richard Jones, or perhaps he's Dr Richard Jonathon Tucker. Who knows? Certainly, he doesn't work at The Medical Ce, but he works at The Medical Centre, Swansea, Wales. (See the note on anonymity in the figure.)

Why isn't there space for the full doctor's name and full address? At least it could get the first line of the doctor's address right, surely?

Instead, the doctor's name and his address are both truncated. The programmer *must have* been told to show where the doctor worked, as the label printer started to print the details, but it never finished. Somehow it was designed *not* to finish printing the full address. What's a name and address good for if it isn't right? What's a name and address label printer good for if it deliberately introduces errors? One wonders whether the barcode has got bits missing as well (the barcode, names, and places I used in the picture are fictitious).

The badly printed blood test form was for me to go and get some blood tests done at the hospital, but when I went to my GP to get the blood results after the tests had been done, I discovered another problem.

Over the months, I've seen several doctors, and they've all ordered various blood tests. So my blood test results are sitting on several databases, and there is no common view. The hospital databases are different from the GPs' databases, and they keep patient data separate. My GP cannot see blood test results unless he ordered them. I'm baffled by this lack of interoperability, since keeping multiple copies of data — with different access security — is a recipe for inconsistent data, and certainly a recipe for never being able to detect problems automatically. These sorts of problems are harder to describe, harder to understand, and much harder for doctors to cope with. The sys-

Fix It: See and solve the problems of digital healthcare. Harold Thimbleby,
Oxford University Press. © Harold Thimbleby 2021.
DOI: 10.1093/oso/9780198861270.003.0025

Part II ◇ Treatment ◇ Finding solutions

Figure 25.1. Part of a form requesting blood tests for me, Harold Thimbleby. Note that my long name is printed correctly, but the doctor's name and the name of his surgery are cut short and printed incorrectly. (For the purposes of this book, I've changed the doctor's and medical center's names, as well as the barcodes, to preserve their anonymity, but the overall effect is unchanged. I've also recently moved house, so my details are obsolete. Sorry!)

tems are not interoperable, but everyone has to live with them, making them inefficient and more likely to make errors.

I want to ask the developers of these systems: When have you sat down and spent all day exploring your systems? Looking for problems? Fixing problems? Looking for splinters, then sanding and polishing your work so it is smooth and shines? If you were a craftsman or other professional — a woodworker, a calligrapher, a climber, an artist, a clinician — you would spend time reflecting on your work so you could get better and safer. Indeed, clinicians in the UK have an entire work program called **quality improvement** (QI):

> Quality improvement is the combined and unceasing efforts of everyone — healthcare professionals, patients and their families, researchers, payers, planners, and educators — to make the changes that will lead to better patient outcomes (health), better system performance (care) and better professional development.[348]

Manufacturers and developers ought to be part of the QI team.

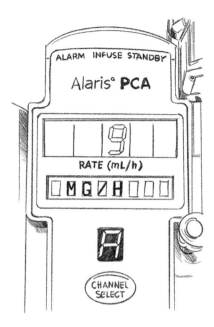

Figure 25.2. An Alaris PC infusion pump module (only part of it has been drawn). The module is permanently calibrated "RATE (mL/h)," but, as shown here, a programmer made it able to display a rate in mg (milligrams) per hour. Will it now deliver drugs at 9 mg per hour or 9 mL per hour? How's the user supposed to know what it's doing?

Part II ◇ Treatment ◇ Finding solutions

———————————■———————————

The Alaris PC is a versatile infusion pump that allows users to attach modules on it so that it can do many different things. The drawing (figure 25.2) shows part of the Alaris PC's PCA module — PCA means "patient controlled analgesia"; it's designed to allow patients to control their painkiller (analgesia) drug dose themselves. On the Alaris, the PCA module permanently and clearly says the drug rate is in milliliters per hour (mL/h), but the programmer has used the LED display to show the rate as MG/H, which means milligrams per hour.

So which units will it use? As shown, nobody knows whether the Alaris is delivering drugs at a rate of 9 mL per hour or at 9 mg per hour.

Note that 9 mL per hour and 9 mg per hour are only the same when the drug concentration is 1 mg per mL. There's no reason why the concentration should be 1 mg per mL. If the drug concentration was actually 0.1 mg per mL, then the two interpretations would differ by a factor of ten, potentially causing confusion that would lead to serious harm to the patient. Whatever is going on, it's confusing.

Confusing medical devices cause errors.

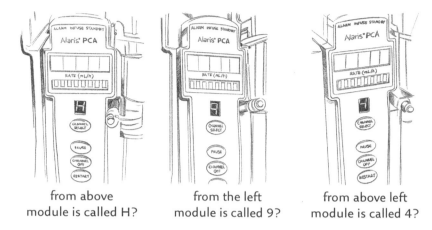

from above
module is called H?

from the left
module is called 9?

from above left
module is called 4?

Figure 25.3. Looked at from three different angles, all very reasonable working angles, *the same* letter A (or perhaps a digit 8?) on an Alaris PC infusion pump module (figure 25.2) also looks like an H, a 9, or a 4. Because the display is deeply recessed inside the infusion pump, the edges of the display get obscured, changing the symbol shown in different ways.

The developers of the Alaris PC made it versatile by using a dot matrix display that can show almost any text, unfortunately even if it's contradictory. Perhaps the programmers never tested their program running on an actual pump? Certainly, it seems that nobody bothered to test it properly using UCD[a] — nor did the regulators do enough to stop a buggy product getting to market. It is, surely, an elementary bug[349] that should have been avoided in the first place. Yet here it is on a pump that is in use — I photographed it in a large hospital, from which the drawings in this book were made.

The Alaris PC has other problems. The manufacturers decided to use a cheaper seven-segment display for the module name, and to sink the display a long way into the case, which can obscure segments and make it impossible to read correctly (figure 25.3). Module codes like A, E, H, 8, 9, and more, are therefore very easily confused.[350]

Fortunately, PCA pumps are generally very safe. Usually the patient presses a button to get more painkiller when they need it, and the hospital will have set limits on how frequently it can be pressed. When they have had so much painkiller they are starting to get sleepy, they are less likely to press the button again and again and get an overdose. Of course the hospital's limit on the maximum dose, programmed into the infusion pump, should stop multiple pressing turning into an overdose even if the patient doesn't go to sleep first.

---

[a] See Chapter 22: User Centered Design, page 301 ←

In 2019, Mobasher Butt, one of the directors of Babylon, a company developing a major medical app, said,

> We're developing and improving our technology and the versions of the symptom checker every two months.[351]

For many products, this would sound exciting and would gain all the benefits of the very latest technologies. But would you take a drug or any other medical intervention from a company that was still updating it every few months? No; you'd ask them to finish developing it, and to get it tested. Once they'd done that, you might appreciate some improvements, but building on top of something that had been rigorously approved.

Despite its regular updates, the Babylon app is already in use, with over 110,000 registered patients in the UK (I discussed the financial impact of this in an earlier chapter[b]). The Rwandan version of Babylon, Babyl, has 2,000,000 registered patients — a sixth of the country's population. It's a huge international project. Yet Babylon's patients are relying on a system a director of the company has said is not yet finished.[352] The app is changing so fast to fix its known problems I'm surprised it was approved for use.

Babylon's system is complex, and, inevitably, like any other digital system, it has bugs. A critical question is: how does it balance pushing an exciting product to market (it would go out of business if it didn't) against essential medical quality, such as ensuring that it is safe and effective (it would unnecessarily harm patients if it didn't)?

In June 2020, Rory Glover was using Babylon to check up on a prescription, but found that Babylon's "Consultation Replays" feature offered him a list of about 50 videos to review. Which he did, of course, but they were videos of other patients consulting with doctors that had been made available to him. Babylon blamed the introduction of a new feature allowing a patient talking to a doctor to change from audio to video during a call for this bug. It's still a serious bug, though, releasing confidential patient consultations to other patients. It's hard to see how software with such flaws meets good regulatory standards; indeed, Babylon reported itself to the UK's data protection authority.[353]

Rory Glover also tweeted about the problem,[354] including a screenshot from his mobile. The videos are called Replay 0, Replay 1, Replay 2, … I'm surprised they don't have more informative labels — like the doctor's name, or at least the date and time of the consultation. Further indication of casual programming.

Babylon has been criticized by Dr David Watkins, a Consultant Medical Oncologist, who used his Twitter handle @DrMurphy11 to tweet examples of its misdiagnoses: he also directly alerted Babylon and the relevant regulators. One of his tweets is reproduced here (figure 25.4). While Dr Watkins

---

[b] See Chapter 18: Babylon patient finance model, page 242 ←

Classic #HeartAttack symptoms in a FEMALE, results in a diagnosis of #PanicAttack or #Depression.

The **Chatbot** ONLY suggests the possibility of a #HeartAttack in MEN!

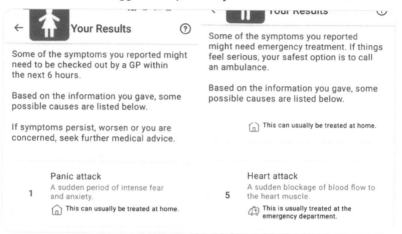

Figure 25.4. Dr David Watkins tweeting a problem he found with the Babylon diagnosis algorithm. With the same symptoms reported, Babylon suggests a man is having a heart attack, usually treated in an emergency department, but suggests that a woman is having a panic attack, which can be treated at home.

has created a media profile on his work,[355] Babylon responded rather critically.[356] There's clearly an argument going on, and I don't know all of the background; nor are the details of it relevant for this book. Nevertheless, I want to pick up on a couple of points from Babylon's press release about their standoff:

> Our technology meets robust regulatory standards [...][356]

Currently, regulatory standards for digital healthcare are inadequate (particularly for AI like Babylon), as I argue throughout this book, and as Rory Glover's video experience confirms.[357] In any case, current regulatory standards don't address the sorts of issues that Dr Watkins has been raising. For example, Babylon has published papers suggesting that Babylon is 100% safe,[358] yet perfection is implausible: 100% says more about the experiment than the safety. Indeed, Rwanda's minister of health claimed that the Babyl app included no questions about malaria, even though it is a major health issue in Rwanda. Babylon disputes this, but if the Rwandan minister for health can't find malaria on it,[359] there are at least some usability problems that need sorting out. Then Babylon wrote in their press release:

So today we're making a big offer: @DrMurphy11 now that
you have stepped out from behind your computer, why not be
part of an open, independent analysis of your AI testing:
publish the entirety of your work, and let the totality of your
data be assessed by any objective expert.[356]

The perspective here seems to be that the data Dr Watkins made needs
independent analysis, and his data needs publishing in its entirety. On the
contrary, he has already published his findings, and they have been reproduced by others. Babylon may be hoping that his full data would show that
bugs are "rare" or "contrived," but I suspect his full data would only say more
about how he finds bugs, rather than how likely patients are to encounter
them.

I think Babylon should be asking themselves whether the bugs indicate
systematic design problems with their approach, and if so, they should start
fixing them, and, even better, start improving their development processes
that result in bugs. Indeed, their press release says, "senior doctors [...] build
our products," when you'd expect senior software engineers to build them.
If software engineers built their system, a good response would have been:
now we know of these bugs from Dr Watkins, we can automate his testing
and do it thoroughly and many times faster — for instance, looking at *every*
possible form of possible gender bias in the system (figure 25.4), we can fix
the bugs and stop them happening again.

Babylon's press release doesn't seem to see the data Dr Watkins *has already* publicly provided as an opportunity, but rather presents it as a public
relations challenge to give Dr Watkins more work, which, obviously, they are
much better placed to do themselves. Babylon ought to be interested in *how*
Dr Watkins repeatedly found bugs *by hand* that they had missed even with
their greater resources. Babylon said their request that he just hand his data
over was a "big offer," but the data is hardly interesting compared to *how* Dr
Watkins found bugs they missed.

It's a shame to be so critical when digital innovators — especially ones
with significant resources like Babylon has — could be encouraging people
to help them improve. The approach here is more likely to put people off
trying. The news is not that there are bugs, but that manufacturers don't
want to know.

To be positive, digital healthcare systems are going to be game-changers
for healthcare. They can relieve work for healthcare professionals, provide
faster care for patients, and have many other benefits on an unheard of scale.
On the other hand, any errors in their design or clinical information, or any
problems in their use, can lead to equally large problems. Even if they only
have a tiny 0.1% error rate, when that's multiplied up by the huge numbers
of users, the impact on patients is significant. In particular, the errors will be
systematic. The way ahead is better regulation — and better programming.

Part II ◇ Treatment ◇ Finding solutions

> **Box 25.1.** Digital internationalization
>
> I've written *Fix IT* about digital healthcare issues, which are international, but I had to make choices: I wrote in English with US spelling. In the UK, we talk about operating theatres, but in the US they're called operating rooms — just changing the spelling of "theatre" to "theater" isn't enough as the whole phrase changes. GP becomes primary care physician. Billion means different things too.[5] But there's more. Anesthetist isn't just the US spelling of anæsthetist — it also changes its meaning.[a] In the UK there's A&E, for Accident and Emergency, but in the US it's ER, for Emergency Room. If I'd written in a language other than English, say Mandarin, I'd have lost many English speakers, even though the digital issues are the same.
>
> Wherever in the world you're reading this, I'm sure you'll be able to take cultural differences in your stride, but for digital systems (technically, this book *is* a program[360]) international issues are critical. There're opportunities for patient harm. Confusing dates (what does 3/4/22 mean?) and mixing up units (e.g., pounds and kilograms) are common problems. Hospitals use international systems, and accidentally import foreign ways of working. Patients travel the world and access their medical records over the internet. The problems arise when people don't spot the differences affecting them.
>
> Handling these problems is called **internationalization**. So if you find confusions in my book's internationalization, think of it as highlighting the problems of internationalizing digital healthcare too. At least you've spotted the problem — but think how a busy nurse might make mistakes when their decisions are driven by a poorly internationalized digital system.
>
> You should ask: how could systems be better internationalized to be safer? Even better: how could healthcare *itself* be internationalized, so the issues dissolve? Mobility and networking of digital don't just highlight problems — they are more positively thought of as drivers for defining and spreading best practice, and hence for improving safety across the world.
>
> ---
> [a] See Chapter 24: Anesthetics training, page 325 ←

Aviation has a very different safety culture to healthcare.

Air Inter Flight 148 flew from Lyon towards Strasbourg. As it neared Strasbourg airport, the pilot commanded the autopilot to descend at an angle of 3.3 degrees. A few moments later, the Airbus A320 flew into the side of a mountain, crashing into woods and killing 87 people.

One cause of the crash was that the pilots had set the autopilot to −33, meaning descend at a *rate* of 3,300 feet per minute, rather than descend at an *angle* of 3.3 degrees, as they had intended. The difference is in the position switch, a small decimal point (does the display show −33 or −3.3), and a display showing V/S (for vertical speed) or FPA (for flight path angle). The most prominent part of the display is the bright number. There is very lit-

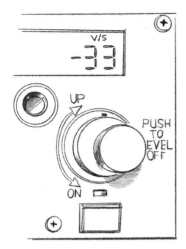 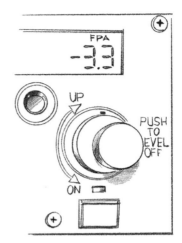

Figure 25.5. Drawing of part of the A320 airplane's autopilot, showing it in two different modes. Imagine trying to spot the critical difference between the displays when you are under pressure. Imagine the consequences of not noticing the decimal point.

tle difference between –33 and –3.3. Indeed, with seven-segment displays, the decimal point is hard to see anyway, because it's so close to the bottom of the 3 that it seems to be part of it.[350]

The pilots never noticed the difference — they had lots of other things on their mind. The mountain was in clouds, and their rapid descent meant they flew into the side of it with no time to recover. Reports of the crash were never controversial; there was no argument. A few months later, Airbus, the plane manufacturer, updated the design of autopilots so a descent rate of 3,300 feet per minute is displayed as –3300 not as the confusing –33. The mix-up can never happen so easily again. I'll talk more about aviation later.[c]

But consider this: in September 2016, when General Motors suspected that they had a software problem with their vehicle airbags that might have killed one person, they recalled over 4 million cars to fix the bug.[361] The reports of the bug weren't controversial. The economic reality is that any crash that might be plausibly blamed on their product designs would be a serious public relations problem, and they quickly move to fix it. It's an interesting contrast to GE Healthcare's handling of their bugs on their Aestiva and Aespire anesthetic machines.[d]

Airbus and General Motors take safety seriously, and they pay serious attention to "small" details. It doesn't matter how big or small the holes in Swiss Cheese are; small holes are still holes.

---

[c] See Chapter 26: Planes are safer, page 347 →
[d] See Chapter 17: Aestiva and Aespire machines, page 213 ←

Aviation safety relies on getting very complex engineering right, and it's getting safer and safer. What can digital healthcare learn from aviation and aviation engineering?

26

Planes are safer

Here's a famous story: a "simple" software bug caused the European Space Agency's Ariane 5 rocket to explode. Less than a minute after its launch, the explosion was spectacular and photogenic. The explosion sent about $7 billion[5] of 1996-valued US dollars up in flames (figures 26.1 and 26.2).

The embarrassing Ariane 5 disaster, with an explosion visible from many miles away, has ensured a lot of attention was paid to why it failed, and how to avoid similar problems in the future. Because space and aviation failures tend to be so spectacular and undeniable, there is now an enormous amount of skill invested in, and attention paid, to software correctness — getting rid of bugs — in aerospace. This begs the question why this successful approach to safe software does not get embraced by digital healthcare.

Error in healthcare isn't photogenic, and everybody is very busy and wants to feel perfect — and manufacturers need to sell things to stay competitive, even if what they sell is not "perfect" stuff. It's hard to get anyone to draw attention to fixing risky software when it's good business not to — it's more profitable to keep selling upgrades, which have more bugs which will mean more upgrades to sell. Like the time of the unsafe cars in the 1960s, we're still in a pre-Ralph Nader world of being excited by digital rather than trying to make it safer.[a]

Consider the classic story of the London Ambulance Service's Computer Aided Dispatch (LASCAD) system failure in 1992: it resulted in at least 30 deaths as well as hundreds of delays.[362] Yet none of it was photogenic like the Ariane 5 explosion (figure). It got less attention because it was harder to understand and it was less dramatic. Even after the lessons of the LASCAD fiasco, the Ambulance Service's digital problems continued on and off: for instance, on New Year's Eve in 2017, one of the busiest nights of the year, another bug meant that control room staff had to rely on pen and paper for several hours.[363]

---

[a] See Chapter 11: *Unsafe at Any Speed*, page 140 ←

Fix It: See and solve the problems of digital healthcare. Harold Thimbleby, Oxford University Press. © Harold Thimbleby 2021.
DOI: 10.1093/oso/9780198861270.003.0026

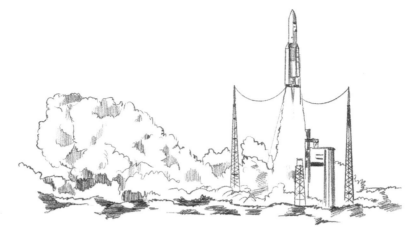

Figure 26.1. The 1996 launch of the Ariane 5 rocket ...
(Continued in figure 26.2.)

Aviation is often held up as a contrasting example to healthcare. Air safety is improving, and it *is* amazingly safe. Sometimes people say it's unfair to compare healthcare and aviation because they are so different (sick patients aren't like predictable planes, for instance), but in this chapter I want to compare their engineering. There are then fascinating, and relevant, comparisons to be made. But aviation wasn't always so safe.

A long time ago, some really serious crashes shocked the aviation industry. I described two crashes to illustrate task saturation earlier.[b] Here's another example:

🚀 In 1977 two Boeing 747 passenger planes collided on the runway at what is now Tenerife North Airport. The crash killed 583 people and had only 61 survivors, making it the most lethal aviation crash ever. It was foggy, and one plane started to take off, while the other plane was about to turn off the runway. They collided. As the Swiss Cheese Model[c] suggests, many things went wrong. There were mutual misunderstandings between the pilots and Air Traffic Control — ATC language has now been standardized.

Leading up to all of these crashes, there was a strong **authority hierarchy** in the cockpit. The pilot was in charge. The pilot was not successfully challenged by more junior members of the crew who were worried about what he — it was always a "he" in those days — was doing. Traditionally,

---

[b] See Chapter 20: Plane crashes, page 262 ←
[c] See Chapter 6: Swiss Cheese Model, page 61 ←

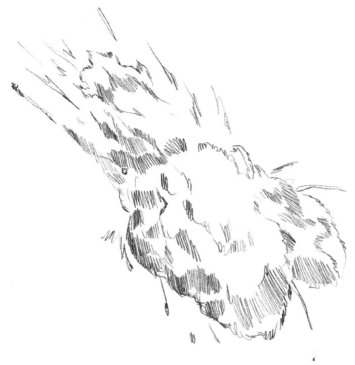

Figure 26.2. ... ended in spectacular failure due to a computer bug.
(Continued from figure 26.1.)

the captain was *the* authority in the cockpit, and the crew had to do what he said, rather than co-operate in solving problems.

After teasing out what was going wrong in these aviation crashes, **crew resource management** (CRM) was developed and has now become standard practice. Crew resource management aims to create an *explicit* culture where authority can be questioned and the decision-makers do not feel threatened by being questioned. There are now standard ways to ask pilots to do things, and standard ways to query instructions, and standard ways to escalate concerns. Air Traffic Control can listen in, and can take over when they recognize conflict. And so on.

But CRM, putting Human Factors into practice in the cockpit — sharp-end stuff — is only one of many approaches that aviation takes. Aviation also takes engineering very seriously: the blunt-end stuff in the Wedge Model.[d] After all, lives depend on both the human crew and the safe engineering of the aircraft and cockpit. In a hospital, we have no idea what software there

---

[d] See Chapter 24: Wedge Thinking, page 325 ←

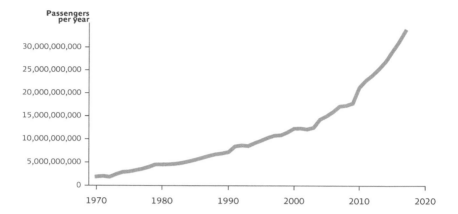

Figure 26.3. Worldwide air passenger numbers are growing exponentially. The graph here shows civil aviation passengers carried per year worldwide, over the period 1970 to 2018.

is or how it is connected; in an aircraft, you can look at a bolt and find out its correct torque, who put it there, what batch, and from which manufacturer it came from. Because it matters.

Paying attention to safety isn't confined to pilots and plane engineers, it is pervasive. Have you noticed, when you, as a passenger, get on an airplane, pretty much the first thing that's said to you is about safety. What you should do if there's turbulence. What you should do if we ditch in water. What you should do to slide down the evacuation chute. How to brace. Put your oxygen mask on first, then help anyone else. The safety instructions are in your seat. This is serious stuff, but it gets airline staff and passengers to engage with safety. It helps improve safety and survival.

Digital bugs are a bit like flight turbulence — random surprises, with unpredictable impact ranging from trivial to disastrous. The analogy is that it would be helpful to regularly remind developers of ways to recognize and control bugs to help improve digital healthcare safety. Maybe *Fix IT* should take on a role like the safety card in every passenger's seat? Please read *Fix IT* before taking off.

The safety improvements achieved in aviation are very impressive. Passenger numbers are growing exponentially, from just under two billion in 1972 to nearly 40 billion in 2017 (figure 26.3), but passenger deaths are dropping dramatically, from 3,346 in 1972 to under 400 in 2017 (figure 26.4).[364] Put another way, the chance of a passenger dying in 1972 was 2 in a million, and in 2015 the chance had dropped to 1 in 100 million — a two-hundredfold improvement per passenger.

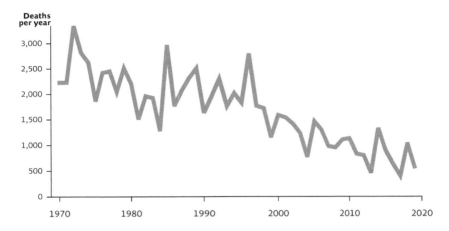

Deaths per year

Figure 26.4. Aviation deaths are falling. This graph shows worldwide civil aviation passenger deaths per year (excluding "routine" passenger deaths inside the plane), over the period 1970 to 2019. Note that the scales of the two graphs (passengers carried in figure 26.3 and passenger deaths in this graph) are different. The chance of dying on a flight is about 1 in 100,000,000. It's very safe, safer than sitting in an armchair.[365] Put another way, every year planes carry four times the world's population, and it goes wrong for just a few hundreds; shouldn't digital healthcare envy aviation's engineering reliability and see what it can learn?

On 15 January 2009, Captain "Sully" Sullenberger was flying US Airways Flight 1549, an Airbus A320, when it flew into a flock of Canada geese. The plane lost both engines, right over the city of New York. With no engine power, they professionally glided the plane to an emergency ditching on the Hudson River. It was an accident that Sully turned into what has been called the "Miracle on the Hudson" — nobody died. He is now a world-recognized safety expert, and writes widely. Here is one of his deep observations:

> In aviation, every rule that we have, everything we know, every procedure we use, we know because someone, or often many people, died. We have learned important safety lessons purchased at great cost, sometimes literally bought in blood. We have an obligation not to forget these lessons and have to relearn them.[366]

In other words, aviation has been getting safer because it has deliberately learned from failures, often from terrible accidents losing lives. As Sully has made clear, he — and all his crew and passengers — survived the Flight 1549 emergency ditching because of years of aviations's deliberate learning to improve safety. You need to seek the learning, and not forget the lessons. One of the best ways not to forget the lessons is to build them into the engineering and procedures and, overriding both, build them into the regulations. How much would healthcare improve if digital systems had Black Boxes and other safety mechanisms inspired by aviation to gather information, and actually *wanted to learn* to apply those lessons in improving healthcare? How much safer would digital healthcare be if the developers prioritized programming safely? There would be no better way to respect all the patients harmed by buggy and dangerous systems.

A very interesting comment following the Miracle on the Hudson was made by Patrick Harten: he said, "the hardest, most traumatic part of the entire event was when it was over."[367] In a later chapter, I'll show how patient (and staff) stories can be used very successfully to both listen to the people affected, and to help share the learning widely.[e]

———————————■———————————

Nine years after the Miracle on the Hudson's example of aviation's safety culture, Boeing's new 737 MAX plane crashed twice within five months. In October 2018, a 737 MAX crashed into the Java Sea killing 189 people, and in March 2019, another 737 MAX crashed and 157 people died. All 737 MAXs have now been grounded, but the 737 MAX story looks like a horrible exception to the consistent trends in aircraft safety (figure 26.4).

So why were there safety problems with the 737 MAX?

The Boeing 737 plane has been in widespread use since 1967, and it's been a popular, very safe aircraft. As the 737 has been developed and modified over the years, its engines have been made more and more fuel-efficient. This has meant that its engines have got larger and larger, as bigger engines are more efficient. The engines chosen for the 737 MAX design were so big that they had to be moved forward from the old engine position under the wings, to be positioned higher to clear the ground when the plane is on the runway.

Moving the engines changed the flight characteristics of the plane. Not just because of increasing the engine power, but the new engine shape and position produces more lift ahead of the wing's center. This tends to raise the nose of the plane, increasing the angle of attack, which makes the plane easier to stall — stalling is a dangerous condition when a plane stops flying and falls like a brick. Boeing's solution was to correct the new flight characteristics with some digital tricks.

Boeing wanted to sell the 737 MAX as, basically, just an improved, more fuel-efficient version of their successful 737 series planes. They therefore wanted to ensure that pilots for the 737 MAX would not need any more training, despite the new software.[368] Pilot training is a major cost for airlines, and cost-saving was part of the sales pitch for the 737 MAX.

In particular, to hide the new software from pilots so the plane seemed like just a 737 to the pilots, that meant that the new software could not be

———

[e] See Chapter 30: How to make Digital Stories, page 422 →

> **Box 26.1.** The scandal of Alternative Summary Reporting
>
> The collusion, often called **regulatory capture**, that occurs between regulators and manufacturers, which was one of the main factors that led to the Boeing 737 MAX disasters, is not unique to aviation. It seriously affects healthcare too.
>
> The FDA, the US medical device regulator, operates the MAUDE (Manufacturer and User Facility Device Experience) database to collect reports on medical device problems and patient harms.
>
> MAUDE is publicly available and makes medical device reports available to patients and healthcare professionals to help them make informed medical decisions. MAUDE is also used in law courts to provide evidence of problems. In the Princess of Wales Hospital case, MAUDE was used to argue that an Abbott XceedPro glucometer was a reliable device and therefore that problems using it must have been the nurses' fault. In fact, the device and its management were at fault, and the nurses were acquitted.[a]
>
> The FDA ran a secret reporting system, the Alternative Summary Reporting (ASR) Program, which enabled manufacturers to bypass MAUDE. ASR collected "exempted" reports of injuries and device malfunctions, so they never ended up in MAUDE. Over six million device incidents were recorded in the ASR, thus giving the misleading impression that many devices were safer than they really were. For instance, in 2016 alone there were 10,000 secret reports of harms recorded in ASR caused by surgical staplers made by Covidien (now part of Medtronic). In the same period, only 84 reports with the staplers were made public in MAUDE.
>
> The FDA disclosed the hidden ASR reports and revoked the exemptions in June 2019.[369]
>
> The controversy has been widely reported.[370] The investigative journalism won Christina Jewett the National Press Foundation's 2020 Feddie Reporting Award.[371]
>
> ---
>
> [a] See Chapter 8: Abbott XceedPro glucometer, page 92 ←

overridden, even if it was doing the wrong thing — if it could have been overridden, then the pilots would need new training to understand how and when to override it. That would be a fine choice if the new software had worked correctly.

The new software relied on a single sensor to detect if the plane was about to stall. To correct a stall, real or imagined, the plane would automatically drop the nose, and the pilot would have to fight against it. Two planes crashed, killing everyone on board.

The full report into the first crash was published in October 2019 — unlike many healthcare incidents, the full report is public and available for free.[372]

Echoing the insights of Swiss Cheese,[f] there were nine faults that contributed to the accident — nine slices of cheese that failed. If any one of them had not occurred, likely the accident would not have occurred. However these are all "what ifs" and at the center of the incident was the digital software.

Gregory Travis's clear discussion of the 737 MAX's problems makes some very important points:[368]

- Safety didn't come first. Money did.

- The ease of using software to modify systems (in this case to correct conventional engineering problems) and the ease of updating software has created a cultural laziness. Less effort is put into getting a design right, since it can always be fixed up by software.

- Software itself is often delivered to the customer unfinished and not properly tested, because it can always be fixed up later to address problems as and when they occur (or maybe after they occur).

- There were pilot training issues — should the pilots have been better trained?

- Cost savings in the way safety is regulated led to serious problems being overlooked. The manufacturers told the regulators that the plane was safe.

- Finally, the 737 MAX software had a **single point of failure**, so when it went wrong, the whole thing failed. There was no redundancy in the software, and no way for it to make the "best" decision when one of its sensor inputs failed.

In summary, software was added to the 737 MAX in the spirit of increasing its safety, but it failed and has now killed people. Boeing works within the aviation regulatory environment, and arguably the core failure was in regulation or in its application.[373] Possibly it was corruption or institutionalized corruption (systematic corruption that is accepted); we don't know yet, and perhaps never will. Investigations are ongoing, but it looks like poor regulation combined with poor management, no doubt "justified" by the amazing track record of safety the industry had had up until that moment, led to failures. It's a common sort of unconscious arrogance, which I'd call **errorgance** — errorgance is the arrogance surrounding an error and the refusal to acknowledge it or to learn from it; errorgance stops people fixing the underlying problems.

The attitude is captured well by Sir Liam Donaldson, champion of patient safety and UK Chief Medical Officer (1998–2010):

---

[f] See Chapter 6: Swiss Cheese Model, page 61 ←

> **Box 26.2.** An aviation analogy
>
> When people get a hip implant or a cancer operation, they rightly spend a lot of time finding out who is the best surgeon to do their operation. When I got neuropathy, I spent a lot of time researching who the best neurologist was.
>
> Yet when we fly on a plane, how much time do we spend worrying about getting a good pilot? We don't even think about it!
>
> The point is: pilots are trained to very high and consistent standards to fly planes safely, but somehow surgeons are far less predictable. If you are a passenger on an Airbus A321, you know the pilots are trained to fly A321s safely. If you need to have a hip implant, you have a lot less assurance that the surgeon is experienced and really good at this particular operation.[374]
>
> When we have a hip implant, we also ought to worry about the quality of the implant,[a] or when we have an infusion, we ought to worry about the quality of the infusion pump, not just our surgeon. The implant or infusion pump will be caring for you a lot longer than the surgeon![b]
>
> When you last took a flight, did you worry whether you were flying on an Airbus A321 or on a Boeing 777? They are both airworthy, and both are safe — they go through airworthiness testing that would put healthcare to shame (because passenger lives depend on ensuring they are safe). Yet infusion pumps vary by a factor of at least two in how safe they are. We ought to be more careful choosing which infusion pumps to use!
>
> ---
> [a] See Chapter 33: The Danger Within Us, page 491 →
> [b] See Chapter 29: Infusion pump evaluations, page 406 →

The most dangerous five words in the world are
"it could not happen here."

The key lessons for digital healthcare are that we need to strengthen *appropriate and effective* regulation (with adequate funding to do a good job of it), and developers must make software systems that are proved safe — relying on upgrading software later is asking for trouble.

If you were admitted to hospital tomorrow in any country, your chances of being subject to an error in your care would be something like 1 in 10, and dying from an error about 1 in 300. Compare this to the risk of dying in an air crash of about 1 in 100 million. The World Health Organization (WHO) points out that healthcare is far riskier than flying.[375]

The United Nations says that out of every 100 hospitalized patients at any given time, 7 patients in developed and 10 patients in developing countries will acquire at least one healthcare-associated infection during their stay.[375] The better rates in some countries proves things could be improved.

I'm arguing that digital healthcare could improve its safety a lot by adopting ideas from aviation engineering and aviation regulation and safety culture. Some people, however, argue that the human sides of aviation and healthcare are very different and should not be compared. I'm not so sure. A heart operation and all its preparation might easily involve a team of 60 people, but this is the same sort of number as needed to run a jumbo jet. In both hospitals and airports there are hundreds of unsung people sorting out problems — sterilizing equipment or handling baggage. There seems to be a lot to learn from aviation systems even if there are differences.

Just like planes are getting safer, so too are many technologies. Car safety has been improving too. There's been much less emphasis on Human Factors with driving cars, but there have been huge innovations in the engineering: air bags, ABS, seat belts, crumple zones, and more. Not only is car safety improving, but we have car safety awards, car safety ratings, and more. There is a car safety *culture*.

Interestingly, bus safety is even better — buses have benefitted from all the improved engineering that car safety benefits from *and* they carry more passengers. So per passenger, they are doing extremely well.

In transport, then, especially planes and buses, engineering for safety has improved dramatically. A lot of that engineering improvement is in the software, in improving the quality of the digital systems.[376]

Aviation and car transport are both highly technical industries. Training engineers for them takes years, and training pilots or drivers is also specialized. Pilots are trained for specific airplanes. Drivers, after training and passing tests, are only allowed to drive specific sorts of vehicles. I am an ordinary domestic driver, and I am not licensed to drive serious professional vehicles like buses, lorries, and diggers. This is so obvious, it's strange to discuss it.

———————————■———————————

Stephen Pettitt was the first patient in the UK to undergo an operation to treat mitral valve disease by robot — in this case, a Da Vinci. He died after the operation at the Freeman Hospital in Newcastle.[377] The coroner, the investigator into the death, said there had been an "absence of any benchmark" for training on the new treatment. Sukumaran Nair, the surgeon, had had no one-to-one training on the Da Vinci robot and had been "running before he could walk." Other experts in the operating room walked out before the operation was finished.

Nobody supervising a pilot or driver would have so little awareness of the importance of training, supervision, competency, and fitness to practice. Nobody is allowed to pilot a plane or drive a car without a license that they have been trained and are competent to do so. Somehow, it seems, healthcare practice focuses so much on the traditional clinical issues that it ignores the new digital risks, like of using robots.

The same oversight has happened in digital development for healthcare. Although a patient's medical data is complicated, the software in planes and cars is even more complex and has to work in real time (very rapidly). Certainly MRI and CAT scanners are complex, but the math behind them is still relatively straightforward. The point is — without starting an argument about the borderline exceptions — the software engineering techniques used to make planes and cars safer would find no trouble making digital healthcare safer.

> ⓓ All the bugs described in this book are avoidable using standard programming practices that are routinely used in other industries — such as aviation and nuclear power — where lives depend on quality programming. Primarily, they use **Formal Methods**,[g] along with a lot of automated tools to help with quality processes, like documentation, version control, and so on.

Getting rid of bugs would make healthcare both easier and safer.

What are Formal Methods? Formal Methods are best explained by analogy with house building. You can get a builder to put up a house, and as it goes up the builder will make many design decisions. We need a steel joist over that window, and let's make it the same size as one I saw in another building. Many houses built like this will stand up and even look cute. The alternative is "Formal Methods," where a structural engineer carefully examines the architect's design, and *calculates* how large the steel joists need to be to hold up the building above the windows. The structural engineer and architect will have some discussions if the architect's plans turn out to be unsafe. For something complicated like a tower block or skyscraper, it would obviously be negligent not to do the relevant calculations, but for many small-scale building projects builders get away with guesswork and adjusting things as they go along.

Playing with programs is very easy, and they are very easy to fiddle with until things *seem* to work. But there may be bugs, just like when your cowboy builder leaves you with a house with structural problems you don't discover until long after the builders disappeared with your money. Indeed, builders are notorious for "plastering over" problems. Programs are no different. Programs can look fantastic, can give persuasive demos, but underneath there is no rigorous engineering to hold it all together. Like building, programming is one of the few things that can be done badly but look successful. Worse, many programmers find it very tempting to add features to make their programs more and more exciting — this is the equivalent of adding windows or knocking out walls: it looks nice, but doing so probably adds more structural problems. The hole the builder made for that new window might have been holding up the floor above.

Many people think programming is really easy. Well, even children can do it, can't they? Well, yes, children can build wonderful things in Lego, but that doesn't mean they are already competent house builders, car designers, or aviation engineers. We all know that real engineering is very different to making Lego models. A skyscraper in Lego looks nice and can be built quite

---

[g] See Chapter 27: Formal Methods, page 379 →

> **Box 26.3.** The Dunning-Kruger Effect
>
> Like building, developing programs can be done badly but made to look good, often extremely good. While this makes programming seem really easy — even children look like they can program well — it creates a potential double-edged problem called the **Dunning-Kruger Effect**:[378]
>
> - Programmers who are weak programmers are unlikely to be aware of *how* bad they are. They will be over-optimistic about their skills, and would see no reason to try to get better. Maybe they will get promoted and start recruiting more staff: and then they won't know how to recruit skilled staff. In short, program quality will be poor, but nobody will realize it, and the problems will be perpetuated.
>
> - Programmers who are good are, for exactly these reasons, often surrounded by weaker programmers. Surrounded by weak programmers — some of whom get promoted — they may not realize how much better they are. They have no reason to realize they are better, possibly *much* better, nor do their managers, and hence they won't have much influence in improving anything.
>
> In contrast, in surgery or anesthesia, or pretty much any area of health-care, if you do something badly it becomes obvious very quickly. Healthcare has therefore evolved strict regulation and tough requirements for training, qualifications, and regular certification to practice.
>
> Despite digital systems being used throughout healthcare, sometimes practically substituting for qualified clinicians, there are no such requirements. Dunning-Kruger explains why. The main solutions are professional training (to increase self-awareness in the relevant skills and meta-skills[379]) and qualifications (to provide objective measurement of skill levels).

quickly, but a real skyscraper needs a lot of serious thought beyond children's abilities. Fire safety. Electrical safety. Earthquake resilience. Wind forces. Lift scheduling. Heating. None of that is needed in a toy Lego skyscraper, however nice it looks.

Somehow these facts about Lego are obvious. We don't go around saying building a skyscraper or bridge is easy because young children can do it in Lego.

Here's a real-life example of this sort of confused thinking about children and programming.

The Times newspaper praised industry for hiring teenagers[380] to test their cybersecurity. Somehow we think children hacking is clever and exciting, but we wouldn't be impressed with their ability to swing sledgehammers and smash their way into a jewelery shop. Surely we'd ask: why didn't the jewelers use professional engineers in the first place? Clearly, if children can break into a jewelery shop, the shop is insecure, so when children break

> **Box 26.4.** Lego workshops
>
> Leanna Rierson has a brilliant idea for running workshops with Lego.
>
> The workshop is divided up into teams, and each team is given a pre-built Lego model, like a car or an airplane. The team writes down on paper the requirements for the model.
>
> This is analogous to writing the requirements for a computer program. You "know what you want" the program to do, so you write requirements so the programmers can construct the program you want. The program should satisfy the requirements, of course.
>
> Then the team takes the model to pieces and puts the pieces and their written requirements into a bag. The bag is passed on to the next team, who will put the model together from the requirements and the bits they are given.
>
> The results are often hilarious, because the end results do not resemble the original models.
>
> In other words, not everyone can write good requirements.
>
> And, these are just requirements for simple Lego models when all the pieces are present in the bag making it easier. Writing effective requirements for real programs, as needed in digital healthcare, is *much* harder, and rarely hilarious.

into a computer system, why do we think the children are clever?

Emphasizing children's amazing computing skills misdirects our attention away from our own struggles with all things digital — and the need for adults to be used to program safely.

Somehow it isn't obvious that safe and secure programming is hard, and if children are programming, then, however imaginative it is, they cannot be doing quality programming.

We are surrounded by very exciting, powerful systems. Amazon would be a good example: it provides a very smooth, very effective experience. It looks very easy. Indeed, it "must be" easy as it is so easy to use. Actually, thinking this is a fallacy. Amazon (and eBay, Facebook, and others) are only so smooth because they put an awful lot of world-leading research and hard work into polishing them. In 2017, Amazon alone invested about $22.6 billion[5] in research and development.[381] They have thousands of highly skilled developers. The end result is something that looks intuitive, but it wasn't intuitive to get there.

This means that when politicians and others look at these wonderful things, they think, wouldn't it be easy to have such nice things in healthcare?

Not unless healthcare has investments comparable to some of the world's richest companies.

Another confusion is with business models. Again, take Amazon as a concrete example. If Amazon makes a mistake, or if you make a mistake

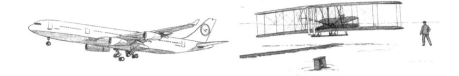

Figure 26.5. What a contrast there is between a sleek modern Airbus 340 plane seating 350 passengers in comfort, and the Wright brothers' simple, flimsy 1903 *Flyer* on its first successful flight! The Airbus's body alone is longer than the entire first flight.

using Amazon, this isn't going to be a big problem, either due to consumer laws or due to Amazon's business philosophy. You can return your faulty product. You can have another one. You can have a refund. There are lots of easy solutions to problems.

Fundamentally, most modern businesses rely on an interesting idea called **fungibility**. That is, things are essentially interchangeable. If my book is damaged, another copy can replace it. If I've lost £10 on a transaction, *another* £10 is just as good, and in fact £12 would be even better. I don't need my original £10 back to be equally wealthy. That's what fungible means.

There is little fungibility in healthcare.

You may be able to replace one drug by another, but if you cut my left leg off by mistake, another leg will not be adequate restitution.[382] Almost every part of my health is *mine*, and very little of it can be exchanged for something else without harming me.

In other words, a company like Amazon has two advantages over digital healthcare. It has huge resources and, if errors happen, it doesn't really matter because they can be easily fixed by financial compensation, if by nothing else. This makes most digital companies very misleading as inspiration for digital healthcare. In healthcare, with fewer resources, you'll have more bugs and more design problems, yet any error has far more serious consequences.

Without enormous investments, which would attract commensurate experience, skills, and qualifications, as well as more and more programmers, the few under-resourced programmers in digital healthcare desperately need competent mentors to open them up to modern programming techniques. This isn't a criticism of them, it's a very hard job, but they need mentors, training, or some other way to get better at safe, dependable programming at the sort of scale needed in healthcare.

Computers look after patients, even directly providing drugs and radiotherapy. Computer companies and hospital IT staff completely specify what computers should do. Healthcare would get a lot safer if IT standards and accountability were improved. Since errors often result in expensive litigation and compensation, improving IT and making IT liable would save healthcare a lot of money as well as making patients safer.

Aviation has improved, and is continually improving. Aviation started off as an exciting but deadly amateur sport when Orville and Wilbur Wright flew the first powered, heavier-than-air craft in 1903.

I think flying a plane in the 1930s was probably about as dangerous as being a patient is now.

The Wright brothers' first flight stalled, but the second flight at Kitty Hawk in 1903 was just 37 meters (120 feet). The 2001 Airbus A340-600 (figure 26.5) is 75 meters long (246 feet) and it can fly 14,500 km (9,000 miles) — a lot further than that first plane! The Airbus A340 is by no means the record holder, but when carrying a full load of over 400 passengers it has a range that's nearly 400,000 times further than the 1903 *Flyer* carrying just the pilot, Orville Wright. It's quite a thought that a modern plane is longer than the first successful powered flight! What's more, the A340 is unbelievably more reliable as well — in fact, what should have been the very first decent powered flight of the *Flyer* stalled after only three seconds.

The A340 and all other modern aircraft are engineered to be reliable because we all recognize that otherwise they'd be too risky to fly. Lives depend on the manufacturers feeling — and being held — accountable for getting safety right, and they do.

Nobody back in 1903 would have thought that "flying" would come to mean sipping wine, watching movies, and reclining in an armchair at 45,000 feet while moving at 600 miles an hour, ideally with a decent internet connection. Neither would the Wright brothers have dreamed that their tinkering with canvas, wire, and wood would transform into a worldwide industry of sophisticated supply chains, computer-aided design, wind tunnels, quality control systems, CRM, Air Traffic Control, loads of technical mathematics — and *loads* of serious regulations. The history of powered flight offers a visible maturing that has yet to occur in digital healthcare: if you could look at many of today's programs, they would seem as flimsy as the Wright brothers' *Flyer*.

———————————■———————————

It took about 70 years — coincidentally, the UK's National Health Service is 70 years old — to turn aviation into a professionally regulated and professionally engineered and very safe form of mass transport.

It's time digital healthcare started to catch up. Catching up will mean addressing culture from the law makers down to programmers and IT maintenance staff. It will take a while, but it will be worth it.

⓵ When you find bugs, don't just fix them. Work out *why* they happened, and improve the processes so that fewer bugs happen in the future.

Safety One thinking is about how we focus on human error and try to get less of it, whereas Safety Two thinking is about focusing on doing more of the right things.[h] Safety One and Two also work well with programming. Safety One is looking for the problems, testing programs, and trying to debug them. Safety Two is avoiding them — following **Correct by Construction** (CbC) practices.[i]

The programming hero Edsger Dijkstra famously said,

> Program testing can be used to show the presence of bugs, but never to show their absence![316]

In other words, just because you can't find a bug doesn't mean there aren't any. Perhaps your bug analysis is not good enough?

Drugs are the dominant treatment in healthcare, and they are tested with trials. We don't know how patients will respond, and we need to try out our drugs on a selection of patients in different circumstances to find out how effective or, maybe, how dangerous drugs are. Patients with other diseases, taking other treatments, or with different genetic makeup, can respond unpredictably.

Software is very different. In principle, we can be certain what it does under all circumstances; trials are necessary (think User Experience, User Centered Design) but not sufficient to establish that it is correct. Thinking — mathematical proof — is required.

If an error arises when several factors combine together, the chances of it being discovered even in a large trial may be vanishingly small. Trials may not last long enough to find all critical bugs. Mathematical proof, on the other hand, will find errors with certainty.

It turns out that mathematical proof is hard (even when computer tools help do it), so other methods are used as well.

Careful programmers will insert temporary, deliberate, subtle bugs to check that their code review processes can at least find some bugs. In fact, if you insert 10 bugs, but the quality control processes only find 9 of them, then you know some useful things about your review process — and you'll probably want to improve it!

Our normal Safety One thinking makes us worry about finding and fixing the bugs, whereas what we should be thinking is *why* did I get that bug — what am I doing wrong that allowed me to introduce or not spot that bug when I was programming it? Can I fix my approach, rather than fix one symptom at a time? Can I avoid the bugs?

Although it's a catastrophe when a building burns down, you don't test whether a building is fireproof by trying to set fire to it. That's Safety One thinking. Instead you *design* it to be fireproof; more precisely, since that isn't strictly possible, you design buildings to contain, limit, and hinder the spread of fire for as long as reasonably possible.

---

[h] See Chapter 12: Safety One & Safety Two, page 145 ←
[i] See Chapter 27: Correct by Construction, page 375 →

Rather than building programs and seeing if they work, you make sure they are well engineered first. That's Safety Two thinking for programmers. Formal Methods helps you do this.

This book emphasizes medical devices, from pacemakers to radiotherapy machines, because they are easier to understand and explain quickly, and I can easily simulate them accurately for research. Unfortunately, big systems that manage patient records and finances, and other complex things are much harder to explain the details of, but they also suffer from bugs. Typically, when the bugs are noticed in these large digital healthcare systems, thousands of people have been affected. Here are some examples:

- Reported in 2016: "Up to 300,000 heart patients may have been given wrong drugs or advice due to major NHS IT blunder" according to the newspapers.[383] The software, SystmOne, was developed by TPP, and is used in 2,500 GP surgeries. The problem occurred when SystemOne incorrectly filled in patient data to use a risk algorithm QRISK. GPs were left with the job of reviewing all the affected patients.[384]

- Reported in 2018: another TPP bug, this time which had remained undetected for three years, meant that 150,000 patients who had opted out of NHS data sharing had their preferences ignored — so their private medical data was then widely shared against their wishes. Although the NHS reassured patients that there was no risk to patient care, there is in practice no way to recover the shared data.[385]

- Reported in 2018: A bug in breast screening software affected up to 450,000 women aged 68 to 71 eligible for breast cancer screening checks. They did not get mammograms as a result of the error, and probably "shortened up to 270 lives" according to Jeremy Hunt the UK Secretary of State for Health and Social Care at the time. Worse (well, worse in the long run) the software was also being used for research,[386] so the bug has also interfered with the debate about whether breast screening (which may cause unnecessary operations) is effective. Interestingly, Hitachi says the problem was not with the software but with what the NHS asked the software to do.[387] That's exactly the sort of problem that Formal Methods can detect, and could have detected at the time the software was written: about ten years before the patients were affected by the missed bug.

The last incident has had a formal review, the *Independent Breast Screening Review*.[388] The review says that the IT systems broadly operated as they were designed to and that the errors were not caused by IT but by errors in using two separate and complicated systems. They say, "5,000 women were not invited for a final breast screening when they should have been because of manual errors in using the unwieldy IT systems to invite women, and a misalignment between a computer algorithm and the way women were being invited to screenings."

The *Independent Breast Screening Review* carries on: "the specific age range of women to be invited was not set out in sufficient detail." What responsible programmer would implement a healthcare system that was not specified properly; why didn't they double-check the specification against the requirements? And "no-one realised or checked that the 2013 Specification was compatible with the existing IT systems." Why not? It is as if everyone thinks IT systems work by magic and there is no need to do hard work to make them work. Moreover, the Review tries very hard to make it sound like the problem was not at least partly the IT itself — as if we cannot question the perfection of IT.

These are IT systems that were being developed since the 1980s. If there have been usability problems, there has been ample time to evaluate the problems and determine good fixes. The "errors in using the systems" are now errors in the design of the systems. The failure to notice that the specifications were incomplete is a failure of using Formal Methods: if the specification is incomplete or inconsistent, you cannot implement a correct program. Formal Methods would have detected this problem, and led to its resolution. In addition, standard practice for developing digital systems requires user interface evaluation and improvement: this clearly did not happen either.

The Review also shows that the systems were owned and overseen by several different organizations. There was no overarching oversight of how they interact and function as a system, so the basic steps such as Formal Methods and good user interface design fell between the cracks.

The *Independent Breast Screening Review* is practically an advert for the systematic approach to safety engineering that aviation uses.

We should program better so that digital healthcare gets safer, which is a Safety Two approach. **Formal Methods** is widely used in safety-critical industries, but not often enough in healthcare. Here's why Formal Methods is needed, and how it works.

27

Stories for developers

Years ago, when I could imagine I was the world's best C programmer (there weren't very many of us back in 1976), Professor Peter Landin — one of my heroes — asked me a simple question. Or so it seemed. It changed my life.

Most computer programs are thousands of lines long. A typical infusion pump — even a simple one — will have hundreds of thousands of lines of program code. The Mersey Burns app has about 15,000 lines of program code *and* that's not counting the code shared with other programs — called the "libraries" and "APIs" (application programmer interfaces, the cool name for libraries). The libraries and APIs are the standard code it relies on, but these are generally written by other people. APIs do things like send email — they provide features that lots of programs need, but there's no point reinventing the wheel and very likely introducing your own bugs to a problem that's been better solved and tested already.

Here's Peter's question … What does the simple program code shown in the box below do?

```
function f(n) {
  for( var i = 2; i < n; f(i++−1) );
  say("*");
}
```

A good programmer will be able to work out exactly what this code does without needing to run it on a computer: how many stars does it print for any value of n?

I've recast Peter's problem into one of the world's most popular programming languages, JavaScript.[389]

🐦 If you're not a programmer, just note how simple this question looks and how simple the program looks. This is a *tiny, tiny, tiny* program

Fix It: See and solve the problems of digital healthcare. Harold Thimbleby,
Oxford University Press. © Harold Thimbleby 2021.
DOI: 10.1093/oso/9780198861270.003.0027

only a few lines long, and it's a very basic question to ask. In comparison, real-world programs are *much* more complex and much more challenging to understand.

> 🔅 It is *very* hard to work out what this very short bit of program does.

> 🔅 If you *are* a programmer, please try answering Peter Landin's question. Try working it out — don't cheat and get a computer to work it out for you!

> 🔅 It's easy enough to work out what f(1) does, what does f(2) do, ... but what does f(n) do in general, for any n?

This deceptively simple problem makes a profound point: if only a few lines of code are so hard to understand, how hard to understand will a typical digital health program of thousands of lines be? And if it's hard to understand, how hard will it be to debug and get right? Nearly impossible.

Therefore we urgently need to increase programming skills in healthcare if we want to have a chance of understanding and managing the risks in digital healthcare. In particular, we needs skills to use computer tools to help us program — programming is too hard to do unaided.

Unfortunately most programmers are unable to work out what this very simple, brief, code does. Or why. This means there are probably many parts of their *real* more complex programs that they do not understand, and which therefore must be deemed unreliable. Most programs are written by teams of programmers. Most programmers have *no idea* what anyone else's code does. \par Have you any idea what my little program does? (The answer is here.[390])

Here's another scary thing. If the word "**var**" is omitted in the code above (or the names "f," "n," or "i" were misspelled), the program will still compile and run happily, but it will do something completely different. *The computer will not notice any such errors*!

JavaScript's failure to help spot errors is one reason why healthcare systems should *never* use JavaScript, because it is hopeless for helping to write safe programs.

Mersey Burns is written in JavaScript. I explored a few of the Mersey Burns app's bugs earlier.[a] To be positive: JavaScript is quick and easy to program in, so if Mersey Burns hadn't used JavaScript we might still be waiting for it. The problem, of course, is to get the right balance between speed and safety, and between seeing Mersey Burns as an exciting and stimulating prototype and as a final, polished product safe for large-scale deployment.

JavaScript isn't the only unreliable and unsafe programming language by a long way, as we shall soon see.

---

[a] See Chapter 10: Mersey Burns app, page 121 ←

Programmers make mistakes they don't notice, just like when I wrote this book I made many spelling mistakes and typos I didn't notice. Fortunately, I worked with careful reviewers and proofreaders who found lots I'd missed.

The Heartbleed bug is a famous story. Heartbleed affected key internet software called OpenSSL, and allowed hackers to access credit card numbers, emails, and other personal data. There was a brief window in April 2014 between the developers admitting there was a bug and people getting their systems fixed — about 17% of the internet's secure web servers were affected. Because of the central role of OpenSSL in internet infrastructure, the scale of the problem was phenomenal. In the six-hour window after the bug announcement, the bug had already led to the Canada Revenue Agency (Canadian tax authorities) losing 600 taxpayers' social security numbers to hackers. A few months later, in August 2014, Community Health Systems — the second-biggest hospital chain in the US — admitted that Heartbleed had enabled hackers to steal security keys from them, compromising 4.5 million patient records.[391]

How did it happen? Robin Seggelmann was a programmer working on OpenSSL, core internet software, back in 2011. He made a trivial typing mistake, which has been famously compared to misspelling Mississippi. He didn't notice that he'd enabled hackers to cause chaos by, as it were, paddling up the wrong river.

There are several astonishing issues here. OpenSSL is about 500,000 lines of code. It is central software used all over the internet. It was being maintained by two volunteer programmers, one of whom was Robin Seggelmann. Overworked volunteers missed this bug for several years. The scary thing is the combination of problems: two volunteers won't be able to spot bugs very quickly, and there is a very large world of hackers out there who are highly motivated to find and exploit bugs. The real mystery is that so little went wrong. Unless we change how we develop software, one day soon we won't be so lucky.

Prof Matthew Green, a cryptographer at Johns Hopkins University, is reported as saying about Heartbleed:[392]

> We have standards for coding in mission-critical systems like the airline industry, but I'm not sure we would want those standards applied everywhere. Such strict standards require programmers to spend significantly more time testing their work — and neither technology companies nor consumers can stomach such delays. I don't think we want to wait 20 years for the next Google and Facebook.

Green's comments about Google and Facebook may seem pretty reasonable. It's a common attitude, after all, but the attitude explains why digital healthcare is so risky. Most healthcare programmers don't know how to work to the sorts of high standards expected in other industries like aviation.[393]

Part II ◇ Treatment ◇ Finding solutions

Would you rather wait "20 years" for something safe, or have something new and exciting tomorrow that, well, maybe isn't as safe as it should be? Of course, the airline industry is different, because lots of people's lives depend on safe programs in airplanes ... so the real problem is that we don't realize, or don't acknowledge, that lots of lives depend on having safe digital healthcare.

Robin Seggelmann's typo got missed — he didn't spot his error, nor did his colleagues until much later. But programmers should not just be relying on humans to check their programming. When programming, the computer itself should also help spot errors. We saw above that JavaScript does not do a very good job of spotting spelling errors; in fact, it just makes things worse by doing unexpected things.

OpenEMR is one very popular patient management system, used by many GP surgeries and hospitals to manage treatment for patients, as well as do administration and finance. It is downloaded about 7,000 times a month. It's used worldwide, from Kenya to the US. In 2018, the cybersecurity group called Project Insecurity found 30 bugs that put at risk the data of 100 million patients worldwide.[394] At the time of writing this book, bug fixes had been released and shared with many — but not all — OpenEMR users. Open-EMR is written in the programming language PHP. PHP is *much* worse than JavaScript.[395]

Here are two examples illustrating how PHP works:

⬥ Healthcare systems need to check numbers. So a program might check that a number x is equal to ten, say, which it would do by writing x==10. Except that in PHP this is always false, even if x is exactly ten (you'd expect x==10 to be true if x was equal to ten) — the problem is, it should have been written $x==10, with a dollar, for it to work correctly.

⬥ If I wrote "$x = 1; echo $x" in PHP, the variable x would first be set to 1, and then its value would be printed, namely PHP would say "1." That seems clear enough, but if I missed out the dollar in the echo, nothing at all would be printed — it just wouldn't work.

In both cases, missing out the dollar sign is an error — perhaps because of a simple typo or spelling mistake — but PHP does not notice and warn me. A safe programming language would complain and stop anyone using a program with such a critical spelling mistake in it.

Amazingly, PHP has a feature, written with just an @ sign, which a programmer can use to force it to *ignore* errors! This feature encourages programmers to write programs that may have errors in them, and just to ignore the errors. This feature certainly saves a lot of time programming, as it completely saves thinking about errors or what to do with them, but it's asking for trouble.

Ironically, you might type @ by mistake and never notice.

It is amazing that the PHP programming language is designed to *encourage* silencing errors, and astonishing that it would then be chosen as an appropriate programming language for any safety-critical systems in healthcare.

I wonder if the programmers who wrote OpenEMR, which, as we discussed above, uses PHP, wrote a computer program to check that @ was *never* used? There are, of course, many other things such a useful program could do to help catch bugs and generally improve quality while it's at it — in contrast, programming languages like SPARK Ada cannot be used without highly developed static analysis tools, so they are much safer.

Far, far, worse than either JavaScript or PHP is the programming language MUMPS,[396] the programming language underpinning many of the world's major healthcare systems. MUMPS underlies Allscripts, EMIS, Epic, and VistA healthcare systems, and many more.

Epic is arguably *the* dominant digital healthcare system,[397] — handling about 200 million patients around the world. The largest digital healthcare system inside the US is VistA, short for the Veterans Health Information Systems and Technology Architecture. VistA is used by about 200,000 staff in 1,000 hospitals, clinics, and nursing homes, managing nearly 10 million patients. It's the US Department of Veterans Affairs (VA) system.

However good a programmer you are, MUMPS allows, no, it *encourages*, errors that it does not help detect. There is a vicious circle: if you use an "easy" language, like PHP or MUMPS, you can recruit cheaper, less competent programmers to work on your systems, and your problems rapidly escalate.

Programs often have to know when something is true; for example, is it true that the user operating the drug dispensing cabinet has an authorized identity? Are they allowed to get drugs out of the cabinet?

In MUMPS, a programmer would write something like

if authorized ...

to test the user's authorization. However if the programmer typed, say, 'if authorised" (with an s) or "if uthorized" (without an a) by mistake the test would not work correctly when the program was used. MUMPS would not notice the typo. More confusingly, if by some slip the programmer just wrote "if," that is, missing out what to test altogether, MUMPS would happily, and silently, use the value of a quirky variable called $test instead. What $test means depends on things done earlier in the program, and it's not very likely the programmer — especially if this is a new programmer joining the team to add code — has much idea what it means. In my view, what MUMPS has done is turn an error into a feature that programmers think is cool, but in reality undermines the safety of the language.

Program tests themselves should always use the values true and false only; nothing else makes sense. However, MUMPS allows *anything*, con-

Part II ◇ Treatment ◇ Finding solutions

verting numbers and strings into true and false following quirky rules of its own. This means that if a programmer makes a mistake, for instance saying **x** instead of **x=0** (is the number equal to zero?), then MUMPS will be completely happy — but do something unexpected. The trouble is that the unexpected, unwanted things MUMPS does *may* be good enough when the program is tested, but may cause a disaster years later.

Here's another way of putting it. Let's carefully check our member of staff knows the correct password to prove they are authorized to take drugs out of the drug cabinet. The correct MUMPS program might say something like

if password="26jumble" ...

but if the programmer misses out a bit, say, writing

if "26jumble" ...

then it will *always* succeed, even though it's nonsense, and regardless of the password the user actually uses.

You might think that is an unlikely error, but with any large enough program this sort of error *will* happen. Systems like Epic are millions of lines of program code, and they are written and maintained by thousands of programmers. One day, one of them will make a mistake, perhaps not understanding exactly what's going on somewhere else in the program — perhaps not even realizing they don't understand.

Silent errors can lie around in a program for years. Who knows what they do? Would clinicians using the MUMPS program notice and realize "their" errors were actually caused by the program? Would the investigators of an incident blame the program and not the "responsible" clinicians?

Putting it more charitably, if a company using MUMPS tries to make safe changes to any program, they will take a long time working out what's going on and how to change it safely — so they will just change it and have to hope for the best. The advantage of being able to write programs quickly thus becomes a serious problem when the shortcuts taken by earlier programmers become unfathomable.

It's a problem recognized by calling it **write-only programming**. Nobody is expected to be able to read and understand write-only programming, and it's often easier to start again and leave old bits of program untouched. Gradually programs collect more and more additions, with nobody ever daring to fix anything in case "fixing" ruins everything else. Write-only programming is a shout of exasperation: "I don't understand this write-only programming! It wasn't written to be read" This is the road to **software rot**, as the problems just get worse and worse over time.

The common problem with JavaScript, PHP, and MUMPS is that the programming languages have tried hard to be concise and quick to use. This

> **Box 27.1.** Epic's daylight saving and Y2K
>
> Twice a year those of us who don't live near the equator change daylight saving, where clocks are changed by an hour to help increase the amount of daylight people have during working hours. The idea was originally proposed in the nineteenth century by George Hudson. It's not a new idea.
>
> Carol Hawthorne-Johnson, a nurse in California, says her hospital doesn't shut down their Epic system during the time change, which means that any patient data entered into Epic between 1 am and 2 am is deleted when the clocks change.[398] An hour's worth of record-keeping "is gone," she says.
>
> Dr Mark Friedberg, is quoted by *USA Today* saying[398] "It's mind-boggling. In 2018, we expect electronics to handle something as simple as a time change. I shudder to think," he said. "What does it do with leap years?"
>
> I wrote about this mess way back in 1991.[399] How is it still a problem when, thousands of years ago, Julius Cæsar sorted out leap years. What we now call 46 BC went down in history as the "last year of confusion." That optimism now looks rather premature!
>
> Problems that get sorted out in the world don't always get sorted out in the digital world. The Year 2000 (Y2K) problem took this to a new height;[a] without a huge worldwide effort, many computer systems would've had problems at the turn of the millennium, on New Year's Day 2000. The problem was that years earlier, nobody had thought computers would work that long, and very few programmers thought to make their software robust enough to survive the date change safely (or possibly managers didn't allow their programmers to spend the time to program more reliably).[400] The year 2000 was hardly unexpected, yet it was a widespread bug. Many of the problems in digital healthcare creep up on us in ways that are very much harder to anticipate.
>
> ---
> [a] See Chapter 4: Millennium Bug (Y2K problem), page 33 ←

makes them popular with many programmers, and soon many useful programs are written in these languages, and then the easiest way to program anything starts off by building on the vast libraries of resources. Thus the community of programmers grows.

Yet none of the languages were designed to be safe. They are unsuitable for healthcare use. I've called such programming languages **heedless**,[401] since they just make programming unsafe, however good the programmers that use them try to be.

MUMPS started life in the 1960s, when it was at the time, arguably, doing a good job with what primitive equipment was available, but now it has left a prehistoric legacy to everything it supports.

Since the 1960s, safe programming has improved beyond recognition. Unfortunately, too few healthcare programmers have caught up with current best practice in safe programming — there are thousands of healthcare programmers caught up in having to program in PHP, JavaScript, and MUMPS to keep old systems working, who haven't had a chance to learn any better.

For a start, unlike JavaScript, PHP, and MUMPS, most modern programming languages require **declarations**, where the programmer has to "declare" they are going to use certain names in their program, like x. If they make a typo and write a name like **xx** by mistake that won't have been declared, then their program cannot even be run: the computer points out the mistake to them so they have to correct it before the program can be run. MUMPS, PHP, and JavaScript do not require declarations, so they cannot even detect such simple typos or help the programmer be safer.

Better modern languages further require names to be **strongly typed**, so that you can't accidentally mix chalk and cheese — I also covered type checking briefly earlier, as it's such a fundamental idea.[b] Strong typing is a bit like requiring every word in this book to be correctly spelled English, and only used in grammatical English sentences — just telling the computer this would pick up more errors that might otherwise have been missed and led to confusion for you, the reader.

For example, with a modern typed language, you cannot accidentally mix up a number and a truth value. While JavaScript and other programmers might find this tedious, it *stops* a wide range of unnoticed errors ever happening. It improves safety, and it's a slight burden on the programmer that is worth it to eliminate bugs.

To go back to my example of trying to get the words in this book spelled right: obviously, I used a computerized spell-checker to check the words were correctly spelled. That's a bit like declaring all my words I use in the book, and the computer automatically checking they are valid English words. In fact, I used the computer *and* human proofreaders to help review this book.

In JavaScript and similar languages, you can do what you like, because they aren't typed like this. Being free from types seems superficially very flexible and convenient, which it sort of is. But if you want to write safe programs — as we need to in healthcare — it's asking for trouble. It's asking for trouble you won't notice until something goes wrong.

It's far better, if you want safe programs, that is, as we surely do in healthcare, to use programming languages that are strict and require declarations and types and assertions and other safeguards — like, for this book, strict proofreaders worried about that what I wrote made good sense in English.[402] Furthermore, we want to move as many checks from run time (for instance, assertions) to compile time — while it's obviously useful to detect errors in a running program when assertions fail, it's even better that programs that may be faulty are never run in the first place.

---

[b] See Chapter 21: Programming with types, page 282 ←

Fortunately, there are much better programming languages available than JavaScript, PHP, and MUMPS, and their friends.[403]

One of the more practical and reliable approaches is to use a system called SPARK Ada. SPARK Ada incorporates Formal Methods and is designed to catch errors, and to stop you writing programs that are badly designed. It is used widely in the aviation industry — because people's lives depend on safe software. It's a great shame it isn't used widely in healthcare — note that you can also write medical apps in it, as it will run on mobile devices.

Another programming language to use is MISRA C (or MISRA C++), which is a safer version of C that is widely used in the car industry. Imagine that you want to program anti-skid brakes; you'll want them to be very reliable to avoid car accidents. MISRA C was developed by the Motor Industry Software Reliability Association (MISRA) to ensure car software is safer than C (and similar languages) can achieve alone. In MISRA C, any programs with simple errors like I've just described above would be rejected and would not even be allowed to be run. It is a much safer way to program. Healthcare doesn't have any equivalent to MISRA to help make digital healthcare safer. Yet.

Indeed, there is much work going on to make safer programming languages. Rust is a new programming language that has been under development for over a decade, and it's starting to become very popular because of its nice balance between safety and flexibility, which programmers like. There's an excellent introductory article on Rust,[404] which I recommend you read because it describes the problems of bad programming that Rust solves — you should about know all these problems, even if you never want to use Rust. However, using Rust (and any of Rust's ideas) would be a huge improvement over conventional digital health programming. A salutary point in the article is that programming safely poses fundamental research questions that are still being addressed — in other words, *any* digital health programming is pushing the boundaries of safety, and one should be extremely careful whatever language you use.

To be realistic, there are all sorts of practical constraints that limit the choice of programming language. In digital healthcare, it's very common that some complex machinery, such as an MRI machine, needs to be controlled and the hardware or, rather, the hardware manufacturers, limit the languages that it can be programmed in. Training programming teams to use new languages is another problem. Or there's a huge, existing, code base that won't work with a new language. In these cases, in fact in all cases, a wise approach is to outline a specification of what the system does in another language, such as Alloy,[405] to explore its design, correctness and safety. By using a formal specification language, you can explore "the big picture" of the program's safety whether or not you use a safer programming language.

It is a bit beyond the scope of this book to explain in detail why MISRA C, SPARK Ada, and Rust are so much better.[406] These programming languages

> **Box 27.2.** Never events and good programming
>
> The healthcare ideas of **never events** and **always conditions** correspond to some important Formal Methods ideas in programming.
>
> **Safety properties** describe things that must never happen; they are theoretical properties that should be proved of programs. For example, if a nurse enters a drug dose to an infusion pump, the pump will never deliver a higher dose.
>
> In contrast, Always Conditions correspond to **liveness properties**. Again, these are theoretic properties that a program must always have. For example, when the `Off` button is pressed twice the device will *always* stop doing whatever it is doing.

are aspects of a programming style called **Correct by Construction** (CbC) – avoid problems in the first place, rather than trying to test and debug to get rid of problems.

People who know SPARK Ada or Rust will also know fifteen other excellent ways of programming; choosing the language itself isn't the only solution. But, here's the thing: if you don't know at least one good approach like MISRA C or SPARK, you should not be programming in digital healthcare, because *your programs will be unavoidably unreliable.* And, as I've emphasized throughout this book, we don't notice our own errors, so a key problem is that you have no idea how unreliable your programs really are. Indeed, almost all programmers are over-confident and have little idea how buggy their own programs are.

I think there are obvious reasons why Formal Methods are good, but those reasons don't necessarily mean that Formal Methods help make safer systems *in practice*. Do Formal Methods work in industry? I reality perhaps too complex for Formal Methods?

As a matter of fact, people have been researching the impact of Formal Methods, and the evidence is that it works very well.

The quality of a program can be estimated by counting bugs, and the standard measure is to count bugs per thousand lines of program code, known as **defects per kLoC** (k here meaning kilo, one thousand). Very good software developers can get down to maybe 10 to 30 defects per kLoC. However, using Formal Methods and CbC methods, one can get down to 0.1 per kLoC *in the same time*. Of course, not all bugs should be counted equally — some are life-critical, some are just a nuisance, some are found quickly, and some may lie dormant for years[407] — so counting or estimating numbers of bugs per kLoC, then, can't be the whole story. What Formal Methods clearly does very usefully is help reduce bugs (and hence the risks to patients) to very low levels, but, crucially, it is a different sort of tool that helps find — and eliminate — bugs that human programmers won't find unaided. Just on that basis,

Formal Methods ought to be required for all digital health development: it works and it complements human programmers.

———————◾———————

The bit of JavaScript program I showed at the start of this chapter[c] is easily translated from JavaScript into the programming language C; it's virtually the same thing, like writing in a different dialect. Interestingly, MISRA C, the safe version of C, will not even let you try my example program at all. Whereas I found it difficult to think about what it does, MISRA C went further and decided that if it's *that* difficult, then it should not even be used. That's how a safety system like MISRA C can help make better and safer systems.

Sensible systems like MISRA C protect us from ourselves.[408]

A long, long time ago, a long time at least in computer terms, Tony Hoare gave a speech to accept his 1980 Turing Award, the Computer Science version of the Nobel Prize. In his speech he famously criticized the bad practices many programmers slip into:[165]

> I note with fear and horror that even in 1980, language designers and [programmers] have not learned this lesson [to check the correctness of their programming]. In any respectable branch of engineering, failure to observe such elementary precautions would have long been against the law.

In the decades since then, programming has become much easier, and it's now far more powerful than in Hoare's 1980. Unfortunately, while programming is easier, programming *safely* has become very much harder. Most people who design programming languages prefer power over safety, and sadly this makes it even harder for programmers to program safely.

Here's a typical example.

Let's say we want to look up a number in a table; to be specific, we want to use a patient's age to look up their risk of having a Down syndrome baby — a serious issue we've already talked about.[d]

In many programs, risk data would be stored in a table called something like dataTable. Each entry in the table is then accessed by writing dataTable[1], dataTable[2], and so on, to look at individual table entries. If a patient is 20 years old, their risk would be found in dataTable[20]. Probably the details would be different — for example, the table might be indexed by weeks instead of years — but this level of detail isn't important for our discussion.

Here is the fundamental tension:

🄐 If you want programming to be *easy*, you will want power, flexibility, and lots of options and choices. So you might use the programming

---

[c] See Chapter 27: Peter Landin's mystery code, page 367 ←
[d] See Chapter 4: Millennium Bug (Y2K problem) and Down syndrome tragedy, page 34 ←

language Python (to take another very popular healthcare programming language to task), which allows you to count from either end of a table, instead of restricting you to one end. So, in Python, dataTable[1] is entry 1, but dataTable[−1] is entry 1 *from the other end.* This may be a convenient feature if you need it, but it means that the accidental error of looking up a negative value in the table is something the programming language accepts as perfectly valid — but it won't mean what you expect.

🔊 If you want programming to be **robust**, forgiving of errors, you want errors to be ignored and for the program to carry on running. So you might use JavaScript, which is a more robust language. If you look up dataTable[−1] in JavaScript, you get the "value" undefined. However, the program carries on running as if nothing has happened, and anything you do with undefined carries on as if it makes sense. You might want to warn the patient if the risk is larger than 0.8, say, which you'd naturally do by writing if(dataTable[i] > 0.9) .... Unfortunately, as JavaScript works, it's false that undefined is greater than 0.9, so the program probably goes wrong — and it goes wrong completely silently, so nobody knows that it's gone wrong.

🔊 If you want programming to be *reliable and dependable*, that is much harder. Every feature that makes a language seem easier, more powerful, and flexible, is also a feature that gives accidental and unintended meanings to your errors. So you don't want cunning features; you want strictness and pedantry. Your boss will think you are a slower programmer, and at the same time your programs will seem to do less. Your programming language is stricter and harder to use, and you have to plan more carefully. Dependable programming *is* difficult.

There is a tension here with **Agile**, an extremely popular approach to quick-and-dirty programming. Agile has been systematized into a whole approach encouraging changing and adapting things quickly and being responsive to customer or user needs.[409]

Agile requires you to build quickly, fail quickly, and improve. Facebook's motto (up to 2014) used to be "Move Fast and Break Things" — a hacker rallying cry that prioritized rapid product development and evolution over everything else.[410] Push out products. If they work, great. If they don't work, learn, update, and push out another version. But at all costs stay ahead in the market. Agile makes things fast, but at the expense of ignoring creating problems on the way to getting there. Agile works for Facebook because its products don't directly harm people if they go wrong. Agile works for Amazon because if something goes wrong, they can send you some credit or send another parcel.

Agile means that developers quickly prototype something, try it out, and improve it — although experimental and iterative design are good ideas regardless of Agile. Despite its popularity in consumer and business systems, Agile is unsuited to healthcare. Agile does not work for healthcare because "Move Fast and Break Things" means it is likely that something will go wrong that might cause somebody irrecoverable harm before you have a chance to improve anything. I make it a rule:

> 🔒 Agile and similar methods are inappropriate for digital healthcare development.

More specifically: Agile is fine for non-critical software, but for anywhere that may have an impact on patients or staff health or welfare, Agile is not appropriate. Inside of healthcare, Agile can be a disaster because systems are used before they are polished, and this is likely to cause problems. Outside of critical areas like healthcare, Agile is fine: it makes developers competitive, racing to provide new features.

In contrast to Agile, Formal Methods requires you to plan carefully, and makes it harder to change, since change can introduce errors with unforeseen consequences. Formal Methods means "build thoughtfully and don't fail." In contrast, Agile celebrates change and adaptation, so *accidental* changes — errors — are hard to manage. Formal Methods are designed to stop accidental change, so the resulting systems are much more reliable. They are different philosophies, with very different benefits. I'll discuss resources for reading about programming at greater length later, including the idea of **flexibility**, which makes Agile easier *and more reliable* to implement.[e]

We ought to be regulating digital healthcare as seriously as equally critical areas of engineering (like aviation, building, radiation, gas, or electricity), just as Hoare said we should. Unless and until regulators start requiring digital safety, reliability and dependability in healthcare won't happen because everyone is too keen on programming being easy and exciting rather than safe.

———————————————■———————————————

When Peter Landin asked me what the program code I showed you at the beginning of this chapter does, my first answer was wrong.

I naïvely thought: "simple program, simple answer."

How wrong I was!

Peter then challenged me to work it out properly. So I spent all that evening on the problem. Finally I got it right (I was young and naïve then; I can do it much faster now). The next day, I met Peter, and I showed him my solution. He then told me how to approach the problem better — my solution wasn't as good as his elegant answer which was *obviously* right, and moreover was obviously a good way of solving many programming problems.

---

[e] See Chapter 33: If you are a developer, page 484 →

My approach really only worked with the particular program; it gave me the right answer but, unlike Peter's answer, it didn't help with solving problems with other, different programs. Put another way: I solved the problem using math, whereas Peter solved the problem using *Methods*, Formal Methods.

It takes a few minutes to do a job well if you know how. It was a formative moment in my career: simple-looking programs are not simple! Now I believe in Formal Methods. What's more, when I write programs, I always put assertions and other rules in them.[f] Just in case I've made a mistake, I always want the computer to help block or help me find my errors. Well ... except when I am over-confident. The trouble is, I never notice when I've fallen into the trap of being over-confident. I usually find out too late. Which is why we need teamwork and all the other help we can get.

I had thought of ending this chapter with a helpful list of programming languages and tools that I would warn you off or that I would recommend. There certainly are unsafe languages to avoid in healthcare (like C, C++, JavaScript, PHP, ...), whereas SPARK Ada is very good. Unfortunately, I don't know what you're trying to do — what you want for an entertainment system will be different from what you want for an MRI scanner or from a telephone exchange. Instead of having a list from me, whenever a programming language or tool is going to be used, make sure there is a professional justification that the choice is safe and appropriate to use for the intended purpose. Make sure the language is well defined and has tools to support its effective and efficient use too. Don't forget that programming languages are a fashion industry, with all the corresponding emotional pressures on us to buy into the latest fashion just to keep the industry going. Remember: digital healthcare (and all the patients and staff depending on it) deserves better, something more thoughtful, than the latest fad.

---

[f] See Chapter 21: Assertions, page 291 ←

Although it helps everything else, Formal Methods isn't enough on its own. Thorough testing is essential to ensure things really work well, especially when things are going to be used in complex environments like healthcare.

28

Finding bugs

Often, programs are tested and demonstrated by people who know what the program is supposed to do, so many bugs are not uncovered — most bugs hit you when you do something the programmer hadn't anticipated.

A famous example of this is when Grete Fossbakk lost a lot of money from her bank account in 2007.

Here's how it happened. Grete Fossbakk used her bank's user interface to try to transfer some money to her daughter. Unfortunately, Grete double-pressed a 0 key, resulting in a longer account number than the correct number for her daughter's account. This number was too long, so it was automatically made shorter, thus obtaining another number. Unfortunately, this number was a valid account number.

Thinking she had keyed the correct number, Grete confirmed the money transfer, despite it actually being to a differently named account. The person who inadvertently received the money was eventually sentenced to prison, but this did nothing to help Grete get her money back — which the lucky chap had already spent.

Grete lost about 500,000 Norwegian krone (which is around $75,000 or £50,000 — a lot of money to lose) because the bad banking system allowed her to type an incorrect bank account number *without blocking her error or warning her.*[55] This is the same sort of failure to help the user we've found in lots of digital healthcare systems. The bank's system must have looked fine to all of the developers who made it, but they'd overlooked a serious problem — which cost Grete a lot of money.

I used a made-up account number in the table (figure 28.1) to make it clear how the problem happened.[411]

The problem is that digital systems can *look* fine, and even do well in user testing, but unfortunately this is misleading: the developers might still have overlooked testing for erroneous user input such as Grete made, or many other forms of error. It's a surprising oversight for a bank to make.

Fix It: See and solve the problems of digital healthcare. Harold Thimbleby, Oxford University Press. © Harold Thimbleby 2021.
DOI: 10.1093/oso/9780198861270.003.0028

Grete Fossbakk's daughter's bank account number. This is the number that Grete intended to type.	87408455566
What Grete actually typed, including an accidental extra 0 digit. I've arrowed the extra digit for clarity. You can also see the incorrect number is now too long.	874008455566 ↑
Instead of blocking the obvious error and warning Grete, the bank just silently ignored the final digit, "correcting" the number into an unrelated but, unfortunately, valid account number for someone else.	87400845556

Figure 28.1. Explaining Grete Fossbakk's bank's mistake. Unfortunately, Grete's typing error was ignored by the bank's computer. Instead of detecting and blocking the error, so Grete could correct it, the bank instead ignored the error. The bank didn't tell her it had changed the number she had typed. Grete then unwittingly transferred money to the wrong account. (All the bank account numbers are just for illustrative purposes.)

I had a look at my own digital bank account, many years after Grete had been caught out, and my bank account still has the same bug. I don't use the same bank as Grete did; this is a general banking problem across the sector. Banks can blame customers for making mistakes that are caused by their programs. I won't tell you my own bank account details, but you can try yours. In other words, anyone today could make an error like Grete made, and still some bank websites won't notice or block it.

A similar error in 2019 lost Peter Teich £193,000 when a sort code was mistyped. Surprisingly, Barclays Bank have several customers with the same account numbers but different sort codes, yet their computer systems do not have redundant checks (such as checking the names match as well as the account numbers). Given that Barclays Bank must know that they have duplicate account numbers, this failure to manage predictable errors seems astonishing. The lucky recipient refused to refund the money, and the bank, even after being notified of the error, allowed them to dishonestly withdraw £193,000, which has now disappeared.[412]

It seems the industry isn't testing code very well, and it isn't using Formal Methods to mathematically specify and check its programs. (More specifically, it isn't using Formal Methods to specify and check a bank's user interface.) Perhaps management thinks a banking system is finished because it looks OK, so why waste more money on testing it? Or they aren't collecting data on how their system is actually used and using the data and real use errors to help improve it. Perhaps the bank did do a cost-benefit analysis on further testing, in which case one could argue that with better programming the testing would be cheaper, and therefore more cost-effective. It looks like

> **Box 28.1.** Don't use bad programming languages
>
> Here is a little bit of program, written in JavaScript:
>
> alert(parseFloat("40.5"));
>
>
>
> There are three steps to this program:
> 1. **"40.5"**   The string of characters 4, 0, dot, then 5.
> 2. **parseFloat**   What is the numerical value of those characters?
> 3. **alert**   Tell the user the value.
>
> The standard JavaScript function **parseFloat** converts the keys you typed into a number, which should of course have the value 40.5. Indeed, the code above will say 40.5 here, as you expect.[55]
>
> It *looks* very easy: the user keyed 40.5 and you've got 40.5. Unfortunately, it's likely that the programmer has overlooked subtleties.
>
> Suppose the user enters "40.5 mcg"; that is, the user specifies the units, micrograms, too. Did the programmer remember to check for that? No. The standard JavaScript code inside **parseFloat** *does not notice*. You will get the same result if the user types mg (milligrams) or kg (kilograms) or even lbs (pounds). None report the error: that important units are being ignored.
>
> You can run this code on a computer and try entering your own imaginative input; the notes at the end of this book give more details on how to do this.[413]
>
> In short, the standard JavaScript code **parseFloat** is a disaster if you want to have a safe program. And if something so fundamental is a disaster, what else is going to go wrong when you use other standard features in a larger program? There is no easy way for a programmer to protect against such built-in bugs. JavaScript should never be used in healthcare.

a head-in-the-sand approach has certainly saved higher development costs too. It's a conflict of interest that shouldn't happen — testing should be done independently and more realistically; it needs a bit of randomization, too, to think out of the box and avoid the developers' preconceptions of what might need testing and how.

Possibly, the developers did use Formal Methods, but they didn't use it on how their program read account numbers. It's likely they used some standard program to read numbers, and they just assumed it worked properly. Uncovering such assumptions is exactly why good testing is required. The testing has to cover what happens "end to end" and not just the bit of code you wrote. It has to cover everything — just as it would be used in the real world by people like Grete Fossbakk.

The trouble is, too many programmers skimp these important things, so their programs end up not being reliable enough for healthcare. Unfortunately, it's very easy to conceal bad programming from managers and hospitals until it's too late — accidentally or deliberately. *Real* programming is very hard, and Formal Methods, and programming languages such as SPARK Ada and similar tools, are a very important *part* of the solution, but companies most likely want to be quick-to-market more than they want to provide high-quality solutions. Since everybody works like this, nobody realizes it is lowering quality across the board. It's a recipe for problems.

Programs must be correct, but they also have to work well for their users. Just because the program is "correct," even if you can prove it is correct, does not mean it *is* correct. You might, for instance, be doing the wrong thing correctly. Correctness as such does not show that a program works correctly in a medical context and is safe and helpful with patients. Just as programming needs code review,[a] Formal Methods, the mathematical specification of the task, also need review. Some of the people reviewing the formal specifications need to come from other disciplines as well, so that there is real input from nurses and others who will use the systems — they will be doing complicated things that the programmers working on their own won't really understand.

Code review supplements Formal Methods. I am surprised how rarely developers make tools to help them do code review systematically.

For example, it's easy to work out all the screens or displays the software can generate, check them off, and record which screens have been correct. When the software is edited, which screens have been changed and need checking again? In principle, that's a very easy question to answer *if* you have a tool to help do it, and *if* you built a program that knows what screens it can generate. If you don't have a tool, then errors will slip through. And if you're writing programs that can't work out all the screens they can display, then that could be worrying.

The lesson that digital healthcare should learn is the fact that something looks great, works (at least up until this moment in time), and even has been tested, means next to nothing. Testing alone is unreliable, and certainly, testing in the lab — although better than nothing — is unreliable and usually misleading. Bugs sometimes take years to surface and affect users, and manufacturers rapidly give up on testing, and then just ship their products and leave it to the rest of us to find the bugs for them.

Formal Methods is not something that can be learned in five minutes, and most programmers will deny they need to use it. Look at all the successful things they have programmed — they didn't use Formal Methods then, so why (they argue) should they need Formal Methods now?

If you are going to be given an infusion, or connected to a ventilator, or given radiotherapy from a linear accelerator, can you — or anyone else — *prove* the program works? Can you prove it is always possible to stop it? Can you prove it will never deliver an overdose? Can you prove it will detect use errors (when users accidentally key in out of range numbers)?

---

[a] See Chapter 20: Code review, page 273 ←

If you can't prove it works, your only reason to believe it is reliable is that when you tested it you found no (or no critical) bugs. But how do you know your testing covered all the possibilities? If some bug is caused by an oversight, how do you know your testing doesn't suffer from the same oversight? How can your testing find types of bugs you don't even know are there?

The answer is to prove your program is correct, which you do through Formal Methods. (You also want to prove your testing covers the relevant parts of the program — **coverage** being a technical problem that should be done rigorously.)

It's important to understand some of the benefits of Formal Methods. Ordinary testing helps improve products and should always be used, but Formal Methods is more thorough at what it does, and it's *much* faster.

Let's say we are using Formal Methods with the banking system that Grete used. Typically there would be a library of standard design properties to check, but a good one might be:

> Pressing the delete key deletes one character of user input
> AND only the delete key deletes input
> AND if there is nothing to delete, it beeps.

... though it would be expressed more mathematically. The notes at the back of the book give ideas for more such properties, and show how to use them to ensure infusion pumps are safe.[414]

Proving a program is correct is difficult, so people usually use computer tools to do it — another aspect of resilience. There are many tools that can help. A Formal Methods tool, given the bank's program to check and the property summarized above, would report that if a user keys more than 8 digits in some parts of the user interface, then some digits get lost — and not because of the delete key being used, but because of a design bug. Formal Methods can report that bug in seconds, but to find it by testing with users would take ages and perhaps it would never be encountered. Not finding a bug during testing never means there isn't a bug!

It's worth noting that as more work is done with Formal Methods, the library of useful things to check gets enlarged with more issues. For example, if UCD testing finds that users often get dates muddled (say, getting month and day number swapped out of order), then these issues can be expressed in a way so that the Formal Methods tool can check the system handles these problems appropriately *everywhere*. In a second, Formal Methods can generalize a UCD insight which, had it continued under conventional UCD investigation, would have taken centuries.

Programmers of digital healthcare should use Formal Methods. The regulators should insist on seeing their homework, and seeing their "working." My teachers used to ask to see my working; I might have what looks like the right answer, but if I don't understand how I got there, perhaps I don't un-

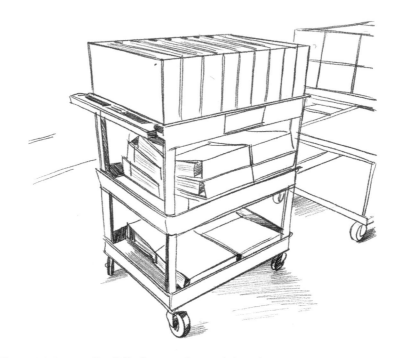

Figure 28.2. A trolley full of a manufacturer's lengthy written response to a regulator's single question.

derstand what I am doing. If manufacturers had to supply why they believe their safety claims, this could be assessed by the regulators or their designated bodies. If manufacturers used Formal Methods, this would be very easy to do — indeed, the regulators could use tools to automatically check the claims.

This is an accurate drawing (figure 28.2) of a huge trolley-load of paperwork a regulator has been sent. In some countries, like the US, the regulator has a limited time to respond to depositions from a manufacturer. It's hard to imagine how diligent regulators can read through such a large quantity of documents fast enough to respond properly, so the system is being gamed. Why has the regulatory process become so disconnected from what it is intended to ensure?

We built a tool that can analyze interactive digital healthcare devices.[415] It can check whether they conform to the US FDA and other safety and usability requirements (figure 28.3).

The picture may not look very exciting, but it allows people to simulate a device (two different devices are shown in the picture) and it is run inside a Formal Methods system that can do all sorts of safety checks. You can click

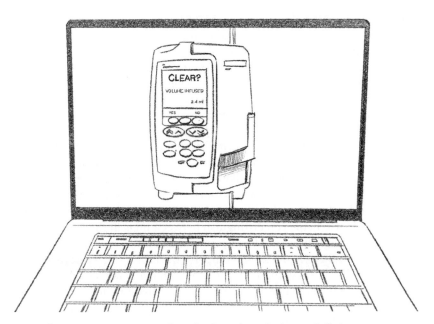

Figure 28.3. Our Formal Methods tool, analyzing an infusion pump.

buttons on the screen, and things happen — the 1.2 and 74 numbers, for instance, were generated by our system and drawn on top of photographs of the systems it is simulating. In its "design mode" you can also move buttons around and add more. What the system does is turn the usually rather mathematical Formal Methods into something that works and can be shown to people and discussed, explored, and tested on clinical tasks. You don't need to be a mathematician to see how useful it is.

If the everyday calculators I criticized[b] had been programmed in SPARK Ada, the computer would have warned that they cannot work correctly with large numbers. You can then *easily* find and fix the problems that Casio and Apple did not notice.

Formal Methods are hard, in that programmers need mathematical skills and training to use them effectively — but I'd argue that a programmer who doesn't know or isn't able to use Formal Methods probably isn't good for digital healthcare, or at least isn't good for the safety-critical parts of digital healthcare — which is most of it. However, there are easier techniques that are still very helpful, and can be used very effectively with Formal Methods.

A very simple and effective approach is **fuzzing**. Instead of, or rather, as well as, testing on users — or, worse, only testing on a few developers — test *on computers.*

---

[b] See Chapter 14: Calculator bugs, page 179 ←

Computers can easily pretend to *be* users, they are cheaper, they are much faster, and they don't get bored or need paying for their time. Huge numbers of tests can be run automatically with virtually no effort.

It baffles me that so many programmers think their programs work so well that they don't fuzz them, not even to check.[416]

We built a simple tool to do fuzzing, so it's easy to collect lots of data and compare alternative designs to see which is better. Data can be collected and then plotted — graphs show trends in the data that can be very insightful. Since the simulated users are behaving randomly, typically you get wiggly graphs, which smooth out as the number of fuzzing trials is increased. It might take a while to generate millions of tests to get smooth lines, but the safety trends are usually very obvious much sooner. In particular, comparing two or more designs is much more insightful than just analyzing one design in isolation. It also helps you distinguish between bugs in the system being tested and any bugs there may be in your simulator.

The graph shown (figure 28.4) compares the user interface of the popular Hewlett Packard EasyCalc 100 (it's similar to many medical devices but is easier to obtain), and a design inspired by the Institute for Safe Medication Practices (ISMP) recommendations for writing numbers reliably (figure 28.5). The details are fully explained in our papers,[417], but in this brief description the details are not as important as seeing that this sort of analysis is very quick, insightful, and easy to do. Any programmer who can generate random key presses can find out all sorts of useful things. Fuzzing quickly finds bugs; random key presses by definition do unexpected things. Fuzzing can compare designs to see how relatively safe they are. Here, fuzzing is making very clear that following the ISMP guidelines would make systems much safer to use.

Failing to do even this basic sort of experiment (and fixing the bugs it uncovers) before releasing products for use in healthcare is negligent, as is any regulation that allows products to be marketed without adequate safety evidence.

———————————————————■———————————————————

A lot of modern software is developed using an Agile process. Agile means that partly working software is quickly developed, trialed, and improved in a repeating process. This approach suits a lot of software development, as often organizations want something "better than nothing" working as quickly as possible. This is what Agile promises and often achieves.[409]

Earlier, we saw how Agile and Formal Methods are opposed,[c] but now we will see that Agile and rigorous testing — as required in healthcare — are opposed. Because Agile and Agile-like methods produce a continual series of rapidly improving prototypes, it is hard to test the systems rigorously, as nothing is finalized. Let's say a statistically reliable test of a new system

---

[c] See Chapter 27: Agile method, page 378 ←

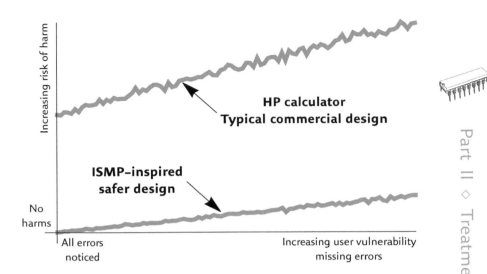

Figure 28.4. A graph summarizing thousands of automatic fuzzing results (simulating user testing) to compare the safety of two devices.[417] As a user misses more errors (increasing their **vulnerability** to error) you'd expect safety risks to increase, as indeed both lines show. However, the HP calculator, with behavior typical of designs commonly found in medical devices, is much riskier to use than the improved design. The plot clearly shows that if the user misses fewer errors (moving left in the plot), the ISMP-inspired design becomes safer and safer, finally becoming completely safe, whereas the common design has residual risks that the user can never avoid, even if they try to correct them. In other words: even if a user notices all errors and tries to recover from all of them, the common design has bugs that could cause patient harm, however careful the user is.

requires 100 users to use it for a day each, but in Agile the system will already have changed before the tests are complete. There is no time with a fixed system to do thorough testing for safety. Agile is fine if you're making something nicer, but if you are trying to make something safer, it's likely that *every* change that is made will affect safety, and therefore every safety test needs doing again when the system changes.

Agile sees bugs as the necessary step to better products, but in healthcare the impact of bugs cannot be dismissed or seen as acceptable side effects of faster development, as Agile assumes. People who promote Agile unconditionally in healthcare are overlooking the need to develop safe products.

Let me justify that important point a bit more.

A lot of effort goes into ensuring drugs are understood and shown to be safe before they are widely used — it's very expensive if problems come to light later, and of course we want to avoid unfortunate or unnecessary side

Reject numbers that have …	Example
A leading zero if the number is greater than 1	05
A trailing zero after a decimal point	5.0
Trailing zeros after a decimal fraction	5.40
A missing leading zero if number less than 1	.5
A decimal point with no digits are after it	5.
More than one decimal point	5..5

Figure 28.5. Rules inspired by the ISMP to pick up and reduce numerical errors.[417] For example, 05 might be misread as 0.5, and 5.0 might be misread as 50, and so on. (Other rules, such as validating that the number value is positive and less than 1,000, are also required.) In contrast, most user interfaces to read numbers ignore all these potential problems, and therefore do not provide adequate support to the user when errors do occur. When these rules were implemented *exactly*, we achieved a safer user interface — which was shown by fuzzing (figure 28.4).

effects. It would be unconscionable to put a drug on the market that had not been shown to be both safe and effective, or whose side effects or other details were not well understood.

The drug development process is broken down into five phases:

Preclinical phase Initial selection, development, and testing of the drug in laboratories, on tissues, or on animals.

Phase 0 How does the drug work? Studies on small groups, about 10 volunteers, usually with tiny doses. Establishes which drugs are most promising to invest in for further phases.

Artificial Intelligence is starting to accelerate these initial phases. The Centaur Chemist AI system took less than a year to design the OCD (obsessive compulsive disorder) drug DSP-1181 ready for Phase I testing, much faster than the typical five-year process.[418]

Phase I Testing of the drug on 20–100 healthy volunteers to test for safety. Patients with serious or terminal diseases may volunteer. Phase I establishes data to balance between safe and effective doses.

Phase II Now known to be broadly safe, larger testing of the drug on 100+ patients to assess efficacy and side effects.

Phase III Testing of the drug on thousands of patients to rigorously assess efficacy, effectiveness, and safety. Sometimes potential new uses of the drug are discovered at this stage (so-called label expansion).

Phase IV Monitoring the drug in public use following regulatory approval for sale. Post-marketing surveillance monitoring the drug's use beyond the manufacturer's control.

Developing a cancer or dementia drug through these phases may take 15 years start-to-finish, and cost around $1 billion.[5] A drug may be abandoned at any phase during the trials, so quite often the development costs are not recovered by future sales. (Often several variants of a drug proceed in parallel through the trials, with only the least promising dropping out.)

Ironically, the ease of modifying digital systems compared to the difficulty of modifying pharmaceuticals means that digital development processes are much more relaxed. The drug development Phases I to IV are treated very crudely, if at all, in the digital world. Because digital systems can be updated so easily at any time, it is cheaper to find and fix bugs in the field after a product has been put on the market than to avoid the problems. Indeed, as bugs are fixed after putting products on the market, gradually digital systems drift into being only loosely related to the original approved systems — figure 16.2 shows an example where post-market product drift seems to be done deliberately to make it easier to get regulatory approval before all the features are added. Regulations like the FDA's 510(k) enable and seem to endorse this.[d] Anything else would be increasing **regulatory burden**, which to some minds is self-evidently a bad idea.

These common habits are often turned into counter-arguments for improving digital healthcare regulation.

Although in digital development a lot of development work goes into the preclinical phases, the only evaluation phase that is routinely done corresponds to Phase 0 (that is, hopefully, by using UCD). Fortunately, post-market surveillance (Phase IV) is being increasingly required. Indeed, Wi-Fi and the internet makes post-market surveillance a doddle, and we can look forward to regulations being improved further.

Drugs are often tested using **Randomized Controlled Trials** (RCTs). RCTs have become the "gold standard" for drug testing and for medical evidence more generally.

What, then, are RCTs?[419]

Put briefly, patients are selected for a study, and some patients are randomly allocated to a **control group** who don't get the experimental treatment, and others are treated with the specified intervention (usually a drug). It's complex to organize an RCT properly, and recruiting all the patients and tracking them throughout the trial is costly. Follow-up may take years, as the effects and side effects of the drug may be slow.

RCTs are **randomized** because people respond differently to drugs, but we don't know how they are going to respond. If we did a trial on students, we might fail to find out what happens with older people or with children — for example, most students are well educated and are healthy, and most older people are already on some drug, which might interact with the drug being trialed. We might inadvertently select patients the drug will do better with,

---

[d] See Chapter 16: FDA 510(k) regulation, page 201 ←

or we may have any number of other systematic biases we are unaware of. So the patients in an RCT are selected from a broad sample of the population, and then randomized to try to avoid any unintentional systematic bias in the trials.

RCTs are expensive, but the thalidomide scandal — or, rather, the desire to avoid another scandal — is sufficient for everyone to agree that they are worthwhile, if not obligatory, for developing drugs, especially when supported by **post-market surveillance** (long-term monitoring of effects after the product is allowed on the market).

When digital systems deliver and even modify drug doses, drug therapy and digital therapy become closely intertwined. The safety and effectiveness of a drug depends on its reliable dosing. In other words, digital healthcare systems need to be developed to comparable standards for drug dispensing, as well as for many other contexts.

Unfortunately, thanks largely to the popularity of Agile thinking,[e] digital systems are often released to patients without large-scale, let alone rigorous testing. There are common arguments for this: Agile is all about **failing fast**; Agile is inconsistent with RCTs; and undertaking proper trials would delay reaping the benefits of the digital innovation — benefits for patients as well as profit for the manufacturers. Agile's failing fast means you can build nice consumer products quickly using iterative design.[f] True, but if — as you would in healthcare — you might harm people by failing fast, the Agile approach is totally inappropriate.

Anyway, Agile enthusiasts argue, by the time any trials are complete, their innovative digital technologies would be obsolete. Which I think is a very devious argument, as it tries to make us feel sympathetic toward avoiding tedious evaluations because we'd miss out on wonderful innovations. Yet if innovative digital products are going to become obsolete so quickly, that's actually a problem, not an excuse to rush their development. It'd be a waste of money buying them if they need replacing so soon.

Certainly, the basic RCT does have a range of problems for digital evaluations. For example, if we're convinced that a new system we've been developing will benefit patients and we want to know how much benefit there is, then an RCT would be a rigorous test — but it will deny some randomly selected people (or hospitals) from the benefits we believe our digital system has.

This worry is expressed as the principle of **clinical equipoise**: we should treat patients fairly. We shouldn't deny people treatments or interventions we know to be effective just because we want to do an RCT. There is a wonderful paper I recommend that illustrates equipoise brilliantly — it describes an RCT evaluating the clinical value of parachutes as an intervention to prevent death when jumping from aircraft.[420]

---

[e] See Chapter 27: Agile method, page 378 ←
[f] See Chapter 23: Iterative design, page 313 ←

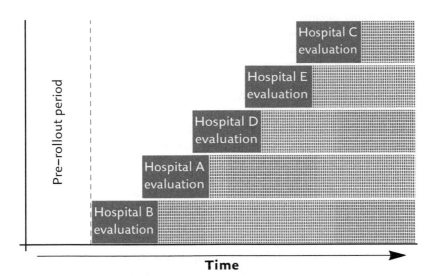

Figure 28.6. An example of a Stepped Wedge Trial (SWT) for five randomly selected hospitals. The hospital test sites are put into a random order, and then the digital system is installed and evaluated at each in turn, illustrated here in the order B–A–D–E–C. The shaded regions, after each individual hospital evaluation, show how you can take advantage of an iterative (or Agile) design process to improve the system as other SWT evaluations proceed.

Not all digital systems need RCT-type methodologies.[421] Lots of research has already found out how men and women interact with computers differently, how people work under pressure, and so on. Digital experiments — especially UCD experiments — typically involve only a few tens of participants, not thousands as in typical drug RCTs. (However, a medical app for mental health would need to be trialed much more like a drug, and for the same reasons — because we don't know how different people respond to new digital therapies.) Furthermore, a lot of the digital system trial phases can be done better and far more easily with digital systems than with drugs, because digital allows for very easy monitoring.

RCTs are slow and expensive, and as most people can't see the bugs and technical defects in digital systems, many people would argue that RCTs are overkill for digital systems. Digital systems *obviously* save money, are faster and more efficient: why do an RCT that's only going to delay the promised improvements? If we are going to roll out our digital systems to every hospital (or to every patient), it isn't possible to deny them to a random selection anyway — they are going to get them eventually.

In other words, RCTs are certainly very good for drug development but they don't work when mindlessly applied in the digital world.[422] Fortunately, there are many variants of RCTs that help get around these problems, and which work well with how digital systems are developed.[423]

As an example, let's suppose we have a digital system we want to evaluate for safe and effective use in hospitals. It might be, say, a back-office administrative system.

The **Stepped Wedge Trial** (SWT) is a form of RCT that works like this: first you write down the hospitals in a random order. Next, in a pre-rollout phase, you measure how well everybody is doing, then you install the digital system in the first hospital on your list. At this stage, this is just like an RCT, but with only one randomly selected hospital, with all the rest being controls. At the next step, you take the next random hospital listed, and install the digital system there. This is like a second RCT — in fact, it's better, because you can start a longitudinal (long-term) study on the first hospital, as it's had the system running for longer. At the third step, you install the system in the third randomly selected hospital. Again, this is like another RCT, with all the remaining hospitals or wards being control groups. And so on.

While you are at it, doing an SWT is a good time to collect evidence of real-world (that is, **post-market**, because it comes after the product has gone to market) effectiveness, not just safety: most organizations are very interested in cost effectiveness, and if you want people to buy your products, safety isn't the only argument that'll be needed.

At the end of the SWT, every hospital has the system. Even better, every hospital ends up with an improved system, and the manufacturers have lots of evaluation information that they can use for meeting regulatory requirements as well as for making further improvements. A diagram illustrating how it would work for just five hospitals is shown in figure 28.6 — the diagram also shows why it's called a Stepped Wedge Trial.

The UK made very expensive mistakes with its national COVID-19 Test and Trace digital system, a system designed to test people and trace back their contacts so that infectious people could be identified and isolate, so reducing the rate of spread of the pandemic. The Test and Trace system went live nationally, but was immediately swamped — exposing many design bugs. It "was beset by technical problems" and the related app, too, was problematic:

> A technical problem [a euphemism for bugs] meant the app
> gave false alerts to users and those who did test positive could
> be left confused as to how long to isolate for, with the app
> giving a different date to the instruction delivered by contact
> tracers.[424]

Because the system was launched on a national scale, the problems very rapidly became overwhelming.

I wonder what would have happened if they'd used a SWT (or similar approach) to roll out the system? If so, they would have found problems with the first small release, fixed them, then proceeded to release the system in another region of the country, and so on. They would have been much less likely to be overwhelmed, and they would have had more resources to focus on fixing the early problems, and keeping it on a much more manageable scale. A crisis would have been avoided, and the incremental evaluations would have improved the system. Who knows? Whatever — even without hindsight, when going into delivering a large, national digital project, surely it's better to plan to evaluate it in phases and to use standard practice iterative design[g] *because* you want to improve. Instead, the UK system was launched as if it worked and needed neither improvement nor evaluation, when plainly it was fatally buggy. People *unnecessarily* caught COVID-19 and some died as a result.

Now the system has got a terrible reputation, it's created a new problem: they now have to recover public trust in any approach. Loss of trust is a huge problem that will undermine other attempts to control the pandemic. Many of the problems would, I am sure, have been avoided by an SWT — and, if not an SWT, by any honest professional approach that acknowledged that digital systems are never perfect and always require evaluation and improvement.

The Agile/RCT/SWT/etc arguments are complex, and for the most part illustrate collisions between very different cultures. To quickly summarize my views, I'll emphasize a few points:

- People say "Digital innovation in healthcare is rushing ahead, and RCTs would slow it down." My view is that this argument only works when you are not interested in one of the main benefits that RCTs offer, namely, empirically assured safety. Since most digital health innovators aren't interested in safety (since it's surely "obvious" that their systems work well[h]), this is a weak argument.

- RCTs are not the best methodology for digital systems that were developed using professional Formal Methods and user interface design practice.

- However, since very few digital healthcare systems were rigorously designed — particularly AI-based systems, which have often learned unknown things from their training data — then doing RCTs or SWTs (or similar) would be a very valuable addition to the evidence for them. This is because randomized trials are especially good when systems are not well defined, as the randomization controls for their unknown features.

- I'd argue that every digital healthcare innovation *must have* solid evidence and arguments for its use, to rigorously assure us of their

---

[g] See Chapter 23: Iterative design, page 313 ←
[h] See Chapter 3: Cat Thinking, page 25 ←

capability, safety, and reliability in *real* use. While Formal Methods can underpin this, RCTs do have the advantage that the healthcare world readily understands them.

🐦 ... if digital healthcare was a mature discipline, we could also add systematic reviews and meta-analyses to RCTs as good things to do, but so far there isn't much of a decent digital healthcare literature to do useful reviews (other than to point out that there aren't many good peer-reviewed papers).

Hindsight is one thing, but what can we learn to use as foresight so we can all have better systems in the future?

The UK's Test and Trace fiasco for COVID-19 showed fallout from the clash between an uncritical rush to implement with the need to have an effective system. We have many other pressures in digital healthcare — to rush into using AI, to rush into connected systems, to rush cybersecurity "solutions," to rush big data ... to rush into all sorts of exciting innovations. So we should learn: SWTs are a really good idea and protect us from small- and large-scale mistakes, and — given human nature — we ought to have regulation to require SWTs (or similar) in all digital healthcare development. And while we wait for regulation, anyone choosing or buying new systems should require SWTs or other evidence that those systems really work as effectively as hoped.

———————————————■———————————————

We started off with the conventional arguments against using RCTs in digital healthcare, and now we've shown how straightforward it is to do digital RCTs. In fact, as figure 28.6 illustrates, you'd definitely want to do iterative design to improve your system anyway, and the SWT version of RCTs lets you do that efficiently *at the same time*, and with the added benefits of rigorous evaluation. You obviously have to decide whether the remaining SWT evaluations use the original design or the improved design; there are advantages and disadvantages of either choice. The obvious solution is to extend the SWT to another set of hospitals after you have finished improving the system with what's been learned during the first trials. When regulators require digital RCTs, the regulations will help make these decisions for you.

Currently many digital systems are exempt from clinical regulation, such as office systems like calculators, email, and word processors. My argument would be that at least parts of these systems must be regulated — I've already made a strong case for calculators and spreadsheets[i] (they are used to calculate drug doses), but even word processors handle patient information, and they must be evaluated to make sure they do not corrupt clinical information. For instance, automatic spelling correction can cause chaos, as shown in box 18.2.

---

[i] See Chapter 14: Risky calculations, page 177 ←

Apart from cutting corners, it isn't obvious why digital systems aren't regulated to the same level as drugs, requiring rigorous evaluations like RCTs and SWTs. Infusion pumps, for instance, deliver drugs, and can aid or ruin drug interventions as much as any poor pharmacological development of the drugs themselves. As I've said before in this book, what's the point of carefully regulating a drug if it can easily be delivered in the wrong doses by buggy software? You need to carefully regulate both.

After this ramble through Agile and RCTs, I, at least, need to remind my-self why we needed the discussion. My argument throughout this book is that we need to improve the quality of digital healthcare, and improving de-velopment and testing is an essential contribution toward that. Ideally digital would be regulated at least as tightly as drugs. Everybody agrees RCTs are the gold standard. Developers argue that RCTs won't work in healthcare, as if digital is somehow an exception. Therefore, they argue, don't regulate us to tighten testing, as it'd just be unproductive regulatory burden that would delay innovation. Aren't we all agreed that digital healthcare needs innova-tion? I think the argument is specious. Even if you think that there might be something (I don't know what) in the argument, I don't think you should concede that digital healthcare doesn't need improving. As the Lancet put it in 2018, "Continuing to argue for digital exceptionalism and failing to ro-bustly evaluate digital health interventions presents the greatest risk for pa-tients and health systems."[425]

Despite the resistance to digital RCTs, especially from the Agile commu-nity, they have in fact been shown to be very valuable in digital healthcare, especially with RCT variants like the SWT. Here's a standard story:

Dr Joseph Smith developed a medical app for virtual therapy and decided to undertake an RCT.[426] His RCT process delayed the product by 30 months and cost him $2 million. However, he now knows his app saves an average of $2,745 per patient. It was worth it. But a disadvantage, he points out, is that his research investment may create a halo around competing products that did not undertake trials.

Here's a quick summary of this chapter's arguments:

- ⓘ Use Formal Methods to specify and help write programs.

- ⓘ Design programs to anticipate and check for bugs — and to attempt to recover from them.

- ⓘ Use or develop your own tools (for instance, for fuzzing) to help test and review specifications and code.

- ⓘ Test programs (once they are known to be safe enough) in the messy reality of hospital wards, or wherever they are intended to be used. There are lots of ways to do this, including SWTs. Don't be put off.

- ⓘ Improve regulation to ensure more of these steps happen.

Part II ◇ Treatment ◇ Finding solutions

Let's have a reliable way of clearly seeing how safe systems are, so that we can make choices based on evidence and improve safety.

29

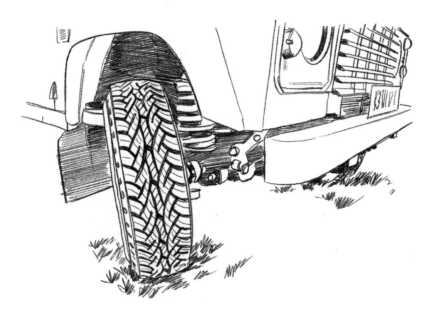

Choose safety

I bought some new tires for our Land Rover. When I went to the garage, they offered me three different makes of tire they had in stock that would fit it. I bought the Continental, as they could do me a deal — I could get it cheaper than the others, so buying it seemed a no-brainer. That's the tire shown on my car in the drawing above.

Tires differ enormously on how safe they are, what their fuel consumption is, and how noisy they are. When you buy a tire, though, you have no idea about any of this, so it's easier to buy on a gut feeling about the brand and the price, and thus probably not end up with the best tire.

The European Union (the EU to its friends) therefore now requires tires to be sold with rating labels. If these labels had been legally required when

Fix It: See and solve the problems of digital healthcare. Harold Thimbleby,
Oxford University Press. © Harold Thimbleby 2021.
DOI: 10.1093/oso/9780198861270.003.0029

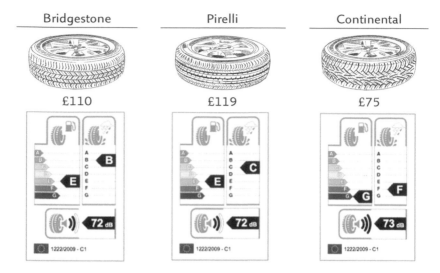

Figure 29.1. EU safety labels for three different car tires.

I was buying my new tires, I would have hesitated about buying the Continental tire (the one on the right in the picture, see figure 29.1), which was noisier, more costly to run, and had a worse stopping distance in the wet. I made a poor choice (given what I wanted) without knowing I was making a poor choice.

The idea is that once consumers *know* the quality of tires, they will tend to buy tires better matching their requirements. In turn, this will encourage the manufacturers to make better tires. More sophisticated consumers might be prepared to pay a premium price for tires that are just what they want; perhaps some people want green, fuel efficient tires?

I personally would prefer safer tires with shorter stopping distances. I think a car that has been in a crash (because it didn't stop soon enough), maybe written off, causes a lot more pollution, with lots of bits going to landfill, than a small saving in fuel and emissions. Perhaps the EU should update the tire label to give an estimate of environmental impact?

Indeed, Michelin, apparently, mentioned that the EU tire label scheme does not assess the lifetime of the tire — Michelin make tires that last a long time. But if the EU assessed environmental impact, then tire lifetime, fuel consumption, and an estimate of scrapped tires and broken cars, because long stopping distances increase the collision rate, would go into the mix of helping consumers make better decisions. While the science behind all the assessment may be complex, the tire rating remains easy to understand.

The EU has used this rating idea on other products, not just tires. In the old days, people would buy white goods (fridges, cookers, washing ma-

Safer

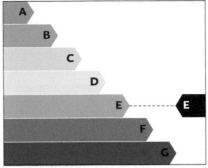

Less safe

Figure 29.2. A simple safety label design based on the EU energy rating label. I was inspired by the EU conventions, so as I've reimagined the label, a *shorter* line represents *more* safety. This might be confusing, so experiments will be required to find out the most reliable way of representing safety, particularly remembering that people may be stressed when they use the label.

chines) on their preferences for looks, brand, cost, and the salesman's patter. Now the EU labels can help consumers choose better energy efficiency.

At first the EU rated white goods with labels G (worst) to A (best) for energy efficiency. But as consumers started preferentially buying more efficient things, now they could see how to, the manufacturers of course improved their products so they could sell more. Soon, more or less everything was rated A. The EU responded by adding tighter criteria — now white goods can be rated A+, A++, A+++, and A++++. And some products are up there.

An important thing is that the EU never told manufacturers *how* to make more energy-efficient white goods (the EU ratings avoid implementation bias). The market pressure encouraged manufacturers to work out how they could do it for themselves.

Wouldn't it be nice if we had EU (or EU-type) safety rating labels for all medical devices and digital systems?

Before you rush in and tell me how impractical an idea this is, note that the Leapfrog Group[427] provides safety ratings for *entire* hospitals, and apparently it's very helpful. Leapfrog has worked out how to do it professionally, with an expert panel, and more. It's worth quoting from the group's website:

> One of the most significant problems with today's health care system is the failure to make safety and quality information available to the public. But the public deserves this information so they can make informed choices about where to receive care. The purpose of the Leapfrog Hospital Safety

Grade is to bring this information to light in a way that is easy for you — the consumer — to use.

Some people do more research on what car to buy than what hospital to go to for medical care. The Leapfrog Hospital Safety Grade provides data and research to help you make informed decisions about a critical aspect of your hospital stay — safety. A hospital may have the best surgeons and greatest technology in the world, but unless it is preventing infections and eliminating errors, it is not delivering on a very basic premise: ensuring the safety of you and your loved ones. The goal of the Leapfrog Hospital Safety Grade is to reduce the approximately 440,000 yearly deaths from hospital errors and injuries by publicly recognizing safety and exposing harm.

The Leapfrog ideas would clearly work equally well with digital health-care.

If safety rating labels stayed on digital systems and devices for ever, then they would become part of everyone's awareness and this would start to change things for the better, as Leapfrog emphasized for its hospital rating system.

I've put a QR code on the safety label in my mock-up (figure 29.3) so that if an incident was reported, it'd be very easy to get the identity of the device into the reporting system. Of course, a QR code is just a clever way of saying something, and it can code for anything — they often code for web addresses — but in the medical area, they should code for **Unique Device Indicators** or UDIs, which are a growing standard of codes. UDIs have expiry dates, and they tie in with a database (the Global UDI Database, GUDID), so while you are at it, many other beneficial things can be achieved.

Sticking safety labels and QR codes on devices permanently will ensure everyone can see them whenever they are used. The codes could also help reduce fraud and other problems (like stealing and reselling expensive devices), and that would improve manufacturers' profits, so they might want to do it regardless of the idea's impact on improving patient safety.

Eventually some incident will occur in the operating room. The clinicians will be more likely to mention the device in their report, especially if it was F or G safety rated! Patients would also put pressure on the system to improve: "why am I getting a B-rated dialysis machine...?"

QR codes have the advantage that they are visible, so they are a visual reminder that they can help report an incident or near miss. Today it might be more exciting to have an active RFID tag inside the label:[428] then using the code would be even easier. However, this would be jumping to conclusions when we need to do experiments. RFIDs are hidden, inscrutable, and they all look the same to the naked eye. Perhaps the invisibility of RFIDs would lead to more errors than they fix? RFIDs might get muddled up without anyone

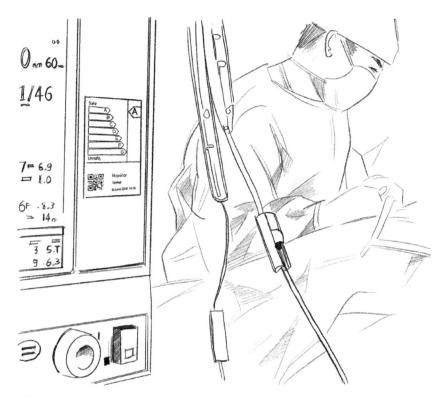

Figure 29.3. My mock-up of using safety labels in a hospital. Perhaps it should also have a hologram to make it hard to forge.

noticing until it was too late, but QR codes can be printed with supporting text.

I and my colleague Patrick Oladimeji helped a hospital procure an infusion pump. They had short-listed 16 pumps and asked us to rate them. Unlike the EU and its tire ratings, we were not sure how to get lots of design features down to a simple "stopping distance" or "energy efficiency" rating. Instead we assessed lots of criteria, 33 in all.

The summary diagram (figure 29.4) doesn't show all the features we evaluated, but it gives the general idea.[429] Each column in the diagram is an infusion pump, and the rows are our assessment of each pump against each of the safety criteria.

Although you may be reading this in black and white, a green-to-red spectrum of colors is used: the colors are copied from our two-dimensional risk assessment (figure 29.6), itself inspired by the international standard IEC 61508, which we will return to again later, in box 32.1. So green means very safe, and red means we think it is very risky. Red means things are ex-

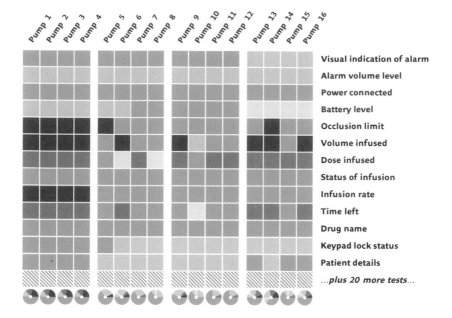

Figure 29.4. Summary visualization of the 33 safety evaluations (each row) of 16 infusion pumps (each column). See figure 29.6 for the explanation of the color scheme, which, unfortunately, may be hard to follow if this picture is reproduced in black and white.

pected to go wrong often and with high, frequent, harmful, impact on the patient. Each column in the table has a summary pie chart (at the bottom), where we just added up all the scores in each column into a simple visual summary. Here, the color coding is very helpful, as the eye can easily assess the dominant colors of the pie chart icons.

One might also want to assess not just risk, as we did, but risk–benefit — here, all the devices were similar infusion pumps, so at face value the benefits are more or less the same. If we were assessing a range of different types of devices, the risks and benefits would need to be compared — for example, with an ambulatory infusion pump the patient can walk around, so it has different benefits than a pump that is big and needs a floor stand to hold it.

Essentially we have rated everything on a 10-point scale, running from 0 to 9. However, we left it to the hospital that was buying the pumps to decide which areas they are most worried about; for instance, they may want different balances of risk in general wards or in intensive care, where there are more staff around and there is more patient monitoring to keep eyes on things. A higher-risk pump might be appropriate in intensive care or the operating room, when it might be unacceptably dangerous in other settings. Or

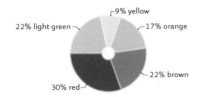
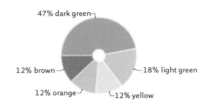

Figure 29.5. Examples of the summary risk pie charts, where each sector indicates the total number of design factors with each risk rating. The meanings of the colors are as described in the matrix figure 29.6. (Colors have been named in case this picture is reproduced in black and white.)

perhaps the operating room can afford to buy more expensive, better pumps, and general wards that need lots of pumps might find that cost is more important than safety. Well, now the hospital can decide on the evidence, whereas before it just bought cute ones or cheap ones, or ones with discounts. Previously it had no idea how safe they were.

It is hard to talk about safety honestly — and we need to talk honestly if there is going to be any chance of making digital health safer.

Digital healthcare industry, on the whole, is resistant to testing and rating safety. Some of the arguments are that testing is expensive and slow, and by the time trials have been done, the technology will have moved on. However, drug manufacturers don't say this, despite drug development — from lab to hospital — being very slow. Sure, pharmaceutical science will have moved on by the time you've finished your trials, but you still want all drugs to be tested before you use them! (With some sensible exceptions for compassionate reasons — for example, if someone is near the end of their life, where hope is important and many potential side effects aren't very relevant.)

Drug testing costs millions, often billions, and the success rate is very low.[430] There isn't this sort of money to invest in digital healthcare trials, let alone the willingness to put up with success rates under 10%. It's a chicken and egg problem. While digital healthcare manufacturers can get away with next-to-no testing, why would anybody invest millions in testing? It'd be money wasted on something that has no competitive value. Although we could start off with a voluntary scheme, it would be far better to change the law so that trials and safety proofs *have to be done.* The money to fund trials would then appear, because there would be no alternative. Regulators are certainly starting to realize the challenge of digital healthcare, but we have a way to go.

As an aside, the scare-mongering of the cost of trials is misleading. Trials would be much cheaper than conventional drug trials. Almost every digital device can record how it is being used and could upload quality data to the internet at virtually no cost (with provisos about patient confidentiality). Given

Part II ◇ Treatment ◇ Finding solutions

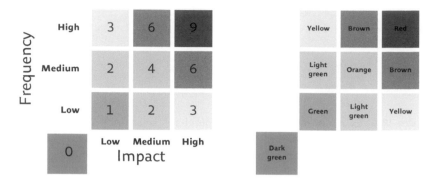

Figure 29.6. Explaining the safety rating color scheme. Something that doesn't happen often and has little impact is colored bright green (bottom left); "minor" things that happen a lot (top left), or terrible things that happen rarely (bottom right), are colored yellow. But things that happen often *and* have a large impact are bright red (top right). The extreme safe case, something that practically doesn't happen and has negligible impact, is represented by the square off at the bottom left, colored dark green.

that stuff is currently rushed to market, a compromise would be to say: you can put new devices and systems on the market today, provided they collect good data on their performance and patient outcomes, and if you can prove they are adequately successful within a year (say), then they can pass their test and will be certified for general use.

Another aspect of scare-mongering is to sow confusion on exactly what needs testing. Clearly, testing everything would be very expensive. But with pharmaceuticals, you don't need to do expensive randomized controlled trials on the packaging or the non-active ingredients. Similarly, when an aircraft is certified for air worthiness, there is no need to waste time testing whether the entertainment systems work nicely. There's a basic principle of Computational Thinking called **separation of concerns**:[a] basically, different parts of programs should be kept separate so they can be thought about independently, and so that they don't interact in unexpected ways with each other. For example, the clinically active and inactive parts of a product are separate things, so keep them separate rather than mixing them up and making them harder to understand. It's a shame the principle isn't very widely used in thinking about digital healthcare systems.[431]

In the meantime, before we get safety labels accepted and working nicely, what can we do?

Many of the examples (not all of them) that we've covered in this book have been about bugs with handling numbers. That's partly because num-

---

[a] See Chapter 13: Separation of concerns, page 169 ←

Part II ◇ Treatment ◇ Finding solutions

Box 29.1. Example evaluation criteria

Feedback: How well is the user kept informed about the state of the device? How clearly does the device communicate the effect of actions to the user? For instance, does it provide clear visual indication of an alarm that can be seen when the aural alarm is turned off?

Adherence to ISMP guidelines: The Institute for Safe Medication Practices produces up-to-date, evidence-based guidelines and recommendations for safer healthcare.[432]

Data entry: What is the probability that the user will notice an error while entering data? For example, a numeric keypad, by design, does not encourage error detection, since the user might not look at the display while entering numbers.[433]

Event Logs: Devices must maintain time-stamped logs in order to support evaluations and incident investigations, and they should be easy to access, review, and learn from. Logs should be in an open format, not limited in size, and should be at a level of detail that allows the accurate replay of user actions that took place at the time the log was recorded.[434] These obvious requirements are rarely met.

Accountability: If the manufacturer provides a strong warranty, this confirms that the product has been professionally designed and built, and that the manufacturer is confident in it. On the other hand, if a warranty has exclusions, it could imply the device or system is unsafe.

Compliance: What relevant ISO, IEC, and other standards does the device adhere to?

---

bers are easy to describe in a book (numbers are very familiar) and partly because numbers are central to digital healthcare: your height, weight, BMI, drug doses, and more are all numbers. Numbers *seem* simple, but the simplicity is deceptive: they often result in bugs and inefficiencies.[55]

There are several popular ways to enter numbers into a system. You can use a number keypad, like the Hospira infusion pump[b] or any of the calculators we've talked about.[c] Numeric keypads are the most familiar approach. You can use up/down keys: you press one button to increase the number, the other button to decrease it. Or, especially on touch screens, you can use rollers.

Of the most popular ways for entering numbers (figure 29.7), which design do you think is safer?

First, what do we mean by *safer*?

Imagine you've been asked to give a patient 2.5 mL of insulin. You need to set up the insulin, and now you need to enter 2.5 into the gadget you are using. There are at least four things that can happen (figure 29.8).

---

[b] See Chapter 5: Abbott AIM Plus infusion pump, page 55 ←
[c] See Chapter 14: Calculator bugs, page 179 ←

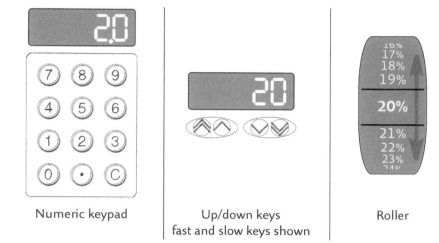

| Numeric keypad | Up/down keys
fast and slow keys shown | Roller |

Figure 29.7. Three common ways to enter numbers. With the numeric keypad, the user concentrates on the *keys* and not on the display; if a mistake happens — like a button bounces and a digit repeats, or the decimal point is pressed by mistake — the error can enter a number a factor of 10 out, but the user is unlikely to notice. With the up/down keys, the mental model is entirely different: the user concentrates on the *numeric display* rather than the keys: they adjust the number up or down until the display is the correct number they want. Users are therefore far less likely to make errors when using up/down keys. Finally, touchscreen rollers (as used on the Mersey Burns app) make it very difficult to enter a number that is a factor of two or more out from the intended value.

If you are using the numeric keypad, it seems easy, as you just press ⬛2 ⬛• ⬛5 , and of course you've entered 2.5.

You *hope*.

If something went wrong — perhaps one of the keys is dodgy — maybe you entered 25 (the decimal point didn't work) or 22.5 (the two got repeated). So you think you entered 2.5, but something else could easily have happened.

We've done eye tracking experiments[435] that show that your eyes spend most of their time looking at the keypad or controls so you know where to press buttons or what to do. That means you don't often look at the number display; you don't pay attention to the number displayed that you have actually entered. If it was wrong, perhaps because of accidentally pressing the wrong button, you probably wouldn't notice.

With the up/down keys, the whole idea is that you keep pressing up or down *until the displayed number is right*. In other words, if you make a mistake, you are going to correct it. You are paying attention to the number displayed. Our eye tracking experiments confirm that you don't spend much

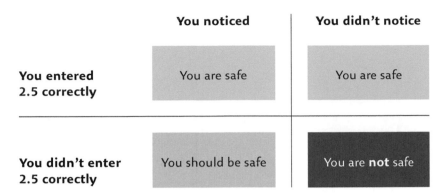

	You noticed	**You didn't notice**
You entered 2.5 correctly	You are safe	You are safe
You didn't enter 2.5 correctly	You should be safe	You are **not** safe

Figure 29.8. The really unsafe case is the combination where you didn't enter 2.5 as you intended *and* you didn't notice your error. That means you will not try to correct the error. Perhaps the wrong number you entered will have serious consequences for your patient.

time looking at the buttons because there aren't many of them and you are concentrating on the number displayed to get it right.

Overall, the up/down design is about twice as safe as the numeric keypad. I'm therefore glad it was the user interface design of infusion pump that was used on me for my doses of rituximab[436] (figure 29.9).

A more dramatic way to put that result is: if across the country 100 people die from wrong drug doses when using an infusion pump with a numeric keypad, then as up/down has half the error rate, 50 would not have died had up/down been used instead.

Our experiments with different ways of entering numbers made some interesting discoveries.[435] Our participants[437] preferred the numeric keypad, probably because it's so familiar, despite it having a worse error rate. We also broke down errors into how serious they were — as a proxy to how harmful they were. The numeric keypad made greater numbers of more harmful errors, and the up/down method made greater numbers of less harmful errors.

If we introduced safety labeling for digital healthcare systems, numeric keypads could get G for safety, and up/down (and four-key) style keypads could probably get an A or B for safety. There are many other factors to rate, including whether the devices have bugs and how significant the bugs are for safety.

I think programmers think numbers are easy, so they overlook problems in programming number entry. Whatever the reasons, numeric keyboards are not only less reliable to use, they often have risky bugs as well. Somehow, though, programmers usually manage to program up/down correctly. That's another reason to prefer up/down keys.

Also, people using numbers are not aware of these subtle but critical differences. Unfortunately, how people behave and what people think are not

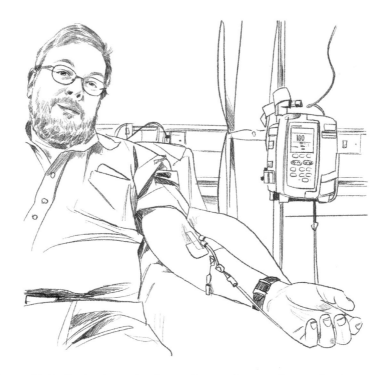

Figure 29.9. I'm having a day-long infusion of rituximab. I prefer the up/down keys on infusion pumps (I'm using an Alaris GP) for my infusions, as our research shows they are twice as safe as numeric keypads. As my dose needed adjusting frequently, I benefitted from the improved safety repeatedly as the dose was adjusted. With many thanks to Katrin, Jenny, Michelle, Chris, and the rest of the amazing nursing team — and with many thanks to the NHS, their cheese sandwiches, and their best filter coffee.

the same thing. It takes careful experiments, like the ones we did, to find out that some designs are safer than others — people are not usually aware of safety. Errors happen infrequently, and they occur most frequently when we are distracted. We are not very clued up over the design features that induce or cause error. On the other hand, we are very aware of "usability," how usable things feel to *us*, but we have little insight (unless we do the experiments) into what the usability to other people is, or what the usability to us really is. If something feels nice we may think it is usable, but an objective measurement might find we are slower or make more errors. We always need rigorous experiments to be sure.

Some designs seem harder to use, and some seem easier. We are very aware of being confused and slowed down by poor user interface design. It seems like every key click is a burden. Why can't the design be easier to use?

Unfortunately, often making things faster — which makes them feel easier — comes at the cost of making them less safe. There is a trade-off.

Abbreviations are unsafe, and the shorter they are, the more problematic they become. Longer abbreviations are safer, but they are more tedious to use. Of course, if the user gets fed up typing long words when they think shorter words would do, their frustration won't help their error rate. In general, careful experiments have to be done to find the best trade-off.

Consider using M and F for mother and father. This makes perfect sense in antenatal clinics, where there are lots of mothers and fathers. Why keep writing or typing **Mother** and **Father** out in full every time, when the much quicker M and F are obviously sufficient?

Now, if the mother's blood is Rhesus negative and the baby's is Rhesus positive, this "Rh incompatibility" is dangerous. It's therefore important to check the mother's and father's blood types.

If the mother is Rh negative and the father is Rh positive, the baby may be Rh positive too, but if it is the other way around, with the mother Rh positive, it doesn't matter what Rh type of blood the baby has. So, it's critical for blood tests to check the mother and father the right way round! However, if the antenatal clinic labels the bloods taken the obvious way as M or F, the blood testing laboratory are very likely to be more conventional and take it to mean Male or Female. That reverses the meanings.

The problem is that M and F are so much easier to write or type than the "long" full words Mother/Male or Father/Female. The single letters are *both* ambiguous. Thus subtle and dangerous errors can arise, especially since neither the antenatal clinic nor the blood lab thinks *their* scheme is remarkable. So nobody thinks through the safety implications: what *they* are doing is safe, so it "is" safe. This is a stark interoperability problem — the computer brings together two incompatible ways of working as the laboratory's conventions appear on the computer screens in the antenatal clinics (and *vice versa*).

People, especially clinicians, often want to reduce the number of mouse clicks they have to do each day, as well as the number of keystrokes. Both clicks and keystrokes are obvious measures of usability — that is, the more clicks to do the same thing, the less usable it is.[438] People want to save time. Unfortunately, reducing mouse clicks makes it *feel* more efficient but, inevitably, the trade-off is that *if it's a critical task* it also makes it more risky. However, when it isn't a useful task, the trade-off of being more efficient is all for the good.

Indeed, *some* clicks just waste time.

Hawai'i Pacific Health has a brilliant project called "Getting Rid of Stupid Stuff."[439] They looked for stupid things. One stupid thing they discovered was that one mouse click their system required was just for auditing purposes. It was: click this if you've walked round the ward to meet each patient. The Getting Rid of Stupid Stuff survey discovered this check was irritating nurses, and the data they were getting was anyway unreliable. It was just a stupid mouse click.

When they looked more closely at it, they found that the clicking took 24 seconds to do. I don't know if these 24 seconds included walking over to the computer and logging in, but it's not an unreasonable figure. The 24 seconds added up to 425 nursing hours per week! If a typical nurse works 35+ hours a week, this question was wasting the four Hawai'i hospitals in the survey the time of 12 nurses — three per hospital.

The Getting Rid of Stupid Stuff work led to fixing the bad design, and effectively increased the number of nurses available without increasing payroll costs. One wonders what other mindless and counter-productive features go into digital systems everywhere else. Projects like Getting Rid of Stupid Stuff are useful!

Menus are often provided to speed up user interfaces. The menu gives the relevant choices and the full phrases, so there is no ambiguity there, but instead of there being abbreviations that are easy to mix up, a menu makes errors happen with a slip of a few millimeters of the mouse. Now, the user can select the wrong thing that the menu has ensured "makes sense." Furthermore, menus usually disappear after the user has selected their choice, so there is a reduced opportunity to notice and correct any error. Possibly the incorrect incident report over Peter Thimbleby's death was an easy menu error rather than the doctor deliberately typing a lie, or perhaps the menu of choices was so restrictive that he slipped and selected the wrong answer?[d] It is very likely that the menu selection happened so fast that the doctor has no clear memory of it.

Earlier, I explained how we found that up/down keys were safer than numeric keypads for entering numbers, by about a factor of two. On the other hand, up/down is safer but it is also slower. Being slower makes it *feel* less usable, and saving a fraction of a second every time you do an infusion seems like a good idea. Unfortunately, clinicians aren't really aware of losing safety, so they are unaware of the trade-off — and it's some trade off to save fractions of a second every time, but more frequently make an error, which will almost certainly take longer to sort out, even if it's possible, than all the saved fractions of a second put together. Visible safety labels would help make the trade-offs explicit and would help bring error rates down — which benefits patients.

Remembering Safety Two[e] — focus on the good, not the bad — it's important not just to expose poor design, but also to have awards and rewards for *good* design. Design awards are common; the Japanese Good Design Award is one internationally recognized example I mentioned earlier.[f] We

---

[d] See Chapter 9: Peter Thimbleby's preventable death, page 109 ←
[e] See Chapter 12: Safety One & Safety Two, page 145 ←
[f] See Chapter 8: Good Design Award, page 96 ←

should extend awards like this to take account of safety, especially in health-care.

We want safer healthcare, and to do that we have to be able to see safety so that we can think more clearly, rather than be driven by our impressions. Safety labels could be the fastest way to improve healthcare safety — and, in turn, they'll drive improvements in assessing safety so the labels are fair, informative, and accurate.

Everybody will benefit.

Part II ◇ Treatment ◇ Finding solutions

We've emphasized problems and solutions to problems, but of course digital can do some fantastic things too. This chapter collects some positive stories about digital successes and how digital can transform lives.

30

Signs of life

If digital healthcare was *only* risky, the simple answer would be to get rid of it all. But we all know that digital healthcare has huge promise and can do amazing things. Instead, then, we need to build on digital health's signs of life; we need to take the bits that work, and make them work in more ways, in more places, more of the time — and of course with far fewer bugs and interoperating together effectively …

There are many inspiring stories to choose from.

The Medal medical app

The Medal medical app[440] has a history going back to 1998, when the company started with a bare suite of algorithms. By 2009, they had over 100,000 registered users of the algorithms. They then put the algorithms into an app: version 1.0 of the Medal app appeared in 2014. The app has now been in use and development for several years. I tried version 2.3 for the iPhone, which I downloaded in May 2016.

As well as iPhones and Androids, Medal can also be used on a conventional PC in a web browser. The features it provides range from simple unit conversions (like converting liters to pints), generic calculations such as Bayes Theorem, and clinical calculations such as determining the dose of potassium iodide following an exposure to radioactive iodine. In some cases, such as estimating blood volume, it provides alternative calculations, as the medical research literature supports many different algorithms.

By 2018 the app already had over 22,000 medical algorithms. Clearly, with so much to check, there should have been an automated test procedure that assured all calculations and user interfaces were implemented correctly. Since there are so many algorithms, I did a "stratified sampling" of the app — I selected a random sample of ten algorithms. Without exception, every algorithm I evaluated had problems impacting safety.

Fix It: See and solve the problems of digital healthcare. Harold Thimbleby,
Oxford University Press. © Harold Thimbleby 2021.
DOI: 10.1093/oso/9780198861270.003.0030

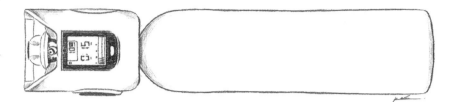

Figure 30.1. A BOC Healthcare oxygen cylinder, showing its digital controller. (The cylinder is 950 mm, just over 3 feet, long.)

Eventually, I found *lots* of bugs.

To be fair, there were so many bugs because there was a common user interface to all the thousands of algorithms. So the same bugs hit lots of algorithms.

I contacted Medal, who responded positively. Rather than tell me I was wrong and I didn't understand their app, Medal met me and we worked towards fixing the bugs by using a more mature software engineering approach. Their current version of the app now has many hundred fewer bugs.

Risky digital healthcare can be improved. Now, Medal wants people to know it is better than a lot of the competition. That's a good story!

Oxygen cylinders and the Internet of Things

Oxygen is one of the most common therapies used in hospitals. Hospitals have thousands of oxygen cylinders, and they need to keep track of them and ensure they are all fully charged with oxygen, ready for use. Cylinders can be hidden in cupboards, may arrive in ambulances, and frequently disappear into homes when patients are discharged or moved to other hospitals.

BOC Healthcare put a Bluetooth transmitter on the top of them, bringing them into the world of the Internet of Things. The transmitter enables every cylinder and its location and status to be very easily tracked centrally.

Another advantage of the computer on the end of the cylinder is that it helps eliminate a common cause of error that can cause serious patient harm.[441] Because of the way it has to be built, the head of the cylinder contains compressed oxygen that can be sufficient to last about 30 seconds. It is possible to check a cylinder and connect it to a patient, but not realize that the brief burst of oxygen is coming from the compressed oxygen in the cylinder head alone, and not from the full cylinder. It's easy to think everything is OK and walk away, leaving the patient to run out of oxygen just after you've left them on their own. The new digital head warns against this error, and helps to stop patients asphyxiating.

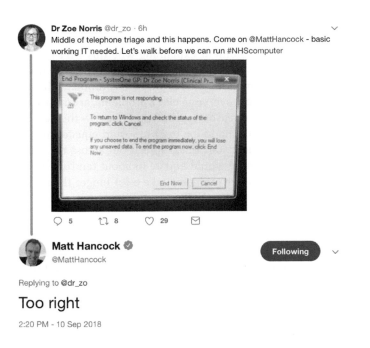

Figure 30.2. Zoë Norris's tweet, and the Secretary of State for Health and Social Care Matt Hancock's quick response to her.[442]

Zoë Norris's tweet

Twitter was founded in 2006. Twitter was a new idea, and by 2009 it was the third-ranking social networking system — though its founders argued it was an information network, not a social network.

In this story, Twitter took minutes to connect a doctor on a hospital ward to the most senior healthcare figure in the country. It started off as yet another everyday symptom of risky digital healthcare: Dr Zoë Norris's hospital computer stopped responding.

Zoë photographed her computer and tweeted (figure 30.2):

> Middle of telephone triage and this happens. Come on @MattHancock — basic working IT needed. Let's walk before we can run #NHScomputer

The UK's Secretary of State for Health and Social Care, The Right Honourable Matt Hancock MP (Member of Parliament) noticed and responded to her, and the conversation then got retweeted to thousands of people, including me. Maybe only one of Matt Hancock's assistants noticed and tweeted for him, but it's still a very good story of how digital improves communication across hierarchies. Let's hope that Matt Hancock and his staff effectively follow up on this tweet.

It's worth spending a moment explaining why this isn't just a random heart-warming computer story: it has far wider implications for digital health. Let's say the NHS has a million general purpose computers. If so, if these bugs, the causes of Zoë's and everyone else's problems, are in each and every computer — and there's no reason to think otherwise — then every minute a doctor or nurse spends trying to log in or to restart equates to a collective million or so minutes of lost staff time, spread out across the whole NHS. Over a year, that loss in time would equate to about ten full five-day jobs, and of course most computer problems take a lot longer than a minute to resolve, so the hidden cost to the NHS is even higher.

Back in the early 1980s, Steve Jobs used to worry about how slow his new Macintosh computer might turn out to be, but he encouraged his staff to design faster computers. He wanted to sell so many of them that speeding them up by only ten seconds would save lives. His thinking was that every Macintosh booting up takes a few minutes out of your life, and if Apple sold millions of them, those precious minutes would add up to wasted lifetimes. Shaving seconds off each Macintosh would — given enough sales! — collectively save lives. Apparently, his encouragement worked.[443] Digital healthcare could save more lives like this, just by eliminating bugs and getting faster at what it does.

Electronic intensive care

The intensive care unit (ICU) provides hospital care for critically ill patients who need life support, close care, and constant supervision. They are very intense places to work, and digital technology is routinely used not just for supporting patients but for monitoring them. If a patient deteriorates, staff are notified and can respond immediately.

Since the digital systems doing the patient monitoring are digital, *they* can be monitored remotely. The idea of an electronic ICU or tele-ICU is that a dedicated room has digital systems that monitor perhaps hundreds of intensive care patients, either in one hospital or spread around a geographical region (figure 30.3).

In a good eICU, the nurses rotate with the staff in the actual ICUs, so everybody gets to see both sides, and then they can help get to implement ways to make the monitoring and help more effective. In particular, rotation avoids any sense that the hands-on staff are being monitored in a negative way.

The evidence shows that eICUs are very effective.[444]

eICUs couldn't be done without digital.

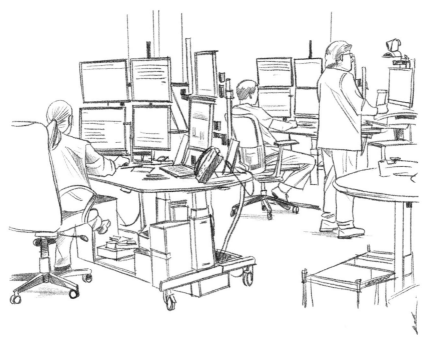

Figure 30.3. Nurses watch over the vital signs of hundreds of patients in critical care. This is the center of an eICU, an electronic intensive care unit.

Unfortunately, the eICU research evidence, like much research in digital healthcare systems, is limited by the small size of the relevant research literature, and that research papers generally want to report positive results rather than problems, or don't want to waste space publishing corrections to previously published works. This is **publication bias**, that the literature is selective. So systematic reviews typically give more optimistic results than are warranted. The published papers also use different methodologies that are hard to compare, and most studies in digital health are rather small, so they have problems with statistics.[445]

If that's the "bad news" about the digital healthcare research in this area, the good news is that digital technologies can help with all of those problems. eICUs work by sharing patient data with a central monitoring facility, and it's then a short step to putting this data online so that researchers can use it. For instance, the **eICU Collaborative Research Database**[446] is a major database that collects data from over 200,000 patient ICU admissions across the US. The database is open access, so anyone (after some formalities) can use it for their research. Even if it's a story that isn't finished yet, this is a very positive sign of life for digital healthcare.

Part III ◇ Prognosis ◇ A better future

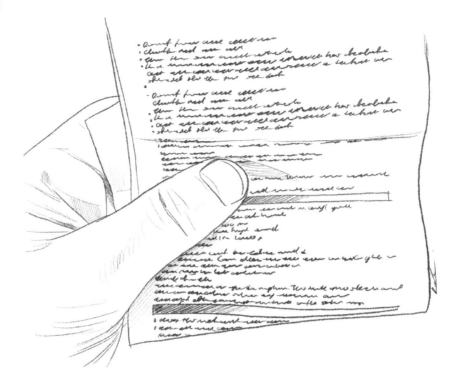

Figure 30.4. It's easy to overlook the many "trivial" advantages of digital. Patient Information Leaflets (PILs) are provided with all medicines, and they are generally complex and very hard to read. Patients are effectively discouraged from reading all the details of how to use their medicines properly and safely. Patients with poor eyesight are extremely disadvantaged. But information on websites and PDF leaflets can be downloaded and scaled to any size, or read aloud by accessibility software.

Digital Stories

After an incident, patients, and relatives may be overwhelmed with grief, but their complaints often encounter "delay and deny" as the hospital handles the complaint legalistically, following set protocols. As complaints fester, more and more causes (used holes in the Swiss Cheese[a]) become apparent, and the possibility of any satisfactory resolution diminishes. Nobody wins.

Digital Stories transform this.

"Digital Storytelling" could mean almost any form of storytelling with digital, but I'll focus on a style of storytelling that is particularly effective in healthcare.

Digital Storytelling gives people a voice through helping them turn their

---

[a] See Chapter 6: Swiss Cheese Model, page 61 ←

story into a two-minute video using voice recording and still pictures. A Digital Story allows patients or staff to find the story that needs telling and get it to an audience.

A Digital Story is a short, usually about two minutes long, simple, and engaging video clip.

Everybody has two minutes to listen!

Digital Stories are told in the first person ("I did this..." etc). The voice recording is edited and put together with photos or drawings using basic video editing software.

The Digital Story communicates powerfully, but equally the person authoring it has to work hard to figure out what their key story is, what story structure it needs to work best, and how to record it clearly. It usually works best with the help of a facilitator who listens and encourages, and deals with the mechanics of recording the story. The listening is a careful, skilled process, which helps focus the story, but also helps develop insights for the story-teller. It's a powerful process even if the story is never heard by anyone else.

It's important to get training in Digital Storytelling to be able to facilitate it well.[447]

I, as a Digital Storyteller, can testify to the effectiveness of the process in distilling what you want to say to maximize effectiveness. My father's story, which I discussed earlier,[b] is online at harold.thimbleby.net/dad; the website also has the hospital's powerful response to the story. The short Digital Story format communicated with the hospital in a really effective way when all of my previous conventional complaints and meetings had failed to communicate.

The Digital Story format originally started in the Berkeley StoryCenter (San Francisco Bay Area),[448] and has been developed and used extensively for healthcare by Prue Thimbleby, who is based in Swansea Bay University Health Board, part of the NHS.[449]

Here, below, are transcriptions of eight Digital Stories, three from members of staff and five from patients and family, all directly experiencing the positive impact of digital healthcare.

Lisa Thomas's story

Lisa Thomas is a ward sister, who explains how her work changed when she started using an iPad to do patient admissions.

Lisa's story ... "Before we had the opportunity to pilot the electronic devices to do electronic admissions, we were averaging between 25 minutes and

---

[b] See Chapter 9: Peter Thimbleby's preventable death, page 109 ←

> **Box 30.1.** Early computer diagnosis
>
> One of the world's first digital healthcare systems was Mickie, which was developed in the late 1960s. Early versions of Mickie used a teletype, a form of computerized typewriter and a telephone line to connect to a large mainframe computer. Mickie had a polite and encouraging computer system; researchers found that alcoholics tested were more truthful about their drinking habits than when talking to real human doctors — they admitted to drinking on average 50% more! The earliest research on the system was published in 1971.[450]
>
>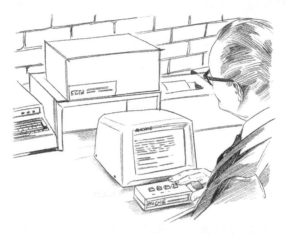
>
> Later versions of Mickie, as shown in the drawing above, used a microcomputer and a simplified keyboard so patients could directly answer "yes," "no," "don't know" and "don't understand" just by pressing buttons. You can see the simplified keypad being used in the drawing.
>
> The system was developed by Dr Chris Evans, an early computer pioneer.[451]

sometimes 45 minutes to do an admission. By having something of an electronic device it reduced the timescale of our admissions. And I think that the ease and use of the devices was really straightforward, very self-explanatory — exactly as our unified assessment is.

Timescale-wise, the time was reduced down to about 12–15 minutes for an admission.

The nature of the surgery that we have here is very sensitive and the patients were having to go back over things that they had already gone over, and they were getting upset through it all the time.

We had one particular lady who came in to us while we were doing the pilot, she was very apprehensive, she was really sort of nervous, lots of problems previously with surgery. So we did what we needed to do, and she was very happy for us to take the information on the iPad, but we were able to spend more time with that lady because of the reduced time spent filling things in on the iPad.

Time-wise with the patient — even though we had shorter times with the patient — doing our paperwork side of things — we were still with patients and supporting them but we didn't have that paper in front of us or the device. We could actually give emotional comfort to the patients if needed.

We had staff here that had never used an electronic device prior to this pilot and they've all gone and bought iPads and various things. They're very happy to use these devices."

Bella Cheham's story

Bella Cheham has pulmonary hypertension.[452] She used to have a very restricted life before she used a digital portable infusion system.

Bella's story ... "I have got idiopathic pulmonary hypertension. I was originally told approximately 50% of people die within five years of diagnosis, and approximately 100% of people die within 10 years of diagnosis, but things are improving all the time, and thankfully it's becoming much more like a chronic condition. The doctor explained that the final, last ditch solution for me is a lung infusion. This involves having a tube put into your lung which sticks out of your chest and connects to a pump which delivers a drug infusion 24 hours a day, 7 days a week, and you can never disconnect the pump.

The introduction of the technology to my life had a number of what I would call side effects, which I didn't expect. The pump needed changing at exactly the same time every 24 hours. If somebody said to me "do you fancy going out tonight?" the answer was, "only if I can be back by half past 10." That's much improved now, as I'm on an improved pump that only needs to be changed every 48 hours.

The other side is that I have been transformed from a person who could not walk up four steps without having to stop and catch my breath; who could not carry my shopping home; who basically was afraid to go out because I wasn't certain that I would maintain consciousness.

Now I can do anything and everything that I want.

I am a lot fitter than most of my friends. I am back to being able to do the gardening, I am back to being able to do singing, dancing, and even playing the recorder, which requires a good deal of breath.

People that do not know that I have pulmonary hypertension would not know that I have pulmonary hypertension, and that is how I like it. I have never in the six years since I have been using the infusion had any lung infections or issues arising from having the pump and the line.

The pump, in my experience, is completely reliable.

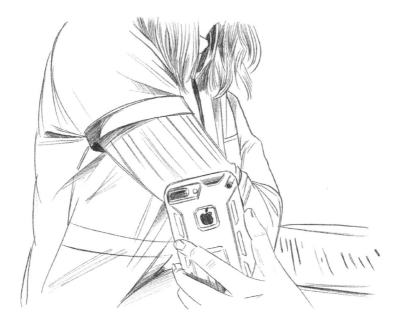

Figure 30.5. Nobody in the café knows Rhian Melita Morris is taking her blood glucose reading.

My pump is reasonably simple and obvious to use, but the bottom line is, it has transformed my life from miserable, depressed, unable to do anything to being fit active and healthy — what is not to like about it?"

Rhian Melita Morris's story

Rhian Melita Morris is a Type 1 diabetic: her body can't make its own insulin. She uses the Abbott FreeStyle Libre sensor to monitor her blood glucose levels.

Rhian's story ... "I'm a Type 1 diabetic, and I've been on an infusion pump for about nine years. Even though the infusion pump can calculate the insulin I need, it doesn't communicate with a device yet that can tell me what my blood glucose is so that it can do that automatically.

They've put me on what's called a FreeStyle Libre sensor, which is a tiny little disk which sticks to your arm where the needle goes in (figure 30.5), and I can scan this with a little blood glucose monitor.

But the best thing is, I've downloaded an app onto my phone which can use it.

My phone can read the scanner, and that for me has been the most useful thing, because in my work I go to regular meetings and to pull out my blood glucose monitor and do a test — it's almost as if I feel the meeting stops and everybody watches what I'm doing! They're holding their breath. Is she OK to continue? You know, especially as people don't understand it.

But with the phone I can just put it up against my arm, and it'll take a reading and nobody even knows what I've done.

This app also has a few analysis tools and graphs so that I can track over days when my blood sugars might rise, so that I can address that on my pump by changing the settings to adjust my insulin. That's been far more helpful than just using the blood glucose monitor which, even though it has graphs and has a tiny screen, whereas I've a 7 inch plus phone. We're all getting older — I can see it much better!

And the technology behind it is much better than on the old device.

By law, UK diabetic drivers have to check their blood glucose levels four times a day, else they may lose their driving licenses. (If you are a bus or lorry driver, you must also store results on a memory meter, and you must have three months of continuous meter readings at an annual medical assessment.) I do it at least four times a day; if I'm poorly, I'll do it at least ten or fifteen times.

So, yes, it's made a world of difference."

Marie Moe's story

Dr Marie Moe is a researcher in cybersecurity, and after having what most of us would call a heart attack (in fact a dangerous type of heart arrhythmia called a "3rd degree AV block") she needed a pacemaker implanted. She is now the world-leading researcher in digital implant cybersecurity. Her life depends on it.[453]

Her life with the pacemaker is so interesting, we've already met her twice before in this book.[c,d] Here's her story of how having the digital implant saved her life.

Marie's story ... "I woke up lying on the floor. I had no idea how I'd got there, or how long I'd been out. I went to the emergency room at the local hospital. It turned out I had fallen because my heart had stopped long enough to cause unconsciousness. Luckily, it started beating again by itself, but the resulting pulse was low and irregular.

I needed to have a pacemaker that would monitor my heart and send an electrical signal directly to it via an electrode to keep it beating.

When I got the pacemaker, it was an emergency procedure. I needed it to stay alive, so there really was no option to not get it. There was, however, time to ask questions.

---

[c] See Chapter 4: Marie Moe's pacemaker bug, page 46 ←

[d] See Chapter 19: Marie Moe's pacemaker and cosmic rays, page 248 ←

I am a security researcher, and at the time that I got this pacemaker my day job was protecting the Norwegian national critical infrastructure from cyber attacks. So I began asking about the potential security vulnerabilities in the software running on the pacemaker and the possibilities of hacking it. The answers were unsatisfying.

It took a few months of trial-and-error tweaking before the doctors could get the pacemaker's tuning right, and this was complicated by a bug in the device they used to adjust the settings. The bug caused the actual settings of my pacemaker to differ from those displayed on the screen that the technician was seeing.

The consequence of this greatly affected my well-being.

The decision to implant a medical device is a risky one. In my case, the benefit of having the pacemaker certainly outweighs the risk, since I don't think I would be alive without it. I've run the New York Marathon with it."

Jelle Damhuis's story

Jelle Damhuis was a typical active 26-year-old guy. He had his own on-line business, played sports, and had a busy social life. And then he was diagnosed with Non-Hodgkin Lymphoma in January 2018. After the cancer diagnosis and chemotherapy treatment, Jelle came across the Untire app (figure 30.6), which has helped him enormously, and he's now an enthusiastic champion for it.

Jelle's story ... "My chemo sessions were a very exhausting period of treatment, but I managed to get through them with a lot of support from friends and family. Fortunately, my doctor gave the good news: everything was gone! What an incredible joy and relief. It was time to celebrate with champagne and a party!

I was excited for my life to return to 'normal,' but no one warned me that this would be the beginning of the most difficult period. As I sat at home, extreme fatigue consumed me. At unexplained moments I was intensely exhausted. This had a huge impact on my daily life. Meeting up with friends became too much to do.

The fatigue was different from tiredness. This cancer fatigue came suddenly, out of the blue, and I would need to lie down. It felt like extreme exhaustion. The fatigue had a huge impact on my quality of life.

Everything changed during a short walk in my neighborhood. Quite by chance, I noticed a company called Tired of Cancer. Once I got home I looked them up, and I found out that this company had developed an app, the Untire app, to specifically address Cancer-Related Fatigue (CRF).

Eureka!

This is what I had been dealing with all along. Why hadn't I heard about this before?

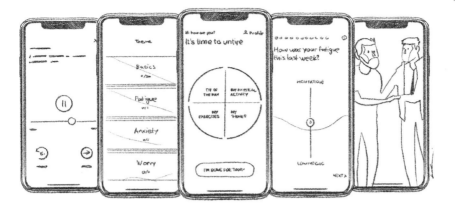

Figure 30.6. The Untire app, used by Jelle Damhuis to help manage his CRF.

I came to find out that 40% of cancer patients and survivors deal with CRF. Immediately, I felt recognition and acknowledgment for my problem. I downloaded the app right away and soon found that it is not one big thing impacting energy, but many little things that impact energy levels.

The Untire app is a free, easy to use, comprehensive self-management program. It helped me to step back and take a good look at what was triggering my fatigue. It helped me gain insight into my behavior, thoughts and symptoms, and it showed me the actions I could take to regain energy.

Because of the Untire app, I am now more aware of my energy and where I get my energy from. I was able to break out of my vicious circle of fatigue, step by step. I started using breathing exercises to regain energy. For instance, if I had dinner plans with friends later in the day I had a few short meditations that would help me re-energize.

Soon, my energy levels improved. After not working for months, I finally felt like I could return to work. I am proud to say that I am now part of the Tired of Cancer team. It gives me a good feeling to be able to contribute from my own experience to help others with fatigue.

Looking back, I realize how much things can change in a short period of time. I can't emphasize enough how important it is to always keep that in mind. A year ago, I would never have pictured my life the way it is now. The periods of illness have cost me a lot, but now I have found a way to gain from it. Through it all, keep moving forward, look ahead, and remember that you will get through it."

Angela Branston's story

Healthcare and social care are intimately connected. As in healthcare, social workers know that they usually only get attention when their work is seen to be substandard or when something has gone wrong. The first instinct of almost anyone is to tell a horror story, to describe poor, mistake-ridden, and bad practice by professionals.

In contrast, the *Signs of Safety* approach was developed in a spirit of appreciative inquiry, asking social workers to describe self-defined and successful practice in difficult situations[454] — this is a Safety Two approach,[e] and has made *Signs of Safety* a powerful tool for driving organizational improvement.

Angela Branston was one of the first social workers to start using a digital version of *Signs of Safety* made by Liquidlogic IT.[455] Her dramatic story is about the radical transformation that good iterative design[f] has on work and morale, and in improving the effectiveness in delivering care.

Angela's story ... "I've got to be honest, I didn't hit the ground running with social work. I found it so, so difficult.

I can really vividly remember sitting in front of my computer all day at work, and not knowing what I was supposed to be writing. The forms were just endless, and they all looked the same.

It was so overwhelming. It really knocked my confidence. I think it actually impacted my mental health. I can remember that period of time just crying, just because I couldn't do it. I felt like such a failure, and my confidence was lower and lower and lower.

I thought 'this new system is going to be great,' and that I could just look at it and all of the stuff will be there, but it wasn't at that stage yet. We'd had all these promises of things, and then here it was, and it wasn't what we thought it was going to be.

The thing that was really fantastic was that people listened, and then they went away and changed the system. The forms drove our practice, but in the parts where they didn't, we could talk to them and tell them, actually this bit doesn't drive our practice, and if it did this instead that it would be better.

Then we saw what they'd done with it.

Now, from being a person who sat and cried and didn't know how to write a plan, I'm advising the managers on what the right thing to do is, and this is the way it's working best. The most exciting part of it is that when we go out and do that with the families, they understand what we're doing."

---

[e] See Chapter 12: Safety One & Safety Two, page 145 ←
[f] See Chapter 23: Iterative design, page 313 ←

Isabel & Jason Maude's story

In 1999, Isabel Maude nearly died. As a result, her father, Jason, was in-spired to develop a digital tool to help improve diagnosis.

Jason called his diagnostic tool **Isabel**, after his daughter.[456]

Jason's story ... "The story starts when my daughter aged three became ill with chickenpox. She was developing fever, diarrhea and was lethargic. So we took her along to the GP. Then she got worse, and that evening we went along to A&E [emergency department], and again it was shrugged off as normal chickenpox. Her temperature was over 40 C [104 F], so they focused on getting her temperature down. They got the temperature down, which they did by using Calpol [Tylenol/paracetamol], and said go home.

She continued to get worse at home. We called up. 'Don't worry — it's normal chickenpox.' There was no thinking about 'could it be anything else'? It was always 'it's just chickenpox.' We got to the point where we thought, 'this is just not right.'

We went back to A&E, and she was seen by a pediatrician, who looked at her and said, 'Oh, she looks a little bit dehydrated. You may have to stay in overnight.' And the nurse who tried to take her blood pressure said, 'Oh dear, the blood pressure machine looks as if it's not working properly,' when in fact her blood pressure was rock bottom.

Literally, about ten minutes later her eyes started rolling, and she went into multi-system failure, and crashed. The crash team was called in. Then it was just chaos.

From that point on, the NHS worked beautifully. The crash team was good. And she was transferred that day by the intensive care retrieval team to St Mary's Hospital, London.

But it needn't have happened.

We actually saw the Medical Director of the original hospital who had been responsible for missing her diagnosis once Isabel had been discharged, and he said, 'I trained at Mary's in infectious diseases. I wrote one of the papers describing exactly what had happened to Isabel: it sits in the proto-col folder.' So all the knowledge was there, but it wasn't in the clinicians that were admitting and assessing Isabel at the time.

That showed in stark relief the problem that needed to be fixed. How do they pluck out the unusual cases within the mass of routine stuff that comes through?

We didn't want to create a tool that diagnosed a patient; the idea was to help the clinician put together a differential to help with clinical reasoning. The problem with diagnosis is there's too much burden on the clinician to remember everything. If you think there are 10,000 diseases in the world, it's just impossible for anybody to remember how those diseases present. And that's what computers are really good at — computers are good at go-

Part III ◇ Prognosis ◇ A better future

ing through mountains of information very, very quickly, and coming up with a shortlist.

So the tool, Isabel, first became available in 2001 — and it worked. When the clinicians tried it, they put in classic cases, and a good list of possible diseases came up. One of our clients recently published a paper, 'Isabel to the Rescue!'[457] They were close to losing the patient. They decided to use Isabel. It prompted them to think of brucellosis, which they hadn't thought about. They asked the patient. Yes, she'd been eating homemade cheese in Mexico. And that's what it turned out to be. They actually said, 'You know, if we hadn't used Isabel, we wouldn't have thought about it — we would've lost that patient.'

You know, Isabel is really a tried-and-tested tool, and is a great contrast to these tools that have not been validated, or proven, or that don't work. Isabel is a tool that's been out there for twenty years. We've had a process of continual validation and development. We cover 6,000 diseases and 4,000 drugs. And today the system is used by over 250 institutions around the world.

In 2012 we decided to make it available to patients. Isabel is a tool to help the patient get much better informed. The better informed patient is the better patient. We're very keen on licensing the tool to other companies that are building health information sites, so for example patient.info has a symptom checker powered by Isabel.

The culture has been our biggest barrier to getting Isabel used, with clinicians not thinking that they need help in this particular area."

Sian Thomas's story

The COVID-19 pandemic made lots of people very sick. All hospital visiting stopped to reduce the spread of infection. Sian Thomas was a Pediatric Occupational Therapist based at Neath Port Talbot Hospital. She was redeployed onto an adult stroke rehabilitation ward to support the most vulnerable patients.

Sian's story ... "It struck me that the patients were going through life changing events. It became quite apparent of the impact of them having no visitors, things like no magazines and no papers on the ward because of infection control. The days were really long for the patients, and they were looking for a lot of reassurance about what was happening. They were really confused about why relatives weren't coming to see them. Why had they been left there? Was anyone coming back for them? It was getting to a point where it started affecting me because I could see the impact. I felt a bit helpless.

I was having a chat with one of the healthcare support workers one day, just talking about our frustrations of the situation and the impact on the patients. She said, 'Oh I've had an iPad donated in the office, it just needs setting up.' So we quickly got it set up, and within half an hour we were on our first virtual call with one of the patients, who hadn't seen his family for weeks. His child was really unwell and was going through their own treatment at home, so he'd a lot of fear about whether they were going to make it, whether they were going to see each other again. Instantly, the connection when we came on the video between the patient and family was just amazing. There were tears in their eyes.

It really struck me: it was an incredibly powerful thing that just reminded me of that basic human instinct that we need to connect, we're social people, and the love just pours through from both ends, you know? It was a really lovely moment. It was such a simple thing to do, really, to just go and get the iPad and make it happen. And we just decided there's no reason we can't carry on doing that.

So we set up a virtual visiting book then. We had to ring some relatives, get some details of what platform they were using.

The difference in some of the patients has been incredible: their mood has changed, they're more motivated to return home, and they can't wait to see their families.

On the other side of it, the relatives had been anxious about knowing about what's going on with their loved ones, and now they've had that daily update it's allayed a lot of their anxieties as well.

So, yes, it's been a really important project, and I think we've learned so much as a therapy team and how we can continue past COVID to make this possible — there's always going to be people in hospitals who can't see their relatives, and the only way is up."

The Patient Experience Library

The 2020 Cumberlege Review, *First Do No Harm*, says:

> Patients often know when something has gone wrong with their treatment. All too often they are the first to know. Their experience must no longer be considered anecdotal and weighted least in the hierarchy of evidence-based medicine.
>
> [Patients] who have been affected have been dismissed, overlooked, and ignored for far too long. The issue here is not one of a single or a few rogue medical practitioners, or differences in regional practice. It is system-wide.[458]

In comparison to the universal respect for medical evidence (such as peer-reviewed research papers in medical journals), patient-centered evidence is under-valued. For example, over the years there have been many patient-facing inquiries and initiatives (the Cumberlege Review is one such)

Part III ◇ Prognosis ◇ A better future

responding to particular incidents, but as each initiative finishes its entire body of learning — and the patient voice — disappears with it.

The Patient Experience Library therefore decided to build a website to promote, curate, and keep patient experience accessible. Their website — www.patientlibrary.net — has many resources, from a weekly newsletter to major reports of patient experience and involvement. As of 2020, the library holds over 60,000 documents.[459]

Even the humble website can be a sign of life to help change the world.

———————————■———————————

There are many, many more stories of the positive impact of digital health-care. I want to collect more stories, particularly with a digital and Safety Two attitude.[g] So if you have a story, please get in contact with me by email at harold@thimbleby.net — if appropriate, we'll then go through a process of recording and editing, and with your consent we'll add it to this book's web-site at **www.harold.thimbleby.net/fixit**

---

[g] See Chapter 12: Safety One & Safety Two, page 145 ←

Part III ◇ Prognosis ◇ A better future

The horrific COVID-19 pandemic has forced healthcare systems to innovate in digital health. Some changes have been amazing, liberating patients, and protecting healthcare staff — but some have been rather worrying. What can we learn?

31

The pivotal pandemic?

Roberta Shelton was the first person to die of COVID-19 in Indiana, USA, on 19 March 2020.[460] Despite being isolated in hospital, she was able to say goodbye to her partner using an iPad.

Hours after his many friends sang Happy Birthday to him using Zoom on an iPad, Thomas Martins fell unconscious and died alone at home from COVID-19, nine days after his mother had died of COVID-19 too.[461]

These tragic deaths, three out of the thousands that have numbed us, were made a little easier to bear because digital technologies eased physical barriers and brought people closer together.

I used to wonder why, with my neuropathy, I had to drive to the hospital, find a parking space, and wait for hours, just to get a brief meeting with the neurologist. The hospital neurologist's computer couldn't even see my blood test results ordered by my doctor. But the pressures of working safely during a pandemic have transformed everything. Last time, my neurologist used Zoom: he worked from his office, and talked to me at home, and I got a prescription fulfilled without even having to visit my GP. Easy. Efficient.

It's awful that it takes a pandemic, but it's proved that improving health-care is possible. We still don't know very much about COVID-19. COVID is the severe acute respiratory syndrome caused by a virus called SARS-CoV-2. COVID stands for COrona VIrus Disease, and the -19 is because COVID was first identified in 2019, where it started in Wuhan in China. Before the pandemic, doctors saw fewer than 1% of patients by video, and now they are seeing over 93%.[462] It "just" needs the political willpower. Until COVID-19 changed the rules, nobody had the permission or funding to seriously think about improving. There was no imperative to change. Now there is.

I'm writing this chapter in 2020, in the middle of the pandemic — sadly, we're now well into its "second wave," and more are to come. In this chapter, I'll cover four central topics relevant to digital healthcare: wearable computers, tracking apps, epidemiological models, and, briefly, ventilators — all ar-

Fix It: See and solve the problems of digital healthcare. Harold Thimbleby,
Oxford University Press. © Harold Thimbleby 2021.
DOI: 10.1093/oso/9780198861270.003.0031

eas where effective digital health innovations are central to the fight against disease, not just COVID-19 of course.

———————————————◼———————————————

COVID-19 is a horrible disease, and as it attacks people they may deteriorate without noticing. If they deteriorate, patients usually have much worse outcomes. Hospitals have to make difficult decisions: they don't want to fill up with patients who don't need in-patient care, yet they shouldn't send patients home if they're going to deteriorate. Instead, it's better to have some sort of early warning system, so patients sent home after initial assessment will know if they start to deteriorate.

Blood oxygenation is a measure of how much oxygen our blood has. When blood oxygenation drops for no good reason, this is a sign that we're deteriorating. Unfortunately, we aren't directly aware of our oxygen levels. There's the problem of "silent hypoxia," where we don't notice as we start to deteriorate. By the time it's noticeable, we may already be in a serious situation.

Hospitals have been sending some at-risk COVID-19 patients home with personal blood oxygenation meters.[463] These are small, cheap devices that clip on your finger or ear lobe, and give you a direct measure of your blood oxygenation. They give an early warning of deterioration if you need hospital assessment. The scheme frees up hospital resources to focus on the patients that need treatment.

This powerful idea raises some interesting points for digital healthcare.

Blood oxygen levels are calculated using computers — tiny, usually specialized computers are sufficient. Blood oxygenation meters are so small, they can be fitted into watches or fitted inside the clips that fit over your finger. You can even buy kits to build your own for a few pounds.[464] I never thought a few years ago that computers would get so small that we'd be sewing computers into clothes — there's now a whole, vibrant, field of Computer Science called **wearable computing** to take these ideas further. It's a powerful testament to how small and ubiquitous digital is.

Because of the versatility of computers,[a] it is now much easier and cheaper to make things with computers in them than not. Gadgets like Apple's iWatch have the oxygen sensor and the computer in them already, and they can do everything a blood oxygenation meter can do and send the data to your phone or healthcare organization. Digital is everywhere, even if we can't see it.

Then there is something more thought-provoking. When computers are hidden — **embedded** is the technical term — inside other devices, the legal position is generally that the device is regulated as a device, not as a digital device. So the oxygenation meter has to work. It's the same if you have a camera or washing machine or car or TV. They come with warranties that

---

[a] See Chapter 13: Computational Thinking, page 151 ←

they will work — as cameras, washing machines, cars, or TVs — yet they have complex software inside them. If, instead, you used the same digital features but on a computer or mobile phone, as we've seen,[b] the manufacturers will go to great lengths to make sure there is no guarantee anything works. In other words, embedded software shows that the non-warranties we are so used to are there for commercial reasons, not for any technical reasons. Digital *can* be made reliable enough for healthcare, but won't be while we let manufacturers get away with it.

Finally, perhaps the most important point for digital healthcare: COVID-19 is forcing us to think and find new solutions. Digital healthcare is up to the challenge. It's now very clear that digital healthcare can do better than merely "computerize healthcare" — it can do a *lot* better.

―――――――――――――■―――――――――――――

One of the problems with COVID-19 is that people can be infectious before they know they're ill, so contact with these people silently spreads the disease. So many people have caught COVID-19 that testing and tracing everybody to find out the sources of infection is impractical in almost all countries. If you can't find the people who are infectious, it isn't possible — at least, without vaccines or other interventions — to limit the spread of disease through the population.

There are proposals for tracking apps.[465] The basic idea seems simple enough. Many of us use mobile phones, and if they are tracked we know where almost everyone is. If we get ill, our phone's location data combined with everyone else's location data can then be used to track our contacts. If lots of people who get ill had previously met me about a week ago, it's likely that I am the person who infected them. Analyzing the big data that track and trace apps collect with powerful digital technology, it's then very easy to focus effort where it'll be most effective.

Big data, powerful digital technology, and *very easy*, are constant refrains of digital healthcare! Examples of complex problems with tracking apps are privacy trade-offs, such as the potential for snooping going beyond epidemiological needs, and interfering with other devices, like diabetes apps,[466] and the sheer complexity of designing programs that have to be very quickly deployed at national and international scales, and which have to fit in with the manufacturers' (primarily Apple's and Google's) sophisticated operating systems — which the rest of the time are designed to *stop* the sort of "undercover tracking" activities that the apps need.[467] Privacy is interesting, because many apps people use enthusiastically, like Facebook and WhatsApp, track us already, but giving data to a system that wants to promote health is a problem? In some countries, like South Korea, it is a legal requirement to be tracked for COVID-19, so the privacy issues don't arise in the same way — except, in all countries, the more willing compliance there is with the app,

―――――――――――――

[b] See Chapter 15: Who's accountable?, page 193 ←

the more successful it will be. And "compliance" — the correct term, but nevertheless a word with horrible overtones — isn't about a technical issue that apps can solve.

An important issue that makes designing apps very difficult is scams. There are many fake text messages, emails (phishing), and websites that convince people they are infected and then need to provide their personal details.[468] How do you design the real systems to assure people they are reliable, and asking for genuine information that will be protected, and at the same time dissuade anyone from the scams?

There are lots of ethical questions. Ethics are not only complex for humans to understand, but they are very complex to program well. Some ethical issues are discussed in box 31.2.

With more data, you can get more certain about the inferences from the data, which is useful medically for managing the disease, but the more data you collect the harder it is to ensure privacy — or to properly regulate the companies running the systems that collect the data.

At this stage of the pandemic and the development of apps, it's impossible to have a definitive view of the issues. Needless to say, at least to mid-2021, the *cost* of apps intended to help fight COVID-19 has been astronomical, and with few clear gains.[469] Some apps failed outright for all the usual reasons: political, legal, and technical. Basically, the developers rushed in and then found insurmountable bugs — in other words, they assumed digital was trivial to get working. They were not professionally prepared for the reality of digital complexity.[470] Clearly, although innovative digital tech sounds easy, successful digital healthcare is much harder than politicians think, especially when (for understandable reasons) people rush in with untested ideas that have not been rigorously developed — issues I've discussed throughout this book.

An example of this "rush in with untested ideas" was England's problem with their Test, Trace, and Isolate systems, which came to public notice in early October 2020.[471] The idea was simple: people get tested for COVID-19; if they are positive (more precisely, if the test says they are positive), then their contacts are traced; people who are deemed likely to have COVID-19 are then asked to isolate so that they do not infect further people. In England, there are lots of places where you can get tested, and lots of places where test samples can be sent to be tested. Finally, the data from all the test centers across the country has to be combined so that people can be traced, as well as to generate local and national summary reports.

Unfortunately, a step in this process of managing the data involved Excel spreadsheets, or, more precisely, it involved files in the Excel format called XLS. XLS is obsolete and not a very good format. When lots of data were combined, because of its limitations, the XLS format lost 15,841 test results, meaning that up to 50,000 people were not warned that they had been in close contact with people with COVID-19 infections. Worse, XLS lost the data silently, and nobody noticed. Losses started to happen on 25 September and continued at least up to 2 October, so it took a week to notice and to start to fix the problem.

Reports of this fiasco largely focussed on the incompetence of using Excel and the old XLS file format.[472] No, the incompetence was designing a system that lost data *and designing in nothing to notice errors.* There was incompetence in pulling Excel (or Excel format files) into a critical healthcare system where it had no place. Nobody noticed the errors until several days in a row of low numbers of tests being reported were obviously a symptom of something going wrong.

This is the same problem that affected the XceedPro glucometers we discussed earlier.[c] In both cases the system was not designed professionally. Any competent programmer expects error: they expect human error, they expect network problems, they expect they themselves will make typos and even have fundamental misunderstandings of the requirements and of the code (especially of code others have written). Therefore, professional programmers use the techniques we've discussed in this book: their programs check that everything is as expected.

> 🛈 The fundamental idea that safe programs *must* continually check their assumptions was explored at some length in the chapters *Computational Thinking*[d] and *Computer Factors.*[e] Indeed, box 21.2, in *Computer Factors*, showed that Alan Turing — arguably the most famous computer pioneer ever — published exactly this idea back in 1947.[308] It's fair to say that developers who build critical systems like a national Test and Trace system without continual checks (including checking the effectiveness of the program for improving public health), and trying to improve it given the insights of testing, seem to be ignorant of routine, professional standards in software. They (or perhaps their managers) unnecessarily put lives at risk.

For instance, if 1,001 COVID-19 test results are sent to another site, the program there *must* check that 1,001 results are received in good order. In the Test and Trace Excel fiasco, there was obviously no such checking. Clearly, the people who designed and built the system implicitly expected it to work perfectly. When it didn't, they had no way of knowing. It hadn't occurred to them that they would need to know immediately if — when — their systems were not being perfect. This is Cat Thinking on hormones.[f]

If you design systems assuming they are perfect, when they fail — as they eventually will — you have nothing to fall back on. You must design systems

[c] See Chapter 8: Disciplinary action against 73 nurses, page 92 ←
[d] See Chapter 13: Computational Thinking, page 151 ←
[e] See Chapter 21: Computer Factors, page 277 ←
[f] See Chapter 3: Cat Thinking, page 25 ←

to fail gracefully.[g] But, in addition to that big failure in design, there were at least four other strategic issues:

🌒 A pandemic is a pandemic because infections are growing exponentially. By definition, then, a national Test and Trace system for a pandemic is going to have to handle lots of tests. To use a data format that can't handle lots of tests was naïve and a failure to understand the basic problem.

🌒 Excel seems so easy to use, that it's tempting to just build systems with it, but we saw earlier that Excel is deceptive,[h] and losing 15,841 tests is a consequence of ignoring that fact. *Involving Excel at any stage doesn't make sense.* Excel is nice because it allows the user to edit and organize numerical data (spreadsheets, in fact) very easily. That is exactly what you do *not* want test laboratories to be doing. If you can edit large amounts of data easily, you can also accidentally edit lots of data too. One slip in Excel and you might delete or mangle thousands of data items; you might delete an entire row or column — who'd know? There should have been a custom design to handle test results reliably, and Excel (and Excel file formats) should have been nowhere near it.

🌒 What training did the people who made the sharp-end mistake get? It seems that laboratories were emailing XLS files — which makes sense if you are using Excel to handle local test data, but as I argued above, using Excel at all was crazy. If any part of a digital healthcare system is crazy, the whole system is crazy.

🌒 We all make errors, and there is no news in that. The thing is, you should never have one programmer develop software of this type working alone. There must be pair programming, code review, and other forms of active teamwork.[i] The basic error wasn't made by one person. It wasn't a mere slip — so where was the team (with the appropriate skills) to spot and block the serious programming slip? Where was the code review? It was a management failure, a failure of management to understand that developing software is not magic.

🌒 It's baffling that a national Test and Trace system costing over £10 billion[5] (not counting the cost of earlier failed apps[470]) didn't have a lot more competent and effective professional input into its design and monitoring. To put the cost of the Test and Trace project into perspective, £12 billion is about a tenth of the *entire* NHS England annual budget. Politicians who plan such large digital health projects

---

[g] See Chapter 21: Graceful degradation, page 292 ←
[h] See Chapter 14: Microsoft Excel, page 182 ←
[i] See Chapter 21: Computer Factors, page 277 ←

simultaneously think digital healthcare is trivial (else there would have been more safeguards against error) and, at the same time, for some reason, think the suppliers of the systems need massive funding.

The solution, of course, is when you are designing a digital healthcare system, in this case a national public health system for Test and Trace during a pandemic, is that you must use competent professional software engineers.

———————————◼———————————

Given that we expect human error and other problems, tracking systems are best designed so that they do not have to be perfect. For app tracking, we shouldn't need everyone to have mobile phones so they can use the app. We just need *enough* people to have mobile phones. We only need to somehow make the **reproduction number** (called R, the increase in the number of cases being generated in the population) go under 1, and then the pandemic will start to die out.

To beat the pandemic, R does not need to be pushed down to a perfect zero, although the smaller it is, the faster the epidemic will die out. In reality, R is an over-simplification — it's an average, so it smooths over the key impact of superspreaders and other dispersion factors, which are particularly relevant for COVID-19.[473]

One way to reduce R is to vaccinate people. In general, we need to reduce infection from one person to another. We can socially isolate people, wear masks, wash our hands, ventilate well, disinfect surfaces ... and we have to test and track down infectious people and quarantine them so they don't infect more people. Tracking infectious people is hard work, especially as so many people are already infected, so it's an obvious idea to use tracking apps to take the laborious work out of tracking.

An app can only help trace infectious people if it knows when people get close to each other, and it can do this using Bluetooth, assuming everyone's mobile's Bluetooth is switched on. In the simplest approach, the app does not need to know who anybody is. Here's how it works: I don't need to know who X is, but if I am close to X, my app records that. Similarly, X's app will record that they are close to somebody, Y perhaps. Later, one of us gets COVID-19 symptoms and we take a test that confirms we do indeed have COVID-19. The test process will include getting our mobile phone data — so the healthcare system now knows how to get in contact with the mobile X owns, even if it still doesn't know who X is as a person. So, X's mobile is told they had a close encounter with somebody who is now ill, and they should go and get tested — they don't need to delay and wait for any symptoms to develop.

The app is useful at this basic level, and not very intrusive, but if it collected a little bit more information, it would be even more use to epidemiologists. The app isn't very motivating for anyone using it; so it needs the

> **Box 31.1.** The 1918 Spanish Flu
>
> Although COVID-19 is not flu, the Spanish Flu pandemic of 1918 is an object lesson in the seriousness of what we face, and what the long-term social impacts might be.[474]
>
> It's possible that more people died of Spanish Flu than were killed in both World Wars combined — the Spanish Flu was a worldwide disaster, killing 20 million in India alone. It killed and orphaned millions of people worldwide who never got counted. Many languages died out.
>
> In 1918 we didn't know anything about viruses — at the time, nobody was able to identify the agent that caused the flu. Although quarantine was well known, people had no alternative ways of working. Nobody had computers or the internet.
>
> Today, managing the COVID-19 pandemic has been made much easier, both by advances in biomedicine and thanks to the internet and mobile communications. In fact, most of the biomedical advances, from the electron microscopes that can see coronaviruses to sequencing the genome of the SARS-CoV-2 coronavirus, are thanks to computers.
>
> Ironically, though, some of the pandemic problems today stem from computers too: the "infodemic" spread of fake news, especially in social media on the internet.

user to be rather altruistic. If you report symptoms, you may have to stay at home and not go to work, so there is a financial penalty for being honest. However, if the app was combined with another app, such as a general healthcare app, it could be made much more helpful to the owner — and, at the same time, provide higher quality information for epidemiological work in managing the pandemic, as the epidemiologists would know things like your age, other illnesses you might have, and so on.

Using Machine Learning on the data is an obvious idea to help enrich the information the app collects — we could identify and better support people who are likely to be more susceptible to COVID-19, for instance — but the Machine Learning will also learn some fascinating things about us (and our contacts) that many would probably prefer to keep private!

The problem is that the tracking information we need is not just helping to fight COVID-19, but it is also *very* valuable data in its own right. Even if we completely trust the motives of the folk collecting and analyzing our data, what if they get hacked? They are sitting on a goldmine that will definitely attract hackers.

At the very least, then, the development of these tracking apps and the storage of the data they collect involves tricky trade-offs, and needs careful oversight. In the UK, the Government gave the secret service (GCHQ) permission to access the data[475] — like everything else with digital technology, this cuts both ways: it means GCHQ can help improve the app's cyberse-

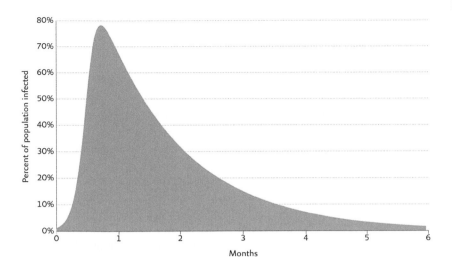

Figure 31.1. My very simple epidemiological model, as run on a computer, showing (given my model's assumptions) how a high proportion of people can get infected, followed by the number of infected people tailing off as people recover or perhaps die. Note how the graph doesn't quite start off at zero, as we need to have some people infected to get the epidemic going. I've made the fully documented code to draw this graph available online.[476]

curity *and* they can monitor personal details of citizens with ease (but they would've been doing that anyway).

People will certainly worry about the use of the data the apps collect. If too many people refuse to use the app, the app won't be very effective. The app's User Centered Design — in the broadest sense of that — will be critical.[j]

It's a trade-off whether privacy is worth risking. Will the information from tracking apps help manage COVID-19 "better" than the risks to privacy? Epidemiological research suggests that COVID-19 will be a disaster unless we *do* make changes, like using apps to track infectious people and isolating those who are infectious. The alternative is that the disease spreads very rapidly, and many people get seriously ill so quickly that health services are overwhelmed. At least, that's what the epidemiological models suggest. It's very important, then, that epidemiological models are accurate, so that the best public health choices are made.

Epidemiological models can be very complicated, and we have to run computer programs to work out what they mean. Computers are needed to work out the results predicting what will happen. Like the rest of digital

---

[j] See Chapter 22: User Centered Design, page 301 ←

healthcare, then, it's important that the epidemiological models are correctly implemented and don't have any serious bugs, otherwise governments will be making policy decisions for the badly informed reasons — they'll keep us locked down for too long, causing economic problems, or release lockdown too soon, causing health problems.

I wrote a short program to estimate infection rates based on the standard, very simple, epidemiological model called susceptible-infected-recovered (SIR).[477] It involves having some data about the population and the disease, and then solving some equations. Using the program, I easily drew a graph from the SIR model (figure 31.1).

If my model had been used to inform public policy, the data driving it would have to be carefully based on what is known about the disease and lots of social factors, like how close people get on public transport, differences between age groups, differences between men and women, how care homes work, the role of children in schools (or not), social deprivation, digital exclusion, and so on. You'd also need to carefully model knock-on problems, like the health issues caused by hospitals filling to capacity with COVID-19 and therefore being unable to handle other problems.

My basic model ignored all those details — it didn't even model the difference between recovery and death. It can't, for instance, predict a second wave of infection if lock down is relaxed too soon because, as it's currently programmed, it doesn't model changes to the infection rate that would be needed to model changes to lock down.

I designed my program so you can run it yourself and see how it works.[476] I wrote it in JavaScript so it"ll run conveniently in any web browser; it just runs a simple model, then draws a graph (figure 31.1). I wrote it in JavaScript to make it easier if you want to play with it, however if I'd been writing it to do real epidemiology to inform public health, with lives depending on the quality of my programming, I would *not* have used JavaScript, C or R (a popular statistics language often used for modeling) but a safer and more robust language, one designed specifically for high-integrity applications, such as SPARK Ada.[k]

I documented the model in case you want to understand how it works. For example, if you decrease the model's assumption about the risks of infecting each other (simulating taking precautions like handwashing or wearing masks), then the model predicts a smaller proportion of the population will get infected.

It's a simple program, and it took just over an hour to document it to the standard I wanted to support this book: documentation is important so that you or anyone can understand how the code works. You might discover I got something wrong. Or if I come back to the code in a few weeks time, it's likely I will have forgotten what some details do — the documentation will

---

[k] See Chapter 27: SPARK Ada, page 375 ←

help me get back to understanding it all.[476] Documentation is always worth the effort of writing it.

My SIR computer model highlights more obvious points:

- The epidemiological model, the data, and all the social assumptions must all be reliable;

- You need to run models on a computer to make predictions; **but** obviously, no predictions are any more reliable than the computer programs used to run them.

- Only if a model is properly documented do you know what it is supposed to do.

Given the critical role of computers in epidemiology, it came as a big surprise to me that many programs used in epidemiological modeling are pretty wobbly.

Neil Ferguson is a world-leading epidemiologist, and his pandemic model influenced particularly the UK and the US in their COVID-19 responses.[478] He tweeted that the code he used is over thirteen years old, was intended to model flu (in fact, H1N1, the same sort of flu as the 1918 Spanish Flu) and not COVID-19, and it is thousands of lines of undocumented C code. He implies he wrote it on his own (figure 31.2).

As Ferguson said in an interview,

> For me the code is not a mess, but it's all in my head, completely undocumented. Nobody would be able to use it ...[479]

I've now read up on lots of epidemiological models and looked at lots of source code, and this relaxed approach to programming seems typical for the field.[480] Public health has the same cavalier approach to programming as healthcare does. I want to emphasize that Neil Ferguson is a world-leading epidemiologist and the epidemiology that he is doing is world leading. But he isn't a software developer. The COVID-19 pandemic has pulled laboratory work out into the world, and it's now having a huge impact on public health policies — so, at the very least, it needs proper documentation.

Poor programming risks lives in epidemiology as it does throughout digital health. It has become a public health issue. Quality software development is essential, as lives are at stake.

I'll explain why Ferguson's approach raises serious problems.

First off, the programming language C is a very poor choice of language for critical epidemiological modeling:

- C has very basic data handling, so you have to do it yourself, and risk getting it wrong. C, then, is a poor choice if your program starts off

Part III ◇ Prognosis ◇ A better future

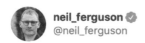

neil_ferguson ✔
@neil_ferguson

I'm conscious that lots of people would like to see and run the pandemic simulation code we are using to model control measures against COVID-19. To explain the background - I wrote the code (thousands of lines of undocumented C) 13+ years ago to model flu pandemics...

9:13 PM · Mar 22, 2020 · Twitter for iPhone

Figure 31.2. Neil Ferguson's statement about his epidemiological model.[481]

by loading lots of data, as a national epidemiological model would certainly do.

🕭 C handles floating point numbers badly. It is very easy to make unnoticed numerical errors in C. C is a poor choice of programming language if you are going to do numerical calculations.

🕭 C ignores many programming errors. For example, if you accidentally store some data in the wrong place, or analyze some data looking in the wrong place, C ignores the errors (and the program may crash later, or — worse — just carry on but generate incorrect results). *Anything can happen.*

These are very well-known problems for professional C programmers.

Of course, a good programmer would use libraries of professional code written by other people to do many things like handling data, searching, sorting, and database things. It's a fine balance: would you trust unknown programmers? Would their code work correctly for your application? Or would you rather just adopt their ready-made code, and get your programming finished sooner?

You could be a disciplined programmer and use a better programming language than C. Using MISRA C or MISRA C++ (even better, using SPARK Ada or another high-integrity language) combined with using Formal Methods would *really* help, as we discussed in earlier chapters.[1]

But Ferguson didn't document his program, and that raises more serious problems:

---

[1] See Chapter 27: Formal Methods, page 379 ←

🜨 After over thirteen years with a program thousands of lines long, there will inevitably be bits of code whose workings or purpose are no longer remembered by anybody. You dare not tidy up or delete these bits of code, because they may be critical for some no longer known reasons. So the code you are using now works in completely unknown ways.

🜨 All programs need debugging. A basic form of debugging is to run a program, spot any errors, and then fix the causes of those errors. If there is no documentation, it is impossible to tell the difference between "fixing bugs" and "fiddling the program to get the results you want." A debugged program may get the results you expect, rather than the results your model would have predicted.

🜨 Over thirteen years, shifting a program from modeling flu (in Thailand) to modeling COVID-19 in a Western country requires major changes. It isn't clear how anyone could reliably keep track of many changes in such a large program without careful documentation and automatic version control.

🜨 If the programmer moves on or gets ill, as may happen, nobody else will have a clue how the program works, how to maintain it, or how to use it. Neil Ferguson says his code is not documented, and he says he's the only person who understands it.[479] He was lucky he didn't get debilitatingly ill from COVID-19 just when he was needed.[482]

🜨 If a program supports research, and science is to be advanced by its insights, it is important that the program is open to peer-review. If a program is not documented, it cannot be reliably reviewed, because nobody will know what it's supposed to do. Indeed, Neil Ferguson has not made his program available in any publication, so it has never been reviewed or put up to independent scrutiny.

🜨 Finally, in science, especially laboratory sciences, it is a normal expectation to keep notebooks.[483] Notebooks are an essential record for all sorts of purposes, from ensuring legal priority to helping plan experiments and to track progress. In programming, computers can keep the lab notebooks almost entirely automatically, so there is no excuse not to keep even minimal documentation.[484]

Ventilators make another controversial digital health story.

A tragic final stage of COVID-19 is respiratory failure, and patients need supporting in intensive care and putting on ventilators to help them breathe. Many countries have experienced a shortage of ventilators as a result, and there has been an understandable push to get more ventilators made to fill the gaps in supply.

> **Box 31.2.** Simple ethical questions?
>
> Ethics makes us ask: how do we ensure people — especially the users — benefit? It isn't yet clear to me what benefits a tracking app gives to the person who uses it. At the very least, a tracking app is going to use up battery, so what does the user get in return for being able to use their phone *less*?
>
> A key concept in ethics is **reciprocity**. If I am going to do something to you, what can you do to rebalance the power? One answer to the probing question might be to quote the Golden Rule: I will treat others as I would like them to treat me.
>
> Before COVID-19, Birmingham and Solihull Mental Health NHS Foundation Trust was already developing a tracking app to assess mental health.[486] The idea is that the app tracks a person's location and calls, and then combines this information to predict mental health crises. Patient tracking data has *already* been given to a foreign private company, Telefonica. Telefonica make money, so what are they giving in return to their vulnerable users? This is a question of **reciprocity**, a basic ethical concept.
>
> In the case of a COVID-19 tracking app, the user of the mobile phone gives away data to the State or to a private company. What do they get back from that relationship? If reciprocity is not thought through, the individual is likely to lose rights — they may lose more data (such as their location and other private data) than they expect, as their data is linked to other information. The new owner of the data gains a lot of power — so much so that the UK Parliamentary Committee on Human Rights said the NHS's design may break the law[487] — so what is reciprocated to the user?
>
> Unfortunately, the more useful an app is made for epidemiologists to help understand a pandemic, the more tempting the data becomes to use for other purposes. Tracking tax evaders or terrorists? And it's very tempting for hackers: if everyone is using the same app on their mobile phones, a hack like WannaCry could bring a country to a standstill.

Imperial College has made the design of their open source ventilator, JAMVENT, publicly available.[485] They are to be applauded for that, but there are qualifications. The UK medical device regulator, the MHRA, has relaxed requirements for approving devices. And Imperial College has not made the essential program available yet, because the team haven't finished it. I'm surprised that the MHRA can approve a device that depends critically on computers (and software) for everything it does, without assessing the computers or their programs at all.

———————————■———————————

As I've shown throughout this book, there's a gap between what we hope digital can do for healthcare, and what we end up actually getting it to do. Healthcare professionals have got much better things to be doing than worrying about the details of digital health. Epidemiologists, too, have better things to be doing. Even ventilator engineers have better things to be doing than programming well and safely. The trouble is, everything depends on software.

A very similar problem happens with ethics.

Few medical scientists have time to think about ethics, so (to cut a long story short) **Ethics Boards** were invented. An Ethics Board is a panel that has some ethics experts sitting on it, and it reviews all proposed research to check it ethically and to approve it. For instance, if an experiment is going to be done on a childhood disease, who is going to look after the children's best interests? Or if a drug is being tested, what are the plans if the drug turns out to be dangerous — or if it turns out to be an amazing cure, and the patients stuck on the control arm of the experiment are not being treated with it? Should the experiment continue, should the problems be ignored, or what?

An Ethics Board makes sure all such questions are raised and appropriately explored. Any project will be delayed until there are satisfactory answers (or the plans are changed to remove the problems). Ethics Boards are standard practice across healthcare systems, research institutions, and government agencies.

Admittedly, some people don't like Ethics Boards, because they can slow things down and they often seem to be excessively bureaucratic. I'm sure there are problems, but some are due to researchers not thinking about ethics until the last moment, and the problems are trivial compared to the alternatives.[488]

I propose that, like Ethics Boards (or Institutional Review Boards), we now need **Software Engineering Boards** to help digital healthcare improve.

A Software Engineering Board would have professional programmers on it, probably senior software engineering professors and programmers from the aviation or nuclear power industries. It would give quality advice.

Software Engineering Boards would help researchers, hospitals, doctors, developers, and, of course, regulators. In short, Software Engineering Boards would help improve digital healthcare.

All research journals would, as medical journals already do with ethics clearance, refuse to publish anything without the clearance of a proper Software Engineering Board. Medical device regulators would require to see evidence of the Software Engineering Board clearance, and medical devices and computer systems would not be approved unless they had proper Software Engineering Board clearance. The pressure of COVID-19 has pressurized many regulators to relax standards, so that solutions can be rushed through, but ultimately, nobody will benefit if programs have bugs. Getting the right balance between thoroughness and speed is tricky, and ideal work for Software Engineering Boards. Indeed, Software Engineering Boards would be able to suggest computerized ways to make software more reliable — asking somebody to program "more thoroughly" doesn't just give them more work

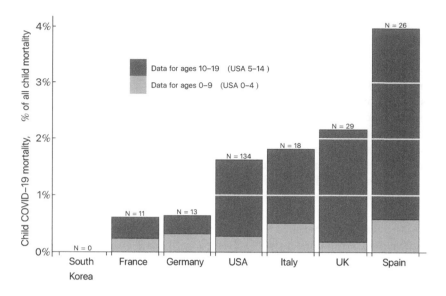

Figure 31.3. It's been said that child mortality in COVID-19 is rare. A 2021 paper published in *The Lancet Child & Adolescent Health Journal* looked at the published data, and found that the Spanish child COVID-19 death rate (in proportion to all-causes child death) was shockingly high compared to other countries. Then the Spanish Government admitted that deaths for people aged 100, 101, 102 ... had been incorrectly classified as deaths for people aged 0, 1, 2 ...[489] — yet, *if* this bug was the explanation, some of the excess must have been from Spaniards aged 110 plus! In any case, the bug is the same as the 20-year-old, very well-known Millennium Bug, discussed at the start of this book.

to do, it can transform *how* they work, so they use more tools and more advanced software engineering techniques.

Obviously details need to be worked out. For example, a Software Engineering Board would have to set proportionate criteria. If something is intended for informing national public health policies, you need to be very thorough. If something is intended for doing Down syndrome calculations, or national mortality (figure 31.3), you need to be very thorough.[m] On the other hand, a pilot research project might not need to be so thorough; perhaps it just needs to be documented enough so that other people can work on it. Again, the right balance is tricky, but Software Engineering Boards could stop people aimlessly drifting from toy programs for research projects into serious safety-critical programming for national emergencies.

In the long run, education is needed so that better and more reliable programming is available and happens in healthcare and in public health. How

---

[m] See Chapter 4: Millennium Bug (Y2K problem) and Down syndrome tragedy, page 34 ←

much should Software Engineering Boards be involved in this? Where will the funding come from? Will their involvement be in monitoring, certifying, policing, or just encouraging? These are important details that need working out some time, but the uncertainties don't all need to be sorted out at once, otherwise Software Engineering Boards will never happen in any form.

One critical detail is getting the right balance. Ethics Boards typically require researchers to fill in forms and to provide details — researchers know if they are doing experiments in petri dishes in a lab or on children at home, for instance, so the forms are relatively easy to fill in (if often quite tedious). On the other hand, few healthcare and medical researchers understand software and programming, so they are not able to fill in software forms on their own. Software Engineering Boards need to know how well engineered the software really is, not how good its developers *think* it is. As typical programs are enormous, Software Engineering Boards are either going to need resources to evaluated programs, or they are going to need to set up independent bodies that can do it for them. There may be other ideas to help make Software Engineering Boards work, but it's clear they are part of the solution and we must not let perfection be the enemy of the good. Software Engineering Boards don't need to be perfect on day one, but they do need to get going in some shape or form to start making their vital contribution to improving digital healthcare.

The economic impact of COVID-19 on the world is astronomical. It has been estimated that the US economy will take a $16 trillion hit — which corresponds roughly to a £1.6 trillion hit for the UK.[490] The predicted economic losses can be viewed as a business opportunity to motivate making positive interventions. Even small improvements to test and trace reliability would have huge economic and health benefits — offering an economic benefit to the country at least thirty times higher than the cost of the investment. Making epidemiological simulations more reliable to better assess different public health strategies would make huge economic and health sense. Yet governments are not investing in making digital health safer or more reliable; in the UK, at least, they have been investing in buying negligently engineered systems that are unreliable and not fit for purpose.

In contrast, as the opening stories of this chapter showed, our human response to COVID-19, particularly transforming how we use digital to relate to and to support patients, shows that we *can* improve digital health when we want to.

The pandemic could be a pivotal moment in so many ways. I suggest that Software Engineering Boards could be one of the positive strategic outcomes from the pandemic — certainly governments urgently need effective Software Engineering Boards.

The next chapter explores more ways in which we can make lasting improvements to digital health.

Part III ◇ Prognosis ◇ A better future

There's a future world where digital healthcare works, and works well. Here's how to get there.

32

Living happily ever after

The day after the car crash that my son Isaac survived,[a] he got to his wedding in one piece. Isaac married Debs, and, as they say in the best fairytales, they lived happily ever after (figure 32.1).

It would be very nice if everyone going into hospital lived happily ever after too. The harsh reality is that people do get ill and that nobody can live forever. But there would be a fairy tale ending if lives were not shortened by unnecessary errors.

About one in ten patients suffer an error in hospital. Every healthcare worker is stressed and overworked, despite, often because of, digital systems. It's time to improve the systems.

I think the digital systems are the best place to start: if we improve those, *everything* will improve, for computers are already everywhere. You can't even book an appointment without one.

Unfortunately, it's too easy to think getting the latest digital solutions is the same as improving things. Computers should be more of an effective team player to help reduce errors, rather than, as we've seen throughout this book, create problems — and often in unnoticed, yet often complex, ways, so the digital systems are then misunderstood and the wrong people blamed.

When things go wrong, as they do, we seek answers by blaming staff. We overlook the digital risks, bugs, and causes. We then dream of buying a new digital system that will magically fix the problems. We are certain it will, for exactly the same reasons we were certain the last one would. Until we change our culture, we are doomed to repeat this cycle.

We need to increase awareness of the risks of digital healthcare, and we need to increase understanding of the solutions.

It's time to take action.

I've divided up the action in this chapter under the following headings: Improving qualifications, training, and education; Improving digital health-

---

[a] See Chapter 11: Isaac Thimbleby's car crash, page 137 ←

Fix It: See and solve the problems of digital healthcare. Harold Thimbleby, Oxford University Press. © Harold Thimbleby 2021.
DOI: 10.1093/oso/9780198861270.003.0032

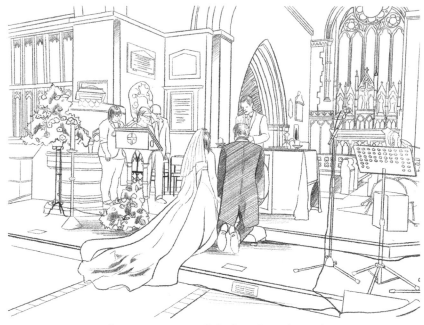

Figure 32.1. How all the best fairytales end.

care regulation; Improving awareness and knowledge; and the final section, Going forward.

It's worth emphasizing that the ideas in this chapter align closely with the Safety Two attitude[b] — they're about improving the quality and safety of digital healthcare systems, rather than worrying about the problems. This chapter therefore collects and organizes the positive ideas, the Safety Two thinking, this book has promoted throughout.

Improving qualifications, training, and education

Risks are not just buggy digital technology, but our — healthcare's — inability to think professionally about complex systems, especially the latest digital ideas.

- Organizations like the IEEE and the ACM — the world's largest computer societies — should provide accreditation and training courses specifically for digital healthcare.

- Hospitals and other healthcare organizations should recruit properly IT-qualified staff for digitally related jobs. Some staff at least should

---

[b] See Chapter 12: Safety One & Safety Two, page 145 ←

have Computer Science degrees. Chief Information Officers should have relevant qualifications, including degrees, and up-to-date training.

🖢 Existing Continuous Professional Development (CPD) schemes need supplementing with digital CPD schemes to ensure Human Factors and digital knowledge is up-to-date in healthcare. Appropriate digital syllabuses (including Human Factors, UCD, and so on) ought to be taught in nursing and medical schools. Developers and regulators need more advanced digital qualifications than healthcare workers.

🖢 Current recruitment in both healthcare and in healthcare industries should involve knowledgeable digital thinkers and leaders (such as university professors) in all stages of the process, from job specification to interview and beyond, to mentoring. I think this simple step would be the best way to start to rapidly improve.

🖢 We need to change healthcare management structures so people with mature digital skills have real roles to play, with mutual trust and shared understanding. A recent advert asks for a nurse to lead national digital transformation. While we absolutely need nurses, we also need people with high-level training in digital — postgraduate, doctoral training, even. The advert makes it clear that healthcare thinks the problem is that digital doesn't understand nursing, so we need a nurse leader. Isn't it equally clear that healthcare doesn't understand digital? I argued for multi-disciplinary *teams* earlier[c] — you can't get effective "digital transformation" skills in one person, and we need structures where multi-disciplinary expertise is respected and nurtured.

All this will take resources, and healthcare is stretched already. Digital enthusiasm is no longer sufficient.

The FBI, well known for its role in US gangster stories, is warning about widespread cybersecurity problems like ransomware targeting healthcare:

> In September [2020], a ransomware attack hobbled all 250 US facilities of the hospital chain Universal Health Services, forcing doctors and nurses to rely on paper and pencil for record-keeping and slowing lab work. Employees described chaotic conditions impeding patient care, including mounting emergency room waits and the failure of wireless vital-signs monitoring equipment.[491]

---

[c] See Chapter 8: Multi-disciplinary teams and skill mapping, page 105 ←

Part III ◇ Prognosis ◇ A better future

The problems go way beyond just the patient-facing healthcare we can see; they also affect international infrastructure, such as path labs and diagnostic labs,[492] the development of vaccines, and more …

> The National Cyber Security Centre (NCSC) dealt with a record of 723 incidents [about 100 a month] with a quarter related to the COVID-19 pandemic. Paul Chichester, the NCSC's director of operations, said cyberattacks by hostile states were focused on vaccine research, while criminal groups were also targeting hospitals and healthcare bodies.[493]

When the attacks are *already* happening, it's clear that healthcare will be on its knees if it does not up its game. Digital healthcare has bugs that cause problems, like harming patients and staff, but in cybersecurity hackers deliberately and systematically exploit these buggy weaknesses. It is no longer a question of one patient and plastering over the consequences with insurance, but *whole* hospitals and regions going under — and, if they are lucky, "only" having to pay massive ransoms to recover (which anyway isn't recommended). Cybersecurity failures are, I hope, very motivating, but don't forget they are just a symptom of buggy digital systems, buggy management of digital systems, and buggy day-to-day running of digital systems (plus a world of nasty people and States willing to exploit those oversights).

It's more strategic and is good business to invest in doing digital healthcare maturely — and seeing it as going beyond cybersecurity, essential as that is, to every topic addressed in this book. This message has to be heard and understood from politicians down.

> 🖊 For every dollar or pound spent on digital, 50% should be spent on digital maturity: primarily human resources — hiring and recruiting properly skilled digital professionals, supporting digital CPD throughout the organization, improving IT support, building multi-disciplinary teams, and so on. It's not a matter of hiring IT technicians — there needs to be qualified dedicated expertise all the way to the top, in directors, managers, and more. You can discuss the 50%, but it needs to be much higher than goodwill.

Improving digital healthcare regulation

Digital systems should be at least as strictly regulated as the clinical procedures they control, collect data for, advise, or prescribe for. However, digital healthcare regulation is not just about clinical effectiveness and safety — there's a lot more that needs to be regulated.

Imagine a hospital thinking of buying an ambulance, a very familiar form of healthcare technology. Obviously, the clinical effectiveness and safety need to be confirmed, and if the ambulance complies with clinically relevant regulations, then buying one will be much easier because those features don't need re-checking.

The hospital will no doubt have some simple requirements: the ambulance needs a siren, the hospital logo painted on it, and space for the first aid equipment. However, the hospital will take it for granted that the ambulance is roadworthy. Roadworthiness covers a lot of technical issues, covered by very detailed regulations. The ambulance won't emit too high a level of greenhouse gases. Its tires will be safe in the wet, and at speeds the ambulance is expected to go. The airbags will work. The windscreen will, in an accident, shatter safely. And so on, through a very long list evolved over more than a century experiencing engineering and safety problems with vehicles. It's so easy to focus just on the clinical requirements alone, and forget about the other critical issues because the regulations for them work so well.

Unfortunately, digital regulations do not work very well, yet the need for them — for effective regulations — cannot be ignored.

Digital healthcare regulation must explicitly cover the reliability of the technology, not just its clinical effectiveness and safety. Indeed, digital healthcare regulation must explicitly cover the reliability of the technology as used in the clinical environment and with patients — including when they are at home and likely have no professional supervision. Will the digital technology be cybersecure? Is there post-market surveillance? What are the contractual terms for fixing bugs? Is patient data sold on by the manufacturer? Does the user interface subtly influence clinical decisions? Is it interoperable? And more. It's possibly a much longer list than the clinical requirements. In fact, this whole *Fix IT* book has been about how the reliability and safety of digital healthcare has been ignored and has caused misunderstood problems. I called it **digivigilance**, or DVig for short,[d] as it's so important I think it needs a catchy name.

Usually regulation is seen as a tricky balancing act between achieving the best outcome (in this case, for patients), the cost of adhering to the regulation, the cost of policing compliance with the regulations, and the potential for stimulating a black market in products that benefit by circumventing regulation. For example, there is a huge market in fake medical devices, because a device that doesn't bother to comply witg regulations can be made very much more cheaply, and hence sold at a huge profit. Sometimes, patients will knowingly buy fake products because they are so much cheaper and they may work well enough (especially if the patient is desperate).

A less conventional approach is that good manufacturers want to make good products, so creating an environment where regulators and manufacturers collaborate is probably going to be much more effective. This is called **co-regulation**.[494] Using social media might be part of co-regulation: man-

Part III ◇ Prognosis ◇ A better future

---

[d] See Chapter 8: Digivigilance, DVig, page 83 ←

Box 32.1. Introducing the IEC 61508 standard

Digital healthcare regulation is a mish mash, spread across many regulators. There are numerous exceptions: medical devices used for law enforcement, sexually transmitted diseases, diagnostic equipment, even office equipment. The overall structure classifies according to medical use: Class I — generally regarded as low risk; Class IIa — generally regarded as medium risk; Class IIb — generally regarded as medium risk; Class III — generally regarded as high risk. But that isn't how software works. For example, spreadsheets are office software, so they aren't covered by medical regulations, yet spreadsheets are *also* used for hazardous medical calculations, such as radiation dosage. Or a spreadsheet used in a hospital might suffer a cyberattack, and open the entire hospital to hackers — the fact that the spreadsheet is classified as "office software" doesn't stop it compromising every medical class.

As this book has shown, lots of awful digital systems are in widespread use, despite regulation. On the other hand, industry worries about the cost of adhering to regulation, the so-called **regulatory burden**, and the potential to stifle innovation if regulation is too harsh. Where is the middle ground?

A different approach would be to start again from *safety*, rather than from the medical traditions that were established long before digital was even on the horizon. We should follow industries where safety is core, such as nuclear power and aviation, where it's recognized that any software has a wide range of components, and therefore has varying requirements for safety. Just because it's an airplane, doesn't mean the entertainment software is safety-critical, nor, conversely, that the autopilot can be treated as lightly as a passenger game. Each *part* of software has a specific risk analysis, and the relevant requirements for it flow from that.

The IEC standard 61508 is a good place to start with a new perspective.[495] Start off with a risk analysis, and (through a process we won't describe here) get to a **safety integrity level**, or SIL. Simply, in regulated industries, the higher the SIL, the more competent and professional the software and its development *must* be.

---

ufacturers want a good reputation, and regulators using social media *with* manufacturers could be of mutual benefit — it would mean disseminating successes as well as failures, and would therefore move regulators away from a Safety One culture (like the FDA MAUDE database, which only reports problems) to a Safety Two culture.[e]

Manufacturers are, by definition, good at manufacturing, so they tend to follow the cutting-edge of the technologies they are using. They know more about digital than the regulators. Co-regulation would therefore help regulators keep abreast of the latest innovations. Manufacturers would be asking "what's the best way *we* can regulate this idea?" Co-regulation, then, is a win-win. The problem is how to transition from regulation to co-regulation

---

[e] See Chapter 12: Safety One & Safety Two, page 145 ←

without losing the safeguards of regulation — it's a bit beyond the scope of my book, but we need to think about the culture of manufacturing and regulation working together so that digital gets fixed, and that fixed digital drives improvement and patient safety, rather than the current culture of reluctantly doing as little as possible to satisfy the regulators.

Organizations like the UK's NAMDET, the National Association of Medical Device Educators & Trainers,[496] which joins members from healthcare and from industry, show how co-operation can begin. They — and international organizations like them — could start getting active members from regulators, and then they would be getting co-regulation off to a good start.

Co-regulation is a new name for an old idea. Many medical regulatory bodies, like the UK's General Medical Council, which was established in 1858 as a statutory body, include practicing medical experts to help in regulating medical experts. Indeed, the GMC needs up-to-date medical expertise in order to regulate medicine knowledgeably and effectively, including setting teaching syllabuses and qualifications. The risk, of course, is **regulatory capture**, when the foxes start running the chicken coop — as happened in the 737 MAX story. One of many standard solutions to this is for different regulatory bodies to review each other's work.

- Regulations will *always* be catching up with technology, and we need to develop "agile regulations," co-regulation, and other methods, like expert panels, to keep them relevant as technology continues to push boundaries. This is an area that needs a lot of good thinking.

  This is not a matter of adding new rules. Like, this year we need new regulations on AI — but what will we need next year? No, it requires research to look ahead and find new, effective, ways to regulate and stay on top of the continual digital innovations.[497]

- Regulators and standards organizations should work together towards developing a safety rating scheme.[f] Meanwhile, safety labeling could be started by a voluntary organization or by individual manufacturers. The best safety labeling would be developed by co-regulation.

- Regulators should review software warranties and have basic standards to revolutionize current practice.[g] Closely related, we must increase accountability for patient harms caused — whether by omission or commission — by digital systems. We need to fix warranties, especially gag clauses and DeWitt clauses. This will no doubt require legislation.

- The incident reports should record details of digital systems that may have contributed to the incident, and the investigation must identify

---

[f] See Chapter 29: Safety rating, page 404 ←
[g] See Chapter 15: Who's accountable?, page 193 ←

systems that should then be improved. This requires a national (ideally, an international) database of all digital systems and where they are used. (Incident reporting systems should pass the **orange-wire test**.)[144h]

⓲ Incident investigation teams need to be multi-disciplinary, and include both Human Factors experts and digital experts.[i] It is notable that the investigation into the Y2K Down syndrome bugs had neither, and it made mistakes, and therefore had negligible generalizable learning that anyone else could benefit from.[23] As with recruitment, the simplest way to fix these problems would be to involve university professors in investigations.

⓲ All healthcare systems should be developed using best practice in UCD and Formal Methods, including being developed in programming languages such as SPARK Ada or others specifically designed for high-integrity applications. Sadly, programming languages designed for healthcare, as I've discussed in this book, have generally failed to be reliable.

⓲ Digital regulation in healthcare should include "office systems" (like spreadsheets and calculators used in hospitals, surgeries and laboratories) that currently escape effective regulation.[j]

⓲ Finally, regulators should require manufacturers and procurers to use and share **safety cases**, which are explicit structured documents that show that the reasons for believing in safety have been worked through carefully. I would argue that if a manufacturer can't produce an adequate safety case for their products, courts should assume their products are unsafe; equally, if a hospital can't produce a safety case for their procurement (that is, that the products, even if assumed to be technically safe, are fit for purpose *within* the particular hospital context they were bought for), then the hospital shares liability.[19]

… A good safety case would be a good antidote to the current practice of providing long unreadable lists of reasons why the manufacturers are not responsible for the safety of their products![k]

Improving awareness and knowledge

When things go wrong in healthcare, the default response is to close down, to delay and deny, and to become secretive, lest any more problems are found

---

[h] See Chapter 12: Orange-wire-test, page 148 ←
[i] See Chapter 8: Multi-disciplinary teams and skill mapping, page 105 ←
[j] See Chapter 14: Risky calculations, page 177 ←
[k] See Chapter 15: Who's accountable?, page 193 ←

and exposed. Besides, isn't this what everybody else does? Nobody wants to talk, in case they implicate themselves as accessories. Serious problems tend to end up in litigation, and everything rapidly becomes confidential.

In contrast, in aviation it is very difficult to hide error. When things go wrong, there is vivid TV and media coverage and there are investigations and public reports. If you want to fly on an A380 — I just picked a random example: you can find and read a complete 285-page report on the failure of one of its Rolls-Royce Trent 900 engines.[227] Furthermore, the report is free for the public to download. The learning is public and available for everyone to see. Every airline worldwide that runs A380s will have read the report and made sure they service the Rolls-Royce engines more carefully. Rolls-Royce have issued a software upgrade to make sure their planes monitor engine speed and don't fail catastrophically. And so on. The world is now a safer place.

The aviation culture is simple: if you want to learn, you need to know.

In healthcare there are a few organizations trying valiantly to spread learning from incidents. In England, there is the Healthcare Safety Investigation Branch (HSIB)[498] which is a statutorily (that is, defined in law to be) independent organization that runs investigations that don't apportion blame or liability.

Crucially, HSIB makes their reports public, and anyone and everyone can learn from them. They have a fascinating website.

We need more organizations worldwide like HSIB. The sad thing is, at the time of writing there were only three countries in the world with organizations like HSIB: Norway, South Korea, and England — HSIB only has a mandate for England, a fraction of the UK. The values that led to the founding of HSIB need spreading around a lot more.

- Funding bodies should fund digital healthcare research, including safety, as fields in their own right. Research in safety hasn't been funded very well — it isn't as glamorous as fighting diseases (like cancer) — but the returns on investment are likely to be much higher. To put it bluntly, a few thousand pounds spent on safety research would make a difference, but a few thousand pounds spent on cancer would hardly be noticed.

- Digital healthcare is an international issue, and funding bodies and organizations like HSIB must collaborate internationally. Although there is funding for exciting digital (AI and big data), there is inadequate funding, and no joined-up funding for digital safety and quality improvement. This must be changed. This book is full of questions and informed guesses, because we don't know the answers: this is unacceptable in an area like healthcare when reliable knowledge is just a bit of funding away from being achieved.

Avoid regulatory burden

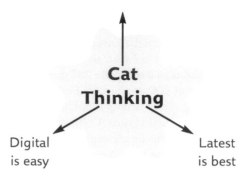

Cat Thinking

Digital is easy

Latest is best

Figure 32.2. The attraction of Cat Thinking is that it's its own reward — the exciting hormones make it so. There's nothing else to do: everything is exciting and easy. We can just rush in, grabbing the latest stuff, and it'll all be exciting. There's no need to make sure it is safe, because it's exciting.

🐾 Lack of awareness of digital health safety and cybersafety is a global problem. We need an international organization for improving digital healthcare. WHO (World Health Organization[499]), IMDRF (the International Medical Device Regulators Forum[500]), or IHI (the US Institute for Healthcare Improvement[501]) may be good places to start; certainly these (and all analogous national organizations) need digital departments, and they are well placed to take leadership.

🐾 We need to raise awareness of the value of good incident reporting. An error may happen just once in our lifetime and we may not think it's significant, but if we report it all, the reports might show the problem is happening "once" everywhere. Without reporting nobody will ever realize there are problems to fix.

🐾 Healthcare and digital need to align and meet half way. Digital is not a solution to a badly thought-through healthcare system, but working out how to align healthcare and digital will improve both. This requires close co-operation between clinicians and developers.

Many people will argue that we already have good enough digital qualifications, and that regulation is getting tighter all the time. Every product has already passed the current regulations, which, they will point out, are already very onerous. All we need to do is to update our computer systems to the latest stuff. Certainly, they'll argue, we don't need the extra burden of safety ratings

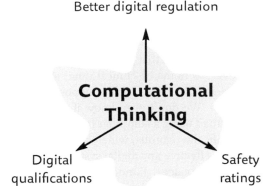

Better digital regulation

Computational Thinking

Digital
qualifications

Safety
ratings

Figure 32.3. The power of Computational Thinking is that it is a solid foundation for rigorous qualifications, regulation, and safety ratings, which applied together will make healthcare safer and more effective.

But after enjoying this book, you now know many tragic stories that prove that people are deceived by Cat Thinking[l] (figure 32.2). The problem with Cat Thinking is that people think everything is obvious and wonderful; they're already perfectly happy on dopamine, so it never crosses their mind to be more rigorous. We need something more professional, and a foundation of that something is Computational Thinking,[m] driving improvements in regulation and in qualifications — in other words, objectively, from *outside* of our hormone-influenced heads (figure 32.3).

Since getting new digital systems introduce new risks, digital systems (including all the devices with embedded computers in them, like infusion pumps, which you may not immediately think of as "digital") you must always do a **safety case**, a rigorous documented analysis of how the new digital stuff will affect safety.[19] Certainly, without a safety case, you do not know what risks you are running — and of course, even with a safety case you may miss risks (safety cases should always be externally reviewed). Crucially, doing safety cases quickly highlights what we don't know — how much of our "safety" really depends on guesswork.

Throughout this book, I've been aware that some of the advice I give is partly guesswork. Take UCD for example.[n] UCD seems, like Cat Thinking, obvious and wonderful, but does it *really* work, and, in healthcare, how should you do it professionally — respecting patient confidentiality and all the other perfectly reasonable constraints of real healthcare? If everything

---

[l] See Chapter 3: Cat Thinking, page 25 ←
[m] See Chapter 13: Computational Thinking, page 151 ←
[n] See Chapter 22: User Centered Design, page 301 ←

to be improved depends on UCD, we need to know how to do it properly. But we don't know how to. Worse, everyone is using different variations of UCD, so all evaluations — whether on usability or safety — are impossible to compare properly.

A recent research paper showed that physicians in hospitals spent 5 hours using computers for every 8 hours of clinical time, and computer time is higher for female physicians.[502] How is this supposed to be an improvement? We have no idea. We don't even know if using a computer for 8 hours is better or worse than using a computer for 7 hours!

Until we have scientifically rigorous, widely accepted methods, we cannot reliably compare how effective any digital systems are, and therefore we cannot improve (except by chance). Funders need to stop saying everyday techniques like UCD and Iterative Design are fine; in healthcare, they aren't. They aren't scientifically sound, they aren't reliable, they aren't standardized, they aren't easy to do. And, while we haven't got any useful qualifications, you have no idea how to hire people who are better at designing, building or buying better digital systems.

Can we start doing *enough* of this to make a difference?

We've got a problem like the movie industry had back in the 1920s. The movie industry was small, disorganized and producing substandard movies. The Oscars, the prizes for the industry, were invented to promote the industry when it was just getting going. Oscars promote both artistic and technical merit — and they have become hugely successful.

Following the ideas of Safety Two, we too must celebrate stories of safety and success, and spread good practice — and make everyone aware of it. In digital healthcare, then, we need ways to raise consciousness — for patients, nurses, technicians, politicians, everyone — of the benefits of high-quality digital solutions. Safety and reliability are achievable.

Prizes, celebrations, and parties are needed. Wouldn't it be nice if healthcare safety successes hit the mainstream news once a year, like the Oscars do?

In some areas, like the cybersecurity of mobile phones, manufacturers already provide **bug bounties**, which are prizes for discovering bugs,[503] yet in healthcare, manufacturers would rather not know.[504] Digital health needs bug bounties, prizes, and competitions for safer and more effective digital healthcare. Prizes for improving digital healthcare would, as a constructive side effect, challenge the "we're not accountable and don't want to know" culture that currently dominates healthcare.°

Professional societies, healthcare organizations, funders, and other bodies could start prizes in digital healthcare improvement.

If we have prizes, we'll raise awareness of the issues and the solutions — but we'll be begging questions about the criteria for the prizes. Those

---

° See Chapter 15: Who's accountable?, page 193 ←

sorts of questions naturally motivate having better evidence for safety and dependability, which in turn underlies the safety rating ideas we discussed earlier.[p] Good ideas work together.

NCAP is the New Car Assessment Program, which I mentioned earlier,[q] and it has worked out how to assess car safety. What can we learn from it?

NCAP started in the US in 1979 and started testing cars the same year. NCAP has been instrumental in making cars safer. Car manufacturers like NCAP because they can show off how safe their cars are getting, and people who buy or sell cars like NCAP ratings because it helps them negotiate and think clearly about safety and quality.

NCAP is so successful, it has gone global. The **Global NCAP** has a nice eight-point mission statement, which I'd like to quote from, except I'm taking the liberty of changing their "safer car" words into "safer digital healthcare" words.[505] So in digital healthcare we need an organization, like NCAP, but to:

1. Support safer healthcare in emerging markets by offering support, guidance, and quality assurance.

2. Provide a co-operation platform for healthcare organizations around the world to share best practice, to further exchange information, and to promote the use of information to encourage the manufacture of safer digital healthcare across the global market.

3. Promote digital healthcare safety with proven effectiveness and encourage its accelerated use across the globe by increasing awareness and, where appropriate, by supporting mandatory application.

4. Support training initiatives in safety regulatory and rating systems to promote policy making capacity, particularly in low- and middle-income countries (LMICs).

5. Promote the use of safer digital technologies by hospitals and healthcare providers in both the public and private sector. This will include competitions and awards for promoting best practice.

6. Recognize achievement in safety, innovation in safety-related technologies and practices, and products through a global awards scheme.

7. Target to halve preventable healthcare deaths and injuries by 2020.

8. Support improvements in evidence-based consumer information to inform patients about the performance of digital healthcare.

---

[p] See Chapter 29: Safety ratings will improve healthcare, page 401 ←
[q] See Chapter 11: NCAP: New Car Assessment Program, page 140 ←

And, as digital healthcare is way behind transport, I need to add these three very important points that NCAP itself doesn't need:

9. Provide digital healthcare qualification frameworks so that digital competence improves, and so that healthcare providers, manufacturers, and healthcare regulators can employ accredited and digitally competent staff responsible for digital leadership. (You could, of course, do this with virtual training academies, enabling universal training and accreditation across the globe.)

10. Once there are qualifications, we must require healthcare providers and manufacturers to be accredited: in order to practice, they must have qualifications at the appropriate level. This, in turn, must be regulated through an appropriate professional body.

11. NCAP takes it for granted that car engineering is good enough and will improve, but digital healthcare needs additional steps. It must explicitly require Formal Methods in software development.

Those last two points are a good place to start. Without digital maturity and competence, everything else will hit inertia and denial.

So NCAP shows it's totally possible and very effective. We could do this in digital healthcare too.

Maybe a leading organization like the WHO should start a "Global NCAP," perhaps called a Global Health IT Improvement Program (Global HITIP)?

If a Global Health IT Improvement Program isn't possible, it's still wide open for any country to take the initiative and get things going. Which country wants to be the world leader? It may be a long-term vision — the car industry's Global NCAP took 40 years to get where it is today — but we know it's achievable.

We just need to start, and this book has given the directions to set off in.

Going forward

If you'd like to make things happen, I give lectures, interactive lectures, and workshops on digital healthcare, and on any and all issues raised in this book. I also mentor people who want to work out how to be more effective — particularly in the digital health area.

I'm building up helpful resources on my website:

www.harold.thimbleby.net/fixit

Please do contact me if you find things that are helpful, if you want to correct errors, or if you have an idea you'd like me to add to the website or to new editions of this book.

By email, contact me on: harold@thimbleby.net

Or if you want everyone to know, tweet me on: @haroldthimbleby

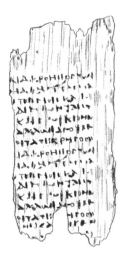

Figure 32.4. *Fix IT* off started with a picture of the oldest surviving written Hippocratic Oath.[1] For centuries, the Oath has framed and motivated the culture of healthcare. It's now time to have a digitally-relevant *Fix IT* Oath.

Here's a first proposal for a *Fix IT* Oath, based on the updated form of the Hippocratic Oath from the World Medical Association's latest Declaration of Geneva:[506]

As a member of the Healthcare IT Profession:

I solemnly pledge to dedicate my life to the service of humanity;

THE HEALTH AND WELL-BEING OF MY SYSTEMS' PATIENTS AND USERS will be my first consideration;

I will ensure I have the most appropriate professional training and qualifications to perform my duties;

I will use the highest standards of program development, following best practice in human factors engineering, user centered design, software engineering, and cybersecurity;

I will use rigorous development processes to ensure my software is safe and helps the patients and staff who may use it;

I will work with diverse multi-disciplinary teams, including relevant clinical expertise and patient representation;

I MAKE THESE PROMISES solemnly, freely and upon my honor.

Can you make a better *Fix IT* Oath to adopt?

This book isn't the end of the story about digital healthcare, and its problems and solutions. This chapter on recommended reading gives lots of suggestions to help take your thinking further.

33

Good reading

If we were having a chat, I'd listen to you and listen to your interests, and maybe I'd say "you need to read *this* book." Sadly, we're not having a face-to-face chat, so this chapter tells you lots of things you could read — but please see it as a conversation: skim the headings and topics, and pick out what you are interested in.

Starting at the beginning and reading through to the end of this chapter isn't really what it's about; please skim this chapter (there is a mini-table of contents to help), then dive into the bits that pique your interest. Pursue your interests and concerns, and temper them with my suggestions of new, interesting things you want to follow up.

This book's aim is to raise awareness of risky digital healthcare and to trigger change. I hope you now want to start doing things, and that my book has left you with lots of questions and wanting to find the answers.

Keeping up with the latest in digital health

Every day something bad happens in digital health. It's a full-time job keeping up.

In just the last week I was working on this book, there was interesting news about the development failures of the NHS COVID-19 tracing app,[507] and about a new widespread cybersecurity problem called RIPPLE20.[508]

RIPPLE20 affects almost all medical devices that have an internet connection; a related bug is known to affect *billions*[5] of devices.[509] These bugs make any devices using them very easy to hack. There are huge problems establishing which devices are *not* vulnerable to RIPPLE20 hacks. It'll be important to monitor internet traffic to see if any hackers are trying to exploit the bugs.

But the point, surely, isn't to keep up with the latest news of problems, but to keep up with the solutions.

Fix It: See and solve the problems of digital healthcare. Harold Thimbleby,
Oxford University Press. © Harold Thimbleby 2021.
DOI: 10.1093/oso/9780198861270.003.0033

You can go on to Google or Wikipedia and search out huge amounts of stuff about anything *that you knew you were looking for*. My list here is brief, obviously tiny compared to the internet, but it's selected to help you answer your questions and, especially, to help raise *new* ideas and questions to explore further. So here's what this chapter covers:

If you are interested in patient safety

By far the quickest way to get into the patient safety area is to watch Mike Eisenberg's 77-minute 2019 film, *To Err is Human: A Patient Safety Documentary*. The film stars the usual suspects this book has already mentioned: Lucian Leape, Albert Wu, Don Berwick, and other experts. The film has a website at www.toerrishumanfilm.com — including links to Amazon and iTunes to watch it. The website also has lots of links to lots more resources and is really worthwhile to explore. The film has had a bit of criticism for being one-sided and overly simplistic,[510] and I'd criticize it for ignoring the role of digital in any error. But it's a very good introduction to the field of patient safety.

There are lots of good books, too, as well as reports and textbooks on patient safety, but here I've chosen a selection of excellent, well-written books that you'll enjoy and that'll give you insights to both support and follow on from my arguments.

Atul Gawande's book about his life as a surgeon, *Complications: A Surgeon's Notes on an Imperfect Science* (Profile Books, 2008) is amazing, and reads like a page-turner, frankly discussing his triumphs, his failures, and errors. It is a very enjoyable way to start thinking your way into real healthcare.

Don Berwick reviewed patient safety following the Francis Report and the Mid-Staffordshire hospital problems. His report, *A promise to learn — a commitment to act: Improving the safety of patients in England*, is powerful and profound. It emphasizes the human side of safety. The report does not explicitly mention digital — but digital must be designed to be the servant to support the culture that Don celebrates. His report is available at

www.gov.uk/government/publications/
berwick-review-into-patient-safety

Suzette Woodward has written two excellent books: *Rethinking Patient Safety* (CRC Press, 2017), and, more recently, *Implementing Patient Safety* (Routledge, 2019). Both of her books are very well-written introductions to, and broad reference works on, patient safety.

Suzette writes from on-the-ground experience. Her books are full of ideas to make safety work. The second book's clear theme is "a balanced approach to safety addressing the culture, conditions, and values that help people work safely." In fact, neither book explores digital system safety in healthcare, so they complement *Fix IT* well.

Suzette has a blog, which in turn points to many other useful resources, and which will keep things up-to-date: suzettewoodward.org

Peter Pronovost and Eric Vohr, *Safe Patients, Smart Hospitals* (Penguin, 2011) gives the full story of Peter's insights into central line infections and working to improve patient safety.[a]

Ross Koppel and Suzanne Gordon, *First, Do Less Harm: Confronting the Inconvenient Problems of Patient Safety — The Culture and Politics of Health Care Work* (ILR Press, 2012) is an excellent edited collection of chapters on patient safety, with a particular emphasis on digital healthcare.

Charles (Chick) Perrow, *Normal Accidents: Living with High Risk Technologies* (Princeton University Press, 1999). Chick's idea is that accidents happen all the time, but most of them do not turn into catastrophes, except by a chance misfortune. So, accidents are **normal**, and we should learn from them, so we can stop the catastrophes happening.

Chick's normal accidents idea is a bit like this book's approach to error. Error is normal (and should be blame-free). Indeed, error is good if we can learn from it. The problem is harm. The other problem is that one of the best ways to reduce harm is to design better systems, especially digital systems, to reduce harm — but for some reason there is too much focus on the sharp-end of error rather than on the Wedge Thinking at the strategic blunt end of designing out error.[b]

---

[a] See Chapter 24: Peter Pronovost, page 330 ←
[b] See Chapter 24: Wedge Thinking, page 325 ←

Perrow is basically expanding on the Swiss Cheese Model[c] — an accident is anything unwanted that gets stopped by any defense, and a catastrophe is when all holes in the defenses line up. In other words, the defenses work most of the time, and the problem is that we tend to ignore the normal working of the defenses and hence learn nothing from their successes. Something went wrong — there was an accident — but instead of thinking about it, we ignored it because there was no catastrophe, such as patient harm.

Perrow has lots of powerful examples of his ideas in practice, from the Bhopal disaster (where 500,000 people were exposed to a toxic gas) to nuclear power station accidents and near misses.

So accidents (in Chick Perrow's terminology) are normal, and we should learn what we can from them to avoid future catastrophes. I've heard medical people objecting to Chick's ideas because they don't like the word "accident," which to them implies an incident is unpredictable and therefore (they say) unavoidable, so in principle nobody is to blame. Most harms in healthcare are preventable, at least in hindsight, which, in contrast, means that somebody must be to blame.[511] The word **incident** (or the terms **adverse incident** or **serious untoward incident**, SUI) are usually preferred in healthcare.

I think words are slippery. If we ban the word "accident" and start using "incident," in a few years' time the word incident itself will come to mean the same thing — it'll become another word we don't like. What is more important than lexical pedantry is to think clearly. Chick Perrow certainly does that, and he makes a very good case for using the term accident.

We can't have a list of safety reading without encouraging you to find everything you can by: Sidney Dekker, Liam Donaldson, Erik Hollnagel, James Reason, and Charles Vincent — these safety leaders have all written or edited classic books as well as lots of research papers you can find on PubMed, Google Scholar, or in digital libraries like the ACM Digital Library — or just do standard web searches. Start here:

- James Reason, *Human Error* (Cambridge University Press, 1991).

- Erik Hollnagel, *Safety-I and Safety-II* (Routledge, 2014).

- Sidney Dekker, *Just Culture* (Routledge, 2016).

- Charles Vincent and René Amalberti, *Safer Healthcare: Strategies for the Real World* (Springer, 2016).

- Liam Donaldson, Walter Ricciardi, Susan Sheridan, and Riccardo Tartaglia, editors, *Textbook of Patient Safety and Clinical Risk Management* (Springer, 2021). DOI: 10.1007/978-3-030-59403-9

---

[c] See Chapter 6: Swiss Cheese Model, page 61 ←

I listed these books in chronological order; the last one, printed in 2021, is both authoritative and excellent in coverage (it has 34 chapters written by numerous world-leaders). It also has the huge advantage of being open access — so it's free to read in PDF or EPUB formats. However, apart from a chapter on UCD, digital healthcare doesn't get a mention.

There are also many good websites.

Check out the Clinical Human Factors website, chfg.org, which has a wide range of resources, including videos and contacts for people who can give lectures or run workshops. Lots of useful resources can also be found at the Institute for Safe Medication Practices, ismp.org, and at the ECRI Institute, ecri.org. Or look at ehrseewhatwemean.org, the US MedStar Health National Center for Human Factors in Healthcare. Once you start searching, there is no real limit — and, of course, your searches will stay up-to-date in a way that this book cannot.

This list of good reads on patient safety would not be complete without mentioning the classic report that started the patient safety movement: *To Err is Human* (US Institute of Medicine, 1999). The report says that the majority of errors are caused by faulty systems that lead people to make mistakes — and that's why fixing digital systems is so important.

———————————■———————————

One of the earliest articles about patient safety is disappointingly anonymous. It's of interest because it is, at least to our ears, so quirky. Written by "F" in 1846, "Some of the causes and sources of error in medicine," was published in the *Boston Medical and Surgical Journal*, **34**:377–380, DOI: 10.1056/NEJM184606100341903

The article points out several valid sources of error, such as having an "improper regard to the authority of professors of medicine," but it also says that ignoring planetary influences and atmospheric vicissitudes causes error! In other words, the article has insights about medical error, yet it mixes them up with old superstitions.

As the Hawai'i Pacific Health "Getting Rid of Stupid Stuff" authors said:[d] everything that we now call stupid (like planetary influences, odd patient safety ideas, or stupid computer system features) was thought to be a good idea at some point. So, what are we overlooking now that will make any of our ideas today seem as stupid in the future? It begs the question, then, what are we doing (such as UCD) to find out what we're overlooking?

If you want to hear from patients

Patient stories are vital. The patient's view is very different from the "institutional view" of healthcare, of doctors, and of nurses. Curiously, patient stories may make little sense unless you've "been there" and seen the strange

---

[d] See Chapter 29: Getting Rid of Stupid Stuff, page 413 ←

world of healthcare from the other side. The following are patient stories that are engaging, profound and, frankly, shocking. I recommend them.

Oliver Sacks was a world-leading neurologist, perhaps most famous for his book *The Man Who Mistook His Wife for a Hat* (Picador, 2011). However, his book, *A Leg to Stand On* (Picador, 1991), is about when he became a patient. He broke his leg, but, more profoundly, he damaged his femoral nerve and had paralysis, and he saw his leg as some kind of alien. To me his book is a powerful exposé of the gulf between the hospital staff's clinical view and the patient's experience.

A Sea of Broken Hearts, by John James (AuthorHouse, 2007). This is John James's book about the death of his son, Alex, who died from inattentiveness and preventable errors. He takes you on a shocking journey, which leads to powerful suggestions for improvements to patient safety legislation and a charter of patient rights. He says that patients should have care based on the best scientific evidence available.

John James is also the author of the important patient safety paper on the rates of patient harms I cited earlier.[110]

I'd like "best scientific evidence available" to include the best computer science evidence as well — computer *science* underpins every area of healthcare. We should not limit our scientific standards and aspirations for best patient care to the conventional sciences (let alone always demanding RCTs when they don't work too well with digital health).

Collateral Damage, by Dan Walter (CreateSpace Independent Publishing Platform, 2010), is the story of a nurse, Dan's wife Pam, who became a patient at Johns Hopkins Hospital after a heart operation that went badly wrong. More details can be found at collateral-damage.net

Joshua's Story, by James Titcombe (Anderson Wallace Publishing, 2015), is about Joshua, who died in Morecambe Bay NHS Trust when he was just 9 days old. His father, James, embarks on the hard pilgrimage of finding out what happened, against the fog and misdirection of unfathomable barriers, denial, and cover-up. It is a heartbreaking read.

The next two books are powerful patient stories that made me cry — a good thing! Like the others here, at first sight they have nothing to do with digital healthcare. Yet if healthcare is so removed from patients, and digital is so removed from healthcare, then digital is far, far too removed from patients. The cure is to get digital experts to connect directly with patients, and understand what healthcare is really all about. This is what digital healthcare is for.

In Shock: How Nearly Dying Made Me a Better Intensive Care Doctor, by Rana Awdish (Bantam Press, 2018). Rana is an intensive care doctor who lost her first child in pregnancy and spent months fighting for her life in hospital. The book is takes us from her dying to her profound insights into compassion, told through her direct first-person stories and her colleagues' stories. It's a stunning book that I can't recommend highly enough. (Rana's book has been mentioned elsewhere in *Fix IT.* [85])

In Shock is, in Rana's own words, "a call to arms for doctors to see each patient not as a diagnosis but as a human being." Indeed, it's a call to arms for all digital developers to see each patient and healthcare professional as a human being. In addition, Rana's book explains the impact of confirmation bias, the confusion of using unfamiliar digital systems, and a few other things we've discussed directly in this book.

Finally, *When Breath Becomes Air* by Paul Kalanithi (Vintage, 2017) can only be described as poetry on the meaning of life as you and your family face death — as we all eventually will. This is a book you cannot forget. Paul Kalanithi was a neurosurgeon who died in 2015, survived by his wife, Lucy, and their daughter. Lucy finished this powerful book.

If you want to know more about healthcare culture

Any list of books about healthcare would be incomplete without these three powerful books:

- Caroline Elton, *Also Human: The Inner Lives of Doctors* (Penguin, 2018).

- Adam Kay, *This is Going to Hurt: Secret Diaries of a Junior Doctor* (Picador, 2018).

  In just the year after it was first published, this book sold 650,000 copies, had been translated into 24 languages, been number one for four months, and was being made into a BBC series. It's very good, and rightly deserves to be so popular.

- Christie Watson, *The Language of Kindness: A Nurse's Story* (Penguin, 2018).

These are all page-turner books. They are worth reading if only to admire the skill of stories and good writing powerfully sucking you in. And, with these books, you'll absorb a lot about the day-to-day life of doctors and nurses.

Healthcare, though, is just a part of the bigger picture of *public* health. It's been a long time since I've read such a relevant and insightful book as Michael Lewis's *The Premonition: A Pandemic Story* (Allen Lane, 2021), a book I strongly recommend. The suspense and urgent problem-solving of the COVID-19 pandemic makes for a gripping thriller. From its first story about 13-year old Laura Glass's school computer project to model pandemics, *The Premonition* is a totally engrossing page-turner.

The Premonition is not just a good book about our response to COVID-19, though, as there are many insights about healthcare culture and digital to be taken from it. Here are a few of my thoughts from it:

🐦 At ground-level, there were many competent and very worried people working on infectious diseases and the pandemic, but the culture at the top, in Government and healthcare organizations, didn't want to upset anyone. People stalled because that seems safer than being decisive.

🐦 Good digital systems — from computerized virus genome analysis to epidemiological models — were absolutely crucial to understand the pandemic and how best to handle it. Unfortunately, some digital systems were awful, yet just having reliable digital systems was only a small part of the story, as there also had to be a competent culture to recognize the value of having *reliable* digital. That was rare.

🐦 One of the bad computer models that misled people was done in Excel. The Excel model misleadingly showed that, even if nothing was done, California's hospital beds could easily manage the pandemic. But Excel shouldn't be used to run computer models that any lives depend on.[e] Indeed, even deciding to use Excel for this purpose says a lot about the dearth of digital skills available to public health advisors. The Excel programmer would have been unaware of their own limited skills, and, in turn, the State relying on the Excel model was unaware of its bugs.

🐦 Here's one more stunning story from the book. With Chan Zuckerberg's support, Joe DeRisi set up free and fast COVID-19 testing, but nobody seemed to want to use it. When Joe's team called the *Zuckerberg* San Francisco General Hospital to find out why even they didn't want free and fast tests, they were told that *their computers* wouldn't allow ordering a zero cost test!

It's possible that the rejection of a zero cost was a deliberate design decision, but I think it's more likely a bug. The program probably treated zero as meaning that the user hadn't entered anything, so it would ask for a number, even if the user had already entered 0. It's a common problem of badly programming interactive numerals.[55] In fact, here it's the standard problem of poor types:[f] "has the user entered a number" and "the value of the number" are values of different types, and if a single numeric variable handles both, there will be bugs, as then zero *ambiguously* also means the user hasn't entered a number. That bug would make it impossible to enter zero.

As I read *The Premonition*, I was shocked by how many decision-makers didn't have a clue about infection control, pandemics, exponential growth —

---

[e] See Chapter 14: Microsoft Excel, page 182 ←
[f] See Chapter 21: Programming with types, page 282 ←

basic stuff, one might have thought. It matters that there aren't adequate scientific skills available at the highest levels. I was struck how this is so like digital healthcare culture, too — so few leaders, who can make a difference, don't have or have access to the professional digital skills they need. It matters that digital has specialist skills, yet everybody rushes ahead as if it is easy and as if they understand everything. As with pandemics, you can only get away with ignorance for so long.

Lastly, Wears and Sutcliffe's book, *Still Not Safe: Patient Safety and the Middle-managing of American Medicine* is a litany of healthcare culture's impact on delaying the development of the patient safety movement. This book stands back a bit, and is really quite an academic look at patient safety culture, but I'll specifically recommend it as really useful for researchers below.[g]

If you are interested in improving

A very accessible article on improving safety in healthcare, and essential reading, is Sir Liam Donaldson's classic "An Organisation with a Memory" (in *Clinical Medicine*, **2**:452–457, 2002). This classic article is more readily available than the full NHS report, *An Organisation with a Memory: Report of an Expert Group on Learning from Adverse Events in the National Health Service*, published by Stationery Office Books in 2000. The full report is at tinyurl.com/yyujuv28

Charles Kenney, *Transforming Health Care: Virginia Mason Medical Center's Pursuit of the Perfect Patient Experience* (Productivity Press, 2010). Back in 2001, Virginia Mason, a failing hospital in Seattle, USA, set out to improve by adopting the Toyota Production System (TPS). The hospital's transformation for the better was dramatic, and proof that to improve you just need to start (and follow a sensible method). The first question they asked was "what are we trying to do?" They got surprising answers, and then pursued improving the quality of what they *really* wanted to do. They have a useful website: www.virginiamasoninstitute.org

A **maturity model** is a way an individual or organization can assess how mature their approach to their work is. There are maturity models in supply chains, software development, cybersecurity, and more. See en.wikipedia.org/wiki/Maturity_model for a good overview. The idea, basically, is by making your maturity explicit you can think about it and then point in the right direction to get better. If you are not assessing your maturity, you aren't mature!

These books are particular ideas, checklists, maturity models, and so on. More generally, healthcare *also* has to change *how* it thinks in order to take full advantage of what digital has to offer. That means manufacturers should

---

[g] See Chapter 33: *Still Not Safe*, page 489 →

not offer exactly what healthcare says it wants, but should offer better things; for instance, things that stretch current practice toward a more interoperable future. This requires what is called **disruptive innovation** — manufacturers should disrupt current thinking, not play along with it.

Clayton M. Christensen has been arguing this for years. His book *The Innovator's Dilemma: When New Technologies Cause Great Firms to Fail* (reprint edition, Harvard Business Review Press, 2016, but first published in 1997) has become a classic. The subtitle of the book might well have been *When New Technologies Cause the Problems of Healthcare to Become Visible*.

The generic business insights of Christensen's *The Innovator's Dilemma* have more recently been focused specifically onto healthcare:

📖 Clayton M. Christensen, Jerome H. Grossman, and Jason Hwang, *The Innovator's Prescription: A Disruptive Solution for Healthcare* (McGraw-Hill, 2009).

———————————————————

Karl Popper transformed science, or at least how we approach and think about experiments.[512] If you plan a successful experiment, and it succeeds, what can you learn? You will have no idea what specifically made the experiment successful. Instead, Popper's insight was that a scientist must develop **risky experiments** that are *intended* to be on the edge of being successful — they may fail. If a risky experiment succeeds, then taking risks has exposed your ideas to rigorous scrutiny, and where you took risks turns out to be right — in other words, the deliberate acceptance of error drives new learning, whereas the avoidance of error — planning to do successful experiments — seriously limits scientific learning.

In a fascinating article,[513] Karl Popper and Neil McIntyre pointed out the many parallels between pre-Popperian scientific thinking and today's healthcare thinking. Healthcare wants to avoid errors, so it has difficulty learning. Errors are concealed, and what is learned has limited value. Instead, they argue to change the ethics of medicine so errors are accepted and learning becomes routine.

Popper and McIntyre's insights about healthcare culture could equally well be leveled at programmers. Most programmers build programs expecting them to work. They do not program defensively, because they underestimate and indeed wish to hide their propensity for error. Instead, a sort of Popperian approach to programming, planning to be fallible, planning to learn from errors — that is, adopting the scientific method to programming — will produce, in the long run, far more reliable programs, and hence safer healthcare. In other words, good programmers should treat programming as an experimental discipline.

I think of myself as a Computer Scientist, and I think that if the field of Computer Science wants to be taken seriously *as a science*, it should take

Popper (and his many successors) seriously, and of course not just Computer *Science* as a field should do this, so should everyday programming and development. Popper and McIntyre's article is a good place to start, provided their mentions of "medicine" are updated in your mind to include "computer science" and "digital healthcare."

If you are doing incident reporting

Learn about incident reporting if you want to learn how *not* to have your systems or staff end up in any incident investigations.

If you are going to do a root cause analysis (in fact, if you are going to avoid doing one, you should know why) — a rigorous analysis of why an incident occurred — you should read the standard IEC 62740, *Root cause analysis (RCA)*, which you can find at webstore.iec.ch/publication/21810

Far and away the best incident report must be Charles Haddon-Cave's review into the 2006 RAF Nimrod plane that had a catastrophic mid-air fire over Afghanistan, which killed the entire crew of twelve as well as two mission specialists — fourteen people in all. Read it, and you'll not only learn about the horrific incident and what failures led up to it, but you'll see a master investigator at work, at the same time also explaining clearly how the investigation is being done and how he's thinking.

> 📖 Charles A. Haddon-Cave, *The Nimrod Review — An independent review into the broader issues surrounding the loss of the RAF Nimrod MR2 Aircraft XV230 in Afghanistan in 2006: A failure of leadership, culture and priorities* (The Stationery Office, 2009).

The Nimrod review introduced the fantastic, pejorative term **Power-Point Engineering**, which means drawing pictures that only *look* technical, but then everyone taking them to be rigorous ideas. It looks like a clear plan, but actually — what nobody notices or questions — is that it's just been drawn to look good. In the Nimrod story, there were plenty of nice PowerPoints. Everybody just assumed that some serious thinking had gone into them and that they made sense and were connected to reality. They weren't.

People often design digital healthcare systems using PowerPoint. It isn't good enough. Some much better ideas are discussed below.[h]

Mitre's Common Vulnerabilities and Exposures database, cve.mitre.org, and the US FDA's MAUDE database are large repositories for reporting and recording problems. MAUDE has a long URL; just Google "FDA MAUDE" to find it easily.

If you are thinking of buying or you are using a device or system, look it up in these systems. If you have an incident, please report it to MAUDE and preferably cve.mitre.org as well as your national system. In the UK, the

---

[h] See Chapter 33: If you are a developer, page 484 →

current system is the NHS National Reporting and Learning System, NRLS, report.nrls.nhs.uk/nrlsreporting

In the UK, in the first instance when you want to report an incident you will probably use your local system, such as Datix; otherwise you should contact the HSIB, the Healthcare Safety Investigation Branch at www.hsib.org.uk for up-to-date and helpful advice.

The UK MHRA has its reporting system too; see www.gov.uk/report-problem-medicine-medical-device. While you can report problems, the website does not cover design problems or bugs; as it says, you can report when someone's injured (or almost injured) by a medical device, either because its labeling or instructions aren't clear, it's broken, or it's been misused. That statement reinforces our culture that once a device is approved for use, it couldn't be problematic, could it?

If you are interested in law and regulation

The authoritative and up-to-date law book on electronic evidence is Stephen Mason and Daniel Seng, editors, *Electronic Evidence and Electronic Signatures* (fifth edition, Institute of Advanced Legal Studies, 2021). It includes excellent discussions of all things digital as they relate to the law and legal procedures. It does not shy away from being critical of the legal system and discussing its deep problems — including various clashes between the legal system and healthcare.

Electronic Evidence and Electronic Signatures is open access, and it's available at humanities-digital-library.org/index.php/hdl/catalog/book/electronic-evidence-and-electronic-signatures

I talked a lot about electronic evidence in the chapter *Side effects and scandals*, especially with the Princess of Wales Hospital and the Post Office Horizon cases.[i] The notes added some more details on the bizarre legal presumption that computers are reliable.[98]

If you don't know about UCD, UX, or HCI

UCD, UX, and HCI are abbreviations for User Centered Design, User eXperience, and Human-Computer Interaction, respectively. All are about ways of putting the user — patient, clinician, manager ... — at the center of computer system design.

UCD is critical for making successful systems, but there is a problem: it is not sufficient for success. You may end up with something that is nice, easy, and pleasurable to use, but it's the wrong thing altogether. You also have to address the larger design issues about *what* to design — and what

---

[i] See Chapter 8: Side effects and scandals, page 81 ←

things need changing — users may be stuck doing things inefficiently, and computerizing things so that they can do what they are already doing better may not be the best thing to do. Computers can improve how organizations work, as well as improving how people do things.

It is obvious that systems should be designed around user needs (UCD and so on[j]): but do you know how to find out what the users' needs are, and what to do when they change as systems are implemented? Do you know what to do when the UCD insights mean re-engineering the healthcare systems rather than the digital systems?

There are hundreds of books in the UCD area, and you should look carefully at several to find which best meet your needs.

🔖 Alan Cooper, Robert Reimann, and David Cronin, *About Face 3* (Wiley Publishing Inc., 2007) is very readable. It's aimed at developing desktop applications, websites, and apps. It's into its third edition, which is a good sign of its popularity.

🔖 One of my own books, *Press On: Principles of Interaction Programming* (MIT Press) covers a lot of user interface design best practice, and is particularly aimed at programmers and producing reliable, dependable, and safe user interfaces. It covers all forms of user interface design, which includes digital healthcare. If digital health systems do not have well-designed user interfaces, then nothing done with them will be safe.

🔖 Ben Shneiderman, Catherine Plaisant, Maxine Cohen, Steven Jacobs, Niklas Elmqvist, and Nicholas Diakopoulos, *Designing the User Interface: Strategies for Effective Human-Computer Interaction* (sixth edition, Pearson, 2016).

Shneiderman's book has got to its sixth edition already, so it's both popular and staying up-to-date. It's always a promising sign when a book runs into many editions: indeed, Shneiderman *et al*'s textbook is, I think, the best general textbook on HCI design.

If you are interested in Human Factors

The best book on Human Factors has a blog site, and you can start exploring it there: hfeinpractice.wordpress.com — the book itself is: Steven Shorrock and Claire Williams, *Human Factors and Ergonomics in Practice: Improving system performance and human well-being in the real world* (CRC Press, 2016).

---

[j] See Chapter 22: User Centered Design, page 301 ←

There's a huge "toolkit" of Human Factors insights for design. The tools have great names like affordance, fatigue, stress, task, leadership, forcing functions, task saturation, and more.

An excellent place to start is Don Norman's fantastic and deservedly popular book, *The Design of Everyday Things*, now in a revised and expanded edition (MIT Press, 2013). The book was originally called *The Psychology of Everyday Things*, but whatever it's called it is *the* classic book on thoughtful design. Do get it and read it.

Sidney Dekker's book *Patient Safety: A Human Factors Approach* (CRC Press, 2011) is directly focused on healthcare and patient safety, acknowledging their complexity. I said it above, but I think it's worth reading everything Dekker writes.

The US FDA has been using Human Factors for over 30 years, and their website has lots of free resources. I won't give specific URLs, as this is a lively area of development — go and have a look and find the most recent white papers and tutorials. Here's the FDA's home URL: www.fda.gov

An important part of Human Factors is cognitive psychology, the Human Factors of how we think. The chapter on Cat Thinking introduced a few ideas,[k] but here are some outstanding books and articles to read more:

- Carol Tavris and Elliot Aronson, *Mistakes Were Made (But Not by Me): Why We Justify Foolish Beliefs, Bad Decisions, and Hurtful Acts* (revised edition, Mariner Books, 2015).[14]

- Daniel Kahneman, *Thinking, Fast and Slow* (Penguin, 2012).[15]

- ... and Elizabeth Kolbert wrote a fun and thought-provoking review of some books and their ideas in "Why Facts Don't Change Our Minds: New discoveries about the human mind show the limitations of reason," *The New Yorker*, 20 February 2017. www.newyorker.com/magazine/2017/02/27/why-facts-dont-change-our-minds

If you are a developer or a programmer

Sometimes programmers just implement the systems they are told to implement. Really, this is called coding; it isn't programming, thinking carefully through how to make things work. Programming means thinking about the requirements and carrying them through to a working implementation, and revising that implementation as experience with how it is really used accumulates.

Thinking like a programmer who is solving problems has become called **Computational Thinking**.[l] It's extremely useful, helps people work out

[k] See Chapter 3: Cat Thinking, page 25 ←
[l] See Chapter 13: Computational Thinking, page 151 ←

better solutions to their problems (before rushing in to program the wrong things). Computational Thinking is under-rated but it's very easy — and fun — to start using it effectively: read Paul Curzon and Peter McOwan's *The Power of Computational Thinking: Games, Magic and Puzzles to Help You Become a Computational Thinker* (WSPC, Europe, 2017).

One of the earliest books that mentions Computational Thinking, and one of the easiest to read, is Seymour Papert's famous *Mindstorms: Children, Computers, and Powerful Ideas* (Basic Books, 1980). Seymour Papert was a hugely inspirational teacher of computing's powerful ideas. This is a book to inspire your (or anyone's!) children to get into computing. It'll inspire you too.

I think no serious book on programming, like *Fix IT*, can fail to praise Donald Knuth's books, which are widely recognized as defining the field of Computer Science. They are quite hard work to read, but if you can cope, they are thorough reference books to help solve any programming problem. They should convince you that programming, properly understood, is a real engineering discipline. They come in a boxed set, along with lots of additional volumes. Read them! Donald E. Knuth, *The Art of Computer Programming* (third edition, Addison-Wesley, 2011).

Knuth's approach to programming assumes that you know that what you are doing is the right thing to be doing; but Knuth does not explore how to program the right things, which is more the concern of Formal Methods (and software engineering more generally). Daniel Jackson's book, *Software Abstractions: Logic, Language, and Analysis* (revised edition, MIT Press, 2011) gives an introduction to his Alloy system as well as a nice overview of alternative approaches. It's a fun, insightful, and very readable book, and comes with a tool that can be downloaded and easily used on real problems. I noted a shorter (and cheaper!) description of Alloy earlier in this book.[405]

You'll seek out books and online sources when you know you've got a problem that you want to solve. If, say, you want a random number, then Knuth has the answer — he's the best source on the planet for every detail in Computer Science. But there is a very different sort of book, one you wouldn't think of reading to seek out an answer to a question: a book that changes how you think. Under this heading, there are a few programming books that will change how you *think*, rather than answer any questions you thought you already had:

- Richard Feynman, *Feynman Lectures On Computation* (Westview Press, 2000). Feynman won the Nobel Prize in physics, and his clear, lucid, fun lectures on computation explain basic concepts in computer science. Suddenly, you realize you never really understood anything until he blew your horizons away.

- Harold Abelson and Gerald Jay Sussman, *Structure and Interpretation of Computer Programs* (second edition, MIT Press, 1996). This book is a hands-on undergraduate course in programming from MIT.

Structure and Interpretation of Computer Programs starts with a famous quote from Alan Perlis,

> it's extraordinarily important [...] that we keep fun in computing

... and it certainly lives up to that exhortation.

🔹 Chris Hanson and Gerald Jay Sussman, *Software Design for Flexibility: How to Avoid Programming Yourself into a Corner* (MIT Press, 2021).

Agile methods[m] encourage continually modifying programs to make them suit user needs, but many bugs arise because we try to modify programs that are hard to modify, and we make mistakes as we change them. Instead, we could design programs to be flexible, and then they would be easy to modify because we intended them to be easy to modify — they would be *flexible*. Domain-specific languages (DSLs) are just one way of being flexible. If you can program in Scheme, this is a *fantastic* book, and if you can't program in Scheme — every programmer should know Scheme! — *Structure and Interpretation of Computer Programs*, mentioned above, is where you should start to learn it — it's a powerful and inspiring language that grows with you.

🔹 DSLs are such a good idea, there are lots of places to read up about them. I recommend exploring DSLs starting with ANTLR, not only because ANTLR is a good place to start and has a very stimulating philosophy about good programming, but it *and its ideas* are also very good tools to have in your programming toolbox. The book on ANTLR is Terence Parr's *The Definitive ANTLR 4 Reference* (The Pragmatic Programmers, 2012).

🔹 Most of us programmers are not as good as we'd like to be. Systems take too long to implement, and have far too many bugs when delivered. Watts Humphrey's *PSP: A Self-improvement Process for Software Engineers* (Addison-Wesley, 2005) provides a powerful way to improve. He also wrote *Winning with Software*, which is the book to get your managers or senior executives to read, so they understand what software is all about. If they don't read this book, then they are likely to drive their programmers with unrealistic goals that will end in failure and in poor products. Maybe getting manufacturing executives and healthcare Chief Information Officers

---

[m] See Chapter 27: Agile method, page 378 ←

to read this book (as well as my own book, *Fix IT*!) will improve healthcare safety more than anything else.

Adacore is a leading international software developer for safety-critical systems. Adacore supplies SPARK Ada and other tools, primarily for safety-critical software for the aviation industry. They could help digital healthcare, too: see **www.adacore.com** and also look up sparkpro on their website. It's fair to say there are many other companies in the area, but Adacore's website is a good place to start looking.

- Nancy Leveson, *Engineering a Safer World: Systems Thinking Applied to Safety* (MIT Press, 2017). This is arguably *the* textbook on engineering safe and reliable systems. The book also covers Nancy's STAMP method. It is full of insightful analyses of real examples and, crucially, methods that work.

- John Knight's book, *Fundamentals of Dependable Computing for Software Engineers* (CRC Press, 2012) is aimed more at programmers. It does a very good job of explaining why safe programming matters and how to do it well.

- Ross Anderson's book, *Security Engineering: A Guide to Building Dependable Distributed Systems* (third edition, John Wiley & Sons, 2021) is the bible for security (including cybersecurity), which is essential for healthcare systems. Cybersecurity changes every day, so get the latest details from Ross's web site at www.cl.cam.ac.uk/~rja14/book.html

If you are a healthcare programmer

If you are a programmer working specifically in healthcare, there are more targeted books than the generic books I summarized above, including these two:

- Peter Spurgeon, Mark-Alexander Sujan, Stephen Cross, and Hugh Flanagan, *Building Safer Healthcare systems* (Springer, 2019).

- David A. Vogel, *Medical Device Software* (Artech House, 2011).

If you want to find out how a serious safety-critical industry, aviation, does its programming, Leanna Rierson's book, *Developing Safety-Critical Software* (CRC Press, 2013) is the best place to start. This book provides a thorough overview of compliance with the aviation standard DO-178C. In my view, the simplest and quickest way to improve digital healthcare would be to require compliance with this standard — at least healthcare organizations should say "we won't pay up until you show you've followed DO-178C." We know it works.

While the DO-178C standard is great, it has a problem. It costs about £250, and that's far too much money to invest when no regulators are requiring its higher standards in healthcare; it's also too much money for training companies or universities to invest in. If we want safety, we need to make safety standards (and this goes for Snomed, HL7, ISO, IEC, BSI, ... too) much cheaper, if not free. Rierson's book, fortunately, is a *lot* cheaper.

It's worth noting that some standards are supported by apps, which makes using them and compliance with them very much easier. For instance, ISO 13485, which is about quality management for medical devices and requirements for regulatory purposes, has an app, Greenlight Guru, which is available at www.greenlight.guru

What about AI? Robotics? Implants? Cybersecurity?

I think digital healthcare's excitement about AI is a bit premature. Certainly, it has lots of potential, but it raises all sorts of unsolved issues, from privacy to introducing new bugs and hard-to-understand errors. Whether AI is an improvement on balance begs some careful experiments, which to my knowledge haven't been attempted yet. That said, Eric Topol's book, *Deep Medicine: How Artificial Intelligence Can Make Healthcare Human Again* (Basic Books, 2019), is a fine place to start. Eric Topol is a doctor, and his excitement in this book is palpable. You can also see the very diverse, almost scattergun, impact AI is *potentially* having. The book palpably conveys the excitement for AI from the medical profession's perspective.

Eric Topol doesn't say much about technologies beyond AI in this book of his — he doesn't explore technologies like robotics, implants, telemedicine, blockchain, or digital security, let alone cybersecurity, and lots more; nor does he say much about the ethics, the harsh realities of market drivers, or the problems of interoperability (getting excited about each AI innovation, rather than fixing integration of all the separate innovations).

Cybersecurity is a dynamic area (there's an entire chapter on it in this book,[n] as well as several discussions of cyber failures), and it's important to get up-to-date advice. Start by going to your national cybersecurity center, such as the UK's National Cyber Security Centre, www.ncsc.gov.uk or the US's National Cybersecurity Center, cyber-center.org or their National Cybersecurity and Communications Integration Center, www.cisa.gov

There's also the US National Cybersecurity and Communications Integration Center at ics-cert.us-cert.gov

However, for focused healthcare cybersecurity, the University of Michi-

---

[n] See Chapter 17: Cybersecurity, page 211 ←

gan's Archimedes Center for Medical Device Security is an excellent source of information. Archimedes is at **www.secure-medicine.org** — they also run regular workshops you might like to attend.

My own article,[87] "Misunderstanding IT: Hospital cybersecurity problems in court" (in *Digital Evidence and Electronic Signature Law Review*, **15**:11–32, 2018. DOI: 10.14296/deeslr.v15i0.4891) not only has lots of useful advice on cybersecurity, but it also has a full description of a major incident that could happen to any hospital.[o] The story will perhaps help the cybersecurity advice to be taken more seriously.

If you are a researcher

For this list of further reading (which will never be sufficiently up-to-date anyway) the best advice is to go online, and look up new health technologies — and be very careful! Avoid misleading, fake information, and see if you can find any randomized controlled trials, systematic reviews, or at least peer-reviewed papers backing up claims before you get too excited. Unfortunately, many papers about digital healthcare ideas are written by the developers and therefore have a conflict of interest. Indeed, if you can find papers that *aren't* written by any of the originators, that at least shows somebody independent is interested in following up on the ideas!

Have a look at **www.chi-med.ac.uk**, which was a large project that inspired much of this book. There's lots more to do.

If you go to the websites of the main research funders for the sort of work explored in this book (in the UK there are the Engineering and Physical Sciences Research Council and the Wellcome Trust): they mostly want to fund new innovation, like AI, and cybersecurity, but — as of the time of my writing this book — they show little interest in making digital healthcare less risky and safer.

Robert Wears was a world leader in patient safety, and his authoritative book,

> 📖 Robert L. Wears and Kathleen M. Sutcliffe, *Still Not Safe: Patient Safety and the Middle-managing of American Medicine* (Oxford University Press, 2020)

is a very substantial history of patient safety since its beginnings. It has some insightful, if depressing, discussion about the statistics of patient safety, the varying estimates of patient harms, a topic we explored briefly in this book.[p]

The emphasis in *Still Not Safe* is how healthcare culture has eaten patient safety and medicalized it — isolating it from the "real" safety professions like Human Factors, Psychology, Safety Science, and Engineering. It's an

---

[o] See Chapter 8: Abbott XceedPro glucometer, page 92 ←
[p] See Chapter 9: The scale of the problem, page 109 ←

ultimately sad book, but it's very telling on how healthcare really works, seen from the inside. It gives many insights into how digital healthcare may be undermined, though there is no mention of digital healthcare as such. There is nothing on the way digital has reified managerialism, despite the book's focus on the forces of professionalism and management. This is strange, because Wears had previously been enthusiastic about using computers to reduce error.[514]

Nevertheless, *Still Not Safe* is fascinating for its mature perspective from one of the leaders of the field. It has numerous key references any serious researcher will wish to explore.

Out-of-the-box thinking

I've **highlighted in bold** key books and papers in the Notes chapter,[q] which, to save space, I will not repeat here.

In addition, please read this classic book:

> 📖 Ralph Nader, *Unsafe at Any Speed: The Designed-in Dangers of the American Automobile* (Basic Books, 1965).

I've mentioned Ralph Nader's book several times,[138] and it's worth getting hold of a second-hand copy (or going to a library), being shocked at how bad the stories he tells are, but being encouraged that so much has improved in car safety since he wrote it.

Unsafe at Any Speed was written well over 50 years ago but, today, reading Nader's classic is just like reading a story about modern healthcare — like my *Fix IT* — if you imagine he's writing about digital healthcare rather than cars. How the car industry has been transformed and become so much safer, and so quickly, should encourage us that we can do the same with digital healthcare.

It's all very well feeling inspired but then not working out how to apply ideas to make change happen. Here are two helpful books to encourage thinking about change and achieving successful change:

> 📖 Anders Ericsson and Robert Pool, *Peak: Secrets From the New Science of Expertise* (Penguin, 2016). If you have heard that you need 10,000 hours to become an expert, Ericsson and Pool show you that it's not the hours you spend, but how you use them.

> 📖 Mathew Syed, *Black Box Thinking: Marginal Gains and the Secrets of High Performance* (John Murray, 2015). Syed's book starts off contrasting the culture of healthcare — with the stories of Martin and Elaine Bromiley[r] — with the culture of aviation improving,[s] learning

---

q See Chapter 34: Notes, page 497 →
r See Chapter 20: Elaine Bromiley tragedy, page 263 ←
s See Chapter 26: Planes are safer, page 347 ←

from accidents and putting that learning into good use.

While both these stories are covered in *Fix IT,* Syed focuses on the reasons why learning does and doesn't happen — and how to ensure it does happen.

Pharma and the medical device industry

None of the following books discuss digital healthcare as such, but they throw a very worrying light on medical research, medical industry, and medical regulation. While it is arguable that digital healthcare needs more resourcing, these three books are a warning that the regulatory incentives (including patent rules) must be very carefully worked out if patients and healthcare providers are going to benefit in the long run.

Ben Goldacre, *Bad Pharma: How Medicine is Broken, and How We Can Fix It* (Fourth Estate, 2013) — Ben's book is a gripping and shocking exposé of the pharmaceutical industry. If all this goes on in the pharma industry post-thalidomide, which Ben documents extremely well, what is going on in digital healthcare, which is even less well regulated than pharmaceuticals?

Goldacre's *Bad Pharma* is primarily about the mess of the science behind pharmaceuticals and how it could be improved. Far more shocking is Jeanne Lenzer's book *The Danger Within Us: America's untested, unregulated medical device industry and one man's battle to survive it* (Little, Brown, 2017). Medical devices like hip implants may disintegrate and lead to mental problems when the metal bits wear down and get into the blood stream and then mess with the brain. It is understandable that if you sell millions of hip implants, there may well be a few awful stories, but the damning thread in Jeanne Lenzer's book is the utter failure of the US regulators to manage medical devices. (Jeanne doesn't cover digital devices or healthcare IT systems.)

Jeanne's book is one of the key sources behind the Netflix documentary, *The Bleeding Edge.*[214] It's really worth reading the book or watching the film: after the damning — and well-written — evidence, it finishes with a chapter with suggestions on what we can do to improve things.

For twenty years Marcia Angell was the Editor in Chief of the world-leading medical journal, *The New England Journal of Medicine.* Her book, *The Truth About The Drug Companies* (Random House, 2005) is a sustained and authoritative indictment of drug regulation, the drug industry, and how doctors typically do their jobs under the influence of commercial pressures. The entanglement of commercial interests and government has led to huge profits and diminishing benefit to patients, particularly older patients — who are typically both poorer and have multiple conditions that need treatment.

It's not all bad news, though. For example, Civica Rx is a new joint hospital and philanthropist-led consortium to develop cheap generic drugs to undercut the huge costs of commercially made drugs.[515] Perhaps similar collaborative business models, thinking outside the small box of the usual business models, could also be developed to drive digital healthcare to scale up and to improve quality.

If you want the big picture of digital health

I tried to ensure that the digital healthcare issues discussed in this book are, at least in principle, common across the world, but healthcare systems vary enormously from country to country, and even within countries. Politics, organizational structures, regulations, managing patients, all vary enormously. International healthcare — digital or not — is hard to understand. My view remains that if we don't get the details right, as *Fix IT* discussed, whatever systems or levels of systems you are concerned with, then digital healthcare will remain unnecessarily risky for everyone involved, patients as well as healthcare professionals.

If you work in any healthcare system, even at the local level, system factors are very intrusive: they affect everything from training, registering patients, treating them, transferring them around the system, to reporting incidents, and, finally, deaths — to say nothing of handling laboratory results, classifying diseases and patient pathways, and much more besides. Typically, there are many computer systems — from many diverse manufacturers — that handle the various phases of getting patients through the systems. They also handle getting paid, and many other things.

If you move jobs within healthcare, you will almost always need to retrain so you know how to do the job you've been doing for years, so now you can do it using different systems. You'll also very likely have fun with your system accounts, as Beth Griffith's story, told in box 33.1, shows.

Fix IT has already hinted at the range of digital problems with discussions on training,[t] interoperability[u] and internationalization (particularly in box 25.1). The increasing popularity of international travel and internet communication ensures system differences often collide without needing to move where you work. Indeed, the regular updates and replacements of digital systems means that your job changes even when you stay still. Often, the old legacy systems, their data, and their habits, will remain and make new technology improvements increasingly quirky, as they compromise to balance keeping the old and benefiting from the new. Fortunately, lots of people have thought deeply about these problems: Marianne Bellotti, *Kill it with Fire: Manage Aging Computer Systems (and future proof modern ones)*, No

---

[t] See Chapter 24: Anesthetics training, page 325 ←
[u] See Chapter 19: Interoperability, page 245 ←

> **Box 33.1.** Digital chaos nearly had a doctor removed by Security
>
> Beth Griffith is an Acute Medicine Registrar. Here's her digital chaos story:[516]
>
> Some NHS hospitals have recently merged, which has led to merging their IT systems over the last few weeks. Because I've moved jobs, I had two accounts. To rectify this, my IT Department deleted one of them — except they deleted the wrong one: the one from my old job, which I hadn't worked at since 2019. So when I tried to log in to a computer in my current hospital, my account had been disabled.
>
> So I rang IT, and asked them to unlock my account, but IT wasn't able to. Somehow, they were confused by my two accounts, and they decided I wasn't allowed to work there because my contract had ended in 2019.
>
> They didn't tell me.
>
> They rang Security.
>
> Security searched the hospital to get me out. However, I'd already gone home, so they decided that I must have "absconded."
>
> The following day, I went to work and my IT account was active again. I had some email from IT saying something about a duplicate account being deleted and all was fine. I thought that was the end of it.
>
> Except that one of the junior doctors had witnessed the security drama, but didn't know it was all a misunderstanding. He'd spent weeks believing I was a fake doctor, and unknown to me, the rumor had spread.
>
> The next thing I knew, when I was seeing a patient, Security came racing in. They've had reports that a fake doctor who'd been escorted off the premises a few weeks ago had come back.
>
> I was excited about the drama. I didn't put two and two together. Then Security called out my name. The "fake doctor" was me.

Starch Press, 2021, is a very readable introduction to properly engineering "system modernization."

For the UK, a brief 150 page summary of digital healthcare in the NHS is Gary McAllister's *An Introduction to Digital Healthcare in the NHS*, second edition, 2021. Gary self-published the book, and it can be ordered easily from Amazon. It quickly introduces topics like Health Level 7 (HL7), Fast Healthcare Interoperability Resources (FHIR), portals, AI, clinical coding, and COVID-19, as well as lots of specifically NHS systems. The book certainly conveys the complexity of national systems, as well as some of the additional politically-imposed complications.

I'm tempted to provide more good reading for other countries — there's plenty of it — but you should really search for what's best for you.

Excitement

Cat Thinking[v] might explain our hormone-driven excitement, but there are also objective reasons to be excited by digital healthcare. Computers have huge potential, and they can transform how everything is done. Computers are now inside many people — they're in heart pacemakers, cochlear implants, insulin pumps, artificial limbs, telemedicine, AI for mental health, and much more. In the future, computers will transform what it means to be human, let alone what it means to be a healthy human. AI is just a small strand. There's robotics, exoskeletons, all the way to androids, VR hologram doctors ... the sort of future that science fiction can only dream of.

There is, of course, tons of stuff to read about exciting futures. I recommend Mark O'Connell's prize-winning book as a good read: *To Be a Machine* (Granta, 2017). Books can't really hope to keep up with the pace of digital innovation, but the magazine *Wired* and its website, www.wired.com, comes out regularly and will keep you up-to-date, in so far as anything will.

Dreams of a future, safer, more effective digital healthcare?

That's a good point to end *Fix IT* on.

---

[v] See Chapter 3: Cat Thinking, page 25 ←

Supporting this book are over 500 notes and references on digital healthcare and patient safety incidents. These notes cover media stories, peer-reviewed cutting-edge research, as well as national and international reports.

Notes in **bold** are especially good sources for further reading.

34

Notes

This chapter collects all the notes from the book. All the notes are cross-referenced back to the pages where they were raised in the book, so you can more easily go backward and forward. Notes highlighted in **bold** are key books and documents that are highly recommended reading.

Many documents referenced in these notes have a DOI, a **digital object identifier**. You can type this identifier into a form on the DOI organization's website, doi.org, or you can write the DOI into a URL directly using doi.org/*identifier*. So for this DOI: 10.1098/rsif.2010.0112, as given in this book, in full you'd type http://doi.org/10.1098/rsif.2010.0112 into your browser (as a URL). In this case, the DOI gets you the full text of the Harold Thimbleby and Paul Cairns open access paper, "Reducing number entry errors: Solving a widespread, serious problem."[51] Of course, if you are using an electronic version of this book, all URLs and DOIs can be clicked on directly.

The idea of DOIs is that they stay the same forever and always refer to the same thing, even if the websites and URLs they refer to get reorganized.[517] In fact you're probably better off taking the title of anything I cite and doing an internet search on it: that way, you'll find all the additional — and later — discussions about it. If you follow the DOI alone, you'll typically only get the original and none of the future improvements.

1 How to read this book

1. Pages 2, 469, 509. Although Hippocrates flourished in around 400 BC, the Edwin Smith Papyrus dates medical insights to much earlier. It's a long ancient Egyptian papyrus scroll, dating from around 1600 BC, covered in medical, not magical, details of injuries and treatment. See en.wikipedia.org/wiki/Edwin_Smith_Papyrus

Fix It: See and solve the problems of digital healthcare. Harold Thimbleby, Oxford University Press. © Harold Thimbleby 2021.
DOI: 10.1093/oso/9780198861270.003.0034

2   We don't know what we don't know

2. Page 15. A good source on Ignaz Semmelweis is K. Codell Carter and Barbara R. Carter, *Childbed Fever*, Transaction Publishers, 2005.

3. Page 15. Christine Hallett, "The Attempt to Understand Puerperal Fever in the Eighteenth and Early Nineteenth Centuries: The Influence of Inflammation Theory," *Medical History*, **49**(1):1–28, 2005. DOI: 10.1017/s0025727300000119

4. Page 18 twice. Practice Fusion is owned by Allscripts Healthcare Solutions Inc.
    A news report on the case is: "In secret deal with drugmaker, health-records tool pushed opioids to doctors," *Los Angeles Times*, 30 January 2020.
    www.latimes.com/business/story/2020-01-30/health-records-company-pushed-opioids-to-doctors-in-secret-deal
    The US Department of Justice's press release on the case is here: "Electronic Health Records Vendor to Pay $145 Million to Resolve Criminal and Civil Investigations Practice Fusion Inc Admits to Kickback Scheme Aimed at Increasing Opioid Prescriptions," Press Release Number: 20-94, 27 January 2020.
    www.justice.gov/opa/pr/electronic-health-records-vendor-pay-145-million-resolve-criminal-and-civil-investigations-0

5. Pages 19, 29, 114 twice, 179, 207, 215, 220, 226 twice, 241, 344, 347, 359, 393, 442, 471. This book tries to be precise about numbers: lives can depend on getting them right. Unfortunately the word "billion" is easily misunderstood, as there are incompatible ways of writing large numbers. For instance, in old British English (pre-1974) and in modern French, billion means a million million, but in modern English, as used throughout this book, the word billion means one thousand million, $1,000,000,000$.

6. Page 19. Twenty-three professors of Computer Science, of whom I was one, ran a campaign. It's now a good few years ago, and starting to get harder to find on the web. Try the *Health Committee Publications, Evidence ordered by the House of Commons*, 22 March 2007: Brian Randell, "Evidence submitted by Professor Brian Randell (EPR 20),"
    publications.parliament.uk/pa/cm200607/cmselect/cmhealth/422/422we64.htm
    and examples like www.bcs.org/content/conWebDoc/18051

7. Pages 20, 245, 298. BBC, "Outdated IT leaves NHS staff with 15 different computer logins," 4 January 2020. www.bbc.co.uk/news/health-50972123

8. Page 20. Gareth Iacobucci, "Government's plan to digitise NHS risks wasting billions, MPs warn," *BMJ*, **371**:m4317, 2020. DOI: 10.1136/bmj.m4317

9. Page 20. Duncan P. Thomas, "The Demise of Bloodletting," *Journal of the Royal College of Physicians Edinburgh*, **44**:72–77, 2014. DOI: 10.4997/JRCPE.2014.117

10. Page 22. The Bill & Melinda Gates Foundation is at www.gatesfoundation.org

3   Cat Thinking

11. Page 25. *Kung Fu Panda* is a fun computer-animated cartoon film by Paramount Pictures, released in 2008.

12. Page 27. David W. Bates, et al, "Incidence of Adverse Drug Events and Potential Adverse Drug Events," *Journal of the American Medical Association*, **274**(1):29–34, 1995. DOI: 10.1001/jama.1995.03530010043033

13. Page 27. Our largely uncritical enthusiasm for computers causes special concern when children get drawn in and are affected socially, and — as usual — our personal experience belies the significance of the scale of what is going on across the world. See, for example, this report of a large US study: *The Common Sense Census: Media Use by Kids Age Zero to Eight*, Common Sense, 2017. www.commonsense.org/research

14. Pages 28, 270, 484. **Carol Tavris and Elliot Aronson, *Mistakes Were Made***

(But Not by Me): Why We Justify Foolish Beliefs, Bad Decisions, and Hurtful Acts, revised edition, **Mariner Books, 2015.**

15. Pages 28, 484. Daniel Kahneman, *Thinking, Fast and Slow*, Penguin, 2012.

16. Page 29. Trisha Greenhalgh, "How to improve success of technology projects in health and social care," *Public Health Research and Practice*, **28**(3):e2831815, 2018. DOI: 10.17061/phrp2831815

17. Page 29. Clayton M. Christensen, *The Innovator's Dilemma: When New Technologies Cause Great Firms to Fail*, Harvard Business Review Press, 1997.

18. Page 29. Boundless Mind's website is boundless.ai
    A good popular article is Haley Sweetland Edwards, "You're Addicted to Your Smartphone. This Company Thinks It Can Change That," *Time*, 13 April 2018. time.com/5237434/youre-addicted-to-your-smartphone-this-company-thinks-it-can-change-that

19. Pages 30, 462, 465. **Safety cases are required in many industries and are being increasingly promoted for use in healthcare. Unfortunately, safety cases don't much help with "unknown unknowns." For example, two recent reports advocating safety cases completely overlook bugs and reliable software engineering — perpetuating the myth, which I hope this book has dispelled, that digital healthcare is intrinsically easy to get right.**
    See: The Health Foundation, *Using safety cases in industry and healthcare*, 2012, www.health.org.uk, which is an excellent introduction to the value of safety cases. However, while it mentions that cybersecurity should figure in a safety case, it overlooks that a case also needs to be made that the software itself is safe and dependable.
    More recently, the UK Healthcare Safety Investigation Branch (HSIB) in reviewing some adverse incidents with so-called smart infusion pumps published *Procurement, usability and adoption of 'smart' infusion pumps*, Report I2019/009, 2020, www.hsib.org.uk
    The HSIB report strongly promotes safety cases to help healthcare proactively manage safety, but, again, the HSIB report assumes that equipment (in this case, smart pumps) is safe, so the issue that's left is for the users of pumps, primarily the hospitals, to make a case that *their* use of the systems is going to be safe.
    It would be better, I think, if any safety case made in healthcare included a statement something like "we have seen and professionally reviewed the safety case made by the vendors" as well, and in turn the safety case for the systems they are procuring should say that the manufacturers have used UCD[a] and rigorous development methods to avoid and manage bugs — in fact, that they can provide a safety case that they have properly addressed all the topics covered in this book.

4   Dogs dancing

20. Page 33. Of course, I'm simplifying when I say I would've been a year old in 1956. Before my first birthday, I wouldn't have been a year old. I was born in July, so I'd be a year old in July 1956, in fact, on my birthday on the nineteenth. Fortunately, the month detail doesn't make any difference to the Y2K problem (or the explanation), and so for simplicity I'm going to ignore it, as if I'd been born on the first day of 1955.

21. Page 34. The Millennium Bug has developed its own conspiracy theory: that huge amounts of money were spent on a non-existent problem. In fact, the problem was solved precisely because huge amounts of efforts and money were directed at solving it.

---

[a] See Chapter 22: User Centered Design, page 301 ←

Martyn Thomas has a short and authoritative article on it: "The millennium bug was real — and 20 years later we face the same threats," *The Guardian*, 31 December 2019. www.theguardian.com/commentisfree/2019/dec/31/millennium-bug-face-fears-y2k-it-systems

22. Pages 34, 287. Northern General Hospital NHS Trust, *Report of the Inquiry Committee Into The Computer Software Error In Downs Syndrome Screening*, undated.

23. Pages 34, 35, 248, 462. How did the Down syndrome calculation go wrong?

Here's how the Down syndrome program worked:

Dates in the program were stored as strings of ten characters, such as 11/10/1970. In itself, this is bad practice (dates should be stored as objects, not as strings — strings can have syntax errors, for instance).

To get the year to do a mother's age calculation, the Down syndrome program extracted the ninth and tenth characters from the string, getting the last two digits of the year of birth. So a date like 11/10/1970 gives the two characters 70. They did the same thing with the current year. So if the year is 2000, the two digits extracted give 00. So in the year 2000, a mother born in 1970 would seem to be aged –70, since the computer would do the calculation 00 – 70 (zero minus seventy = minus seventy), rather than doing the correct calculation 2000 – 1970 (= plus thirty).

There is no justification whatsoever (such as limited computer memory) for only extracting two digits when four are needed. The program is already storing dates as long ten character strings — so, clearly, there's plenty of memory. There is also no justification for a program not to check that a calculated mother's age falls within a sensible window, say 12 to 60 years, which would immediately trap invalid, indeed insane, ages like –70. It should always be standard practice to build such **sanity checks** into programs, just in case they have unknown bugs. This program had bugs and clearly did no useful sanity checks.

In fact, there was another bug in the program, detected earlier, in 1994, that involved the program failing to notice it was doing incorrect calculations with mothers with an impossible zero weight. Unfortunately, the programmer didn't learn from this earlier incident that checks are standard programming practice.

The obvious fix to the Y2K bug is to extract all four year digits from a date. Then a date like 11/10/2000 would give 2000 rather than 00, and the age calculation would be correct. The Inquiry report explains how this works using the example date 3/4/2000, for which the seventh to tenth characters are 00 and not 2000 — did you notice that the report used 3/4 and not 03/04? This is surely an ironic bug for an inquiry into bugs, but it does illustrate why it is such bad practice to store dates as strings of characters (after all, the string 3/4/2000 is as good a string as 03/04/2000 is).

The obvious fix to a program's problems, however, is distracting. A much better fix is to ask: why are we even doing this? Repeatedly parsing strings to extract dates is a symptom of poor programming. Instead, the user interface should use a standard, properly developed API to convert the date to a timestamp, and the program would never need to covert dates, as it would all be done in the standard, accredited code throughout the program.

It's a shame that all critical healthcare software and documentation is not **open source**, and therefore available for the wider community to check and improve. If the Down program had been made open source, the community would have helped improve it — and it's clear from the Inquiry that it had many avoidable bugs. Moreover, with open source, every hospital would have been able to use the improved system, so bugs in other hospitals would also have been better managed.

24. Pages 35, 286. Bill Goodwin, "Hospital software failure shows Y2K bug can still bite," *Computer Weekly*, 27 September 2001, www.computerweekly.com/feature/Hospital-software-failure-shows-Y2K-bug-can-still-bite

This article also says the program was written in Basic, which is a totally inappropriate programming language to use.

25. Page 35. Martin Wainwright, "NHS faces huge damages bill after millennium bug error," *The Guardian*, 14 September 2001.
www.theguardian.com/uk/2001/sep/14/martinwainwright

26. Page 35. Bill Goodwin, "Y2K hitch exposes NHS skills deficit," *Computer Weekly*, 20 September 2001. www.computerweekly.com/news/2240042406/Y2K-hitch-exposes-NHS-skills-deficit

    The NHS has a publication *Risk Calculation Software Requirements for Down's Syndrome Screening* (by Dave Wright, Barry Nix, Steve Turner, David Worthington, and Andy Ellis, published in 2013), but it baffles me. There are so many vague ideas: it does *not* provide useful requirements for software engineers wanting to implement Down syndrome calculations reliably. There is *nothing* in the requirements about error, proving programs correct, or signing off projects; there is no reference to professional software engineering practice at all. There is not even any mention that a mother's age must be positive — so the errors of the Y2K could get through again. In other words, bugs in software can extend much wider — here, there are bugs in the software's requirements and management.

    Later chapters, particularly Computer Factors[b] will give some positive ideas for solutions.

27. Page 36. I made a video of the simulation which is available at www.youtube.com/watch?v=brNbDWnHDVs — "Problems with a syringe pump," YouTube, 2008. The general methodology, and in particular the simulation of the Graseby syringe driver, is described here: Harold Thimbleby, "Interaction Walkthrough: Evaluation of Safety Critical Interactive Systems," *Proceedings International Workshop on Design, Specification and Verification of Interactive Systems — DSVIS 2006*, Lecture Notes in Computer Science, **4323**:52–66, Springer-Verlag, 2007. DOI: 10.1007/978-3-540-69554-7_5

28. Pages 40, 41, 42. Yong Y. Han, Joseph A. Carcillo, Shekhar T. Venkataram, Robert S. B. Clark, R. Scott Watson, Trung C. Nguyen, Hülya Bayir, and Richard A. Orr, "Unexpected Increased Mortality after Implementation of a Commercially Sold Computerized Physician Order Entry System," *Pediatrics*, **116**:1506–1512, 2005. DOI: 10.1542/peds.2005-1287

    My graph is based on the paper's figure 1, but unfortunately the paper provides no exact data for each quarter. An erratum appears in *Pediatrics*, **117**(2):593–594, 2006.

29. Page 41. Sam Sachdeva, "Testing times for Epic at Cambridge," *digitalhealth*, 25 November 2014.
www.digitalhealth.net/2014/11/testing-times-for-epic-at-cambridge

30. Page 41. There are many papers to carry on reading. Here are two:

    Mary G. Amato, Alejandra Salazar, Thu-Trang T. Hickman, Arbor J. L. Quist, Lynn A. Volk, Adam Wright, Dustin McEvoy, William L. Galanter, Ross Koppel, Beverly Loudin, Jason Adelman, John D. McGreevey III, David H. Smith, David W. Bates, and Gordon D. Schiff, "Computerized prescriber order entry-related patient safety reports: Analysis of 2522 medication errors," *Journal of the American Medical Informatics Association*, **24**(2):316–322, 2017. DOI: 10.1093/jamia/ocw125

    Gordon D. Schiff, Mary G. Amato, T. Eguale, J. J. Boehne, Adam Wright, Ross Koppel, A. H. Rashidee, R. B. Elson, D. L. Whitney, T-T. Thach, David W. Bates, and A. C. Seger, "Computerised physician order entry-related medication errors: Analysis of reported errors and vulnerability testing of current systems," *BMJ Quality & Safety Online*, **24**(4):264–271, 2015. DOI: 10.1136/bmjqs-2014-003555

31. Page 42. Raj M. Ratwani, Michael Hodgkins, and David W. Bates, "Improving Electronic Health Record Usability and Safety Requires Transparency," *Journal of the American Medical Association*, **320**(24):2533–2534, 2018. DOI: 10.1001/jama.2018.14079

32. Page 43. "Bawa-Garba: timeline of a case that has rocked medicine," *PULSE*, 13

---

[b] See Chapter 21: Computer Factors, page 277 ←

February 2018. www.pulsetoday.co.uk/news/gp-topics/gmc/bawa-garba-timeline-of-a-case-that-has-rocked-medicine/20036044.article

33. Page 43. Lyvia Dabydeen, Hilary Klonin, Nigel Speight, Sethu Wariyar, Sanjay Gupta, and Sanjiv Nichani, "An account by concerned UK paediatric consultants of the tragic events surrounding the GMC action against Dr Bawa-Garba," 54000doctors, 54000doctors.org/blogs/an-account-by-concerned-uk-paediatric-consultants-of-the-tragic-events-surrounding-the-gmc-action-against-dr-bawa-garba.html

34. Page 44. BBC News, "Hadiza Bawa-Garba: Medics rally behind struck off doctor," 29 January 2018. This article has the text of the letter: Nick Bostock, "More than 5,000 GPs sign Bawa-Garba protest letter," GP Online, 29 January 2018. www.gponline.com/5000-gps-sign-bawa-garba-protest-letter/article/1455743

35. Page 44. There is far more to this case than the IT failure. Please also read University Hospitals of Leicester NHS, Investigation Report, Final Report re: ██████, Unexpected Death, Incident Report Form Ref No W65737, STEIS Log No 2011/3518, 24 August 2011/updated 3 January 2012. See also much discussion in the *BMJ*, e.g., Deborah Cohen, "Back to blame: the Bawa-Garba case and the patient safety agenda," *BMJ*, **359**:j5534, 2017. DOI: 10.1136/bmj.j5534 and lots of discussion on the Twitter handle #IAmHadiza

36. Page 44. The NHS has an excellent — and brief — Just Culture guide, "A just culture guide: Supporting consistent, constructive and fair evaluation of the actions of staff involved in patient safety incidents," which can be found on the Just Culture web pages at www.england.nhs.uk/patient-safety/a-just-culture-guide

37. Page 45. MCG Health Inc., *COMPUTERIZED PROVIDER ORDER ENTRY Superuser Reference Manual*, 2008. paws.gru.edu/pub/cis/training/documents/pdfs/manuals/cpoesuperuserreferencemanual09_26_08.pdf

38. Page 45. Rachel Clarke, "Hadiza Bawa-Garba could have been any member of frontline staff working in today's overstretched NHS," *BMJ*, 8 December, 2017. blogs.bmj.com/bmj/2017/12/08/rachel-clarke-hadiza-bawa-garba-could-have-been-any-member-of-frontline-staff-working-in-todays-overstretched-nhs

39. Pages 45, 117. *The Mid Staffordshire NHS Foundation Trust Public Inquiry*, chaired by Robert Francis QC (February 2013), www.gov.uk/government/publications/report-of-the-mid-staffordshire-nhs-foundation-trust-public-inquiry

40. Page 45. Clare Dyer, "Bawa-Garba is free to practise again without restrictions after tribunal ruling." *BMJ*, **374**:n1690, 2021. DOI: 10.1136/bmj.n1690

41. Page 46. Dr Marie Moe works at the Norwegian University of Science and Technology (NTNU). She's got YouTube movies, including a great 2016 TEDx talk, "Can hackers break my heart?" at www.youtube.com/watch?v=W1YWpVMpPi8

    Marie has also written some very interesting articles on her experiences. See lots more on her web home page: www.ntnu.edu/employees/marie.moe

42. Page 46. Payam Safavi-Naeini and Mohammad Saeed, "Pacemaker Troubleshooting: Common Clinical Scenarios," *Texas Heart Institute Journal*, **43**(5):415–418, 2016. DOI: 10.14503/THIJ-16-5918

43. Page 47. See our paper: Yi Zhang, Paolo Masci, Paul Jones, and Harold Thimbleby, "User Interface Software Errors in Medical Devices," *Biomedical Instrumentation & Technology*, **53**(3):182–194, 2019. DOI: 10.2345/0899-8205-53.3.182

5   Fatal overdose

44. Page 49. AIM stands for Ambulatory Infusion Manager.

45. Pages 49, 50. Nurses *program* infusion pumps to deliver a specific dose, typically by pressing buttons on them. Confusingly, the same word, "programming," is also used when programmers *program* infusion pumps by writing their software. The main difference in usage is that the nurse's programming will change as needed for each

occasion, but exactly the same software programming is intended to work in all circumstances (barring bugs).

46. Pages 49, 50, 54, 63. Institute for Safe Medication Practices Canada, *Fluorouracil Incident Root Cause Analysis*, 2007.
www.ismp-canada.org/download/reports/FluorouracilIncidentMay2007.pdf

47. Pages 51, 503, 517. Harold Thimbleby, "Calculators are Needlessly Bad," *International Journal of Human-Computer Studies*, **52**(6):1031–1069, 2000. DOI: 10.1006/ijhc.1999.0341
    A more mathematical analysis, using matrices (which is much easier than it sounds), of some of the crazy problems of calculators can be found in: Harold Thimbleby, "User Interface Design with Matrix Algebra," *ACM Transactions on Computer-Human Interaction*, **11**(2):181–236, 2004. DOI: 10.1145/1005361.1005364

48. Page 51. When somebody makes an error because they thought they were doing the right thing, this is called an **intentional error**. Here, if the nurses thought 28.8 was the right rate, then not dividing by 24 would have been an intentional error. Had they thought 28.8 was a daily rate and therefore that they needed to divide by 24, but they made an error and didn't divide by 24, then that would be a **slip**. In other words, the same error and outcome have different formal descriptions, depending on what the people were intending.
    I don't like the term intentional error. In healthcare, it's a dangerous term: nobody *intends* to make an error. The term makes it sound like that making the error was intentional! The nurses didn't intend to make any errors; they intended to do the right thing, but what they did happened to be an error, whether they thought they were doing the right thing, whether it was a slip, or had some other cause.

49. Page 52. The app is open source and written in HTML5, so you can see how it works if you want to. A description of the app and its motivation is available at: Harold Thimbleby, "Ignorance of Interaction Programming is Killing People," *ACM Interactions*, 52–57, September+October 2008. DOI: 10.1145/1390085.1390098

50. Page 53. Over the years I've written a lot about calculators: see note 47 for some of my papers. A paper on the design and analysis of a calculator (as a simple finite state machine) is: Harold Thimbleby, "Contributing to Safety and Due Diligence in Safety-critical Interactive Systems Development," *Proceedings ACM SIGCHI Symposium on Engineering Interactive Computing Systems — EICS'09*, 221–230, ACM, 2009. DOI: 10.1145/1570433.1570474

51. Pages 53, 497. Harold Thimbleby and Paul Cairns, "Reducing number entry errors: solving a widespread, serious problem," *Journal of the Royal Society Interface*, 7:1429–1439, 2010. DOI: 10.1098/rsif.2010.0112

52. Page 55. Abbott Laboratories, ABBOTT a*i*m *plus*, System Operating Manual, List 13967-04 (Rev 2/96), 1996.

53. Page 55. Institute for Safe Medication Practices (ISMP), *List of Error-Prone Abbreviations*, 2017.
www.ismp.org/recommendations/error-prone-abbreviations-list

54. Page 56. ISMP Canada, "Death Associated with an IV Compounding Error and Management of Care in a Naturopathic Centre," *ISMP Canada Safety Bulletin*, **18**(1), 4 January 2018.
    Other examples include Gary Bradshaw, who died after handwriting a lab technician misread calcium as cancer: George Greenwood, "Lost notes and illegible records risking lives of NHS patients," *The Times*, 16, 2 October 2019.

55. Pages 57, 182, 190, 285, 383, 385, 409, 478. **Everybody should know about "interactive numerals," whether you use numerical systems (nurses do all the time) or you are a programmer of digital healthcare systems. Harold Thimbleby and Paul Cairns, "Interactive numerals," *Royal Society Open Science*, 4:160903, 2017. DOI: 10.1098/rsos.160903**

56. Page 58. The quotation in the text uses my emphasis for "took an exceptional step." The original source is: ISMP, "Fluorouracil Error Ends Tragically, But Application of Lessons Learned Will Save Lives," 20 September 2007. www.ismp.org/resources/fluorouracil-error-ends-tragically-application-lessons-learned-will-save-lives

    A short follow-up report has a good summary of the recommendations: ISMP Canada, "Fluorouracil incident RCA: follow-up," *ISMP Canada Safety Bulletin*, **7**(4):1–4, 2007. www.ismp-canada.org/download/safetyBulletins/ISMPCSB2007-04Fluorouracil.pdf

    An alternative source is Matthew Grissinger, "Fluorouracil Mistake Ends With a Fatality Applying the Lessons Learned Can Save Lives," *Pharmacy & Therapeutics*, **36**(6):313–314, 2011. DOI: 10.1007/s10389-020-01371-3

6 Swiss Cheese

57. Page 62. More details of the Swiss Cheese Model are in Good reading,[c] as well as in this paper: Yunqui (Karen) Li and Harold Thimbleby, "Hot Cheese: A Processed Swiss Cheese Model," *Journal of the Royal College of Physicians Edinburgh*, **44**(2):116–121, 2014. DOI: 10.4997/JRCPE.2014.205

58. Page 63. Here's a systematic review of double checking: Alain K. Koyama, Claire-Sophie Sheridan Maddox, Ling Li, Tracey Bucknall, and Johanna I. Westbrook, "Effectiveness of double checking to reduce medication administration errors: A systematic review," *BMJ Quality & Safety*, 2019.

59. Page 63. The story is taken from Medical Malpractice Lawyers.com, "Pharmacy Error Was The Cause Of Chicago Infant's Death," 15 April 2012. www.medicalmalpracticelawyers.com/blog/pharmacy-error-was-the-cause-of-chicago-infants-death

    Some more details, including a video, can be found here: Alex Perez, "Couple Says Park Ridge Hospital Killed Their Baby," *NBC 5 Chicago*, 5 April 2011. www.nbcchicago.com/news/health/genesis-burkett-malpractice-suit-119272599.html

60. Page 64. This book promotes SPARK Ada as a powerful, flexible, and dependable language for all healthcare applications. Many readers will question this — there are many alternatives — but please remember that this book is not a programming course, and there isn't the space to present and discuss lots of alternatives, so I focused on one or two.

    While readers may have their own preferred programming language preferences — C++, Eiffel, Erlang, Go, Haskell, Kotlin, ML, Rust, Scala, Swift, to name but a few — the point of this book is not preferences as such, but dependability in the complex environment of healthcare. Do the programming languages you like and would promote make the programs you write more reliable? Easier to analyze? Easier to maintain? Easier to document? Easier to get qualified professional support? What you are good at and like isn't necessarily what *is* good, unfortunately — and that's surely true of my own ideas too. Keep thinking, when I use Ada as a recurring example: how does your favorite language compare?

    The index entries "Programming language" and "Programming tools" are pointers to the programming language discussions to be found in this book.

61. Page 65. Cliff Kuang with Robert Fabricant, *USER FRIENDLY: How the Hidden Rules of Design Are Changing the Way We Live, Work, and Play*, Penguin (WH Allen), 2019.

62. Page 65. Brian MacKenna, Seb Bacon, Alex J. Walker, Helen J. Curtis, Richard Croker, and Ben Goldacre, "Impact Of Electronic Health Record Interface Design On Unsafe Prescribing Of Ciclosporin, Tacrolimus and Diltiazem: A Cohort Study In English NHS

---

[c] See Chapter 33: James Reason's *Human Error* book, page 474 ←

Primary Care," *Journal of Medical Internet Research*, in press, 2019.
preprints.jmir.org/preprint/17003

7   Victims and second victims

63. Page 69. Arthur M. Johnston, *Unintended overexposure of patient Lisa Norris during radiotherapy treatment at the Beatson Oncology Centre, Glasgow in January 2006*, Scottish Executive, 2006. The URL for The Beatson West of Scotland Cancer Centre is www.beatsoncancercharity.org/about-us/the-beatson-west-of-scotland-cancer-centre

64. Page 71. Richard I. Cook, Christopher P. Nemeth, and Sidney Dekker, "What went wrong at the Beatson Oncology Centre?" edited by Christopher P. Nemeth and Erik Hollnagel, *Resilience Engineering Perspectives*, **1**: Remaining Sensitive to the Possibility of Failure:225–236, Ashgate Publishing, 2008.

65. Page 71. Daily Mail Reporter (anonymous), "Mother-of-four dies after blundering nurse administers TEN times drug overdose," *Daily Mail*, 23 February 2011. www.dailymail.co.uk/health/article-1359778/Mother-dies-nurse-administers-TEN-times-prescribed-drug.html

66. Page 74. Details of the beam calculation came from *Investigation on an accidental exposure of radiotherapy patients in Panama. Report of a Team of Experts*, 26 May–1 June 2001, International Atomic Energy Agency. For a nice article on problems with software quality, including a good analysis of the Panama incident, see: D. Cage and J. McCormick, "We did nothing wrong: Why software quality matters," *Baseline*, 2004. www.baselinemag.com/c/a/Projects-Processes/We-Did-Nothing-Wrong

67. Pages 74, 177, 561. Albert Wu, "Medical error: The second victim," *BMJ*, **320**:726–727, 2000. DOI: 10.1136/bmj.320.7237.726

68. Page 74. Cobalt 60, ^{60}Co, is a radioisotope that emits gamma rays. Cobalt 60 has a half-life of five years, and therefore requires frequent replacement: the short half-life, and the problems of managing the radioactive waste, is one reason why cobalt machines are being replaced by linear accelerators.

69. Page 79. **Nancy Leveson and Clark Turner's famous article about the Therac-25 should be required reading for anybody using, buying, designing or manufacturing radiotherapy systems, or indeed any critical digital healthcare systems. This is the classic paper all programmers should read: Nancy G. Leveson and Clark S. Turner, "An Investigation of the Therac-25 Accidents," *IEEE Computer*, 26(7):18–41, 1993. DOI: 10.1109/MC.1993.274940**

   If you can't easily get hold of their paper, Nancy Leveson's book, *Safeware: System Safety and Computers* (Addison-Wesley, 1995) is fantastic and has a full description of the Therac-25 problems.

70. Page 79. Nancy G. Leveson, "The Therac-25: 30 Years Later," *IEEE Computer*, **50**(11):8–11, November 2017. DOI: 10.1109/MC.2017.4041349

8   Side effects and scandals

71. Page 81. Sunday Times Insight Team, *Suffer the Children: The Story of Thalidomide*, Viking Press, 1979.

72. Page 82. Thalidomide Society, Thalidomide FAQs, www.thalidomidesociety.org/what-is-thalidomide, 2017; see also *The Guardian* article, "Thalidomide: how men who blighted lives of thousands evaded justice," by Harold Evans, www.theguardian.com/society/2014/nov/14/-sp-thalidomide-pill-how-evaded-justice, 2014.

73. Page 82. James Badcock, "Spain's forgotten Thalidomide victims see glimmer of hope," www.bbc.com/news/world-38386021, 2016.

74. Page 83. Morton Mintz, "Heroine of FDA Keeps Bad Drug Off of Market," *The Washington Post*, 15 July 1962.

75. Page 84. In 2019, Gosport War Memorial Hospital's website has since disappeared; Wikipedia has an entry that should be up-to-date: en.wikipedia.org/wiki/Gosport_War_Memorial_Hospital

76. Page 84. The Right Reverend James Jones, *Gosport War Memorial Hospital The Report of the Gosport Independent Panel*, Her Majesty's Stationery Office, 2018. www.gosportpanel.independent.gov.uk

77. Page 85. Nick Carding, " 'Disregard for human life' — 450 patients killed by painkillers at hospital, report says," *Health Service Journal*, 20 June 2018. www.hsj.co.uk/patient-safety/disregard-for-human-life-450-patients-killed-by-painkillers-at-hospital-report-says/7022705.article

   There are huge ongoing criminal investigations into the Gosport tragedy. See: Clare Dyer, "Gosport: new criminal investigation is launched into hundreds of deaths at hospital," *BMJ*, **365**:l1991, 2019. DOI: 10.1136/bmj.l1991 and "Gosport hospital deaths: Inquiry reviews 15,000 death certificates," BBC, 15 March 2021, www.bbc.co.uk/news/uk-england-hampshire-56404256

78. Page 85. Note that I have no idea why Anne Grigg-Booth committed suicide — she was certainly under pressure and would have felt in the focus of blame. She may have committed suicide for many reasons; perhaps because she felt she was going to be exposed as guilty, or because of the pressure, which there certainly was on her.

   See Paul Stokes and Nigel Bunyan, "Nurse's suicide leaves mystery of how many patients died at her hands," *The Telegraph*, 31 Aug 2005. www.telegraph.co.uk/news/uknews/1497300/Nurses-suicide-leaves-mystery-of-how-many-patients-died-at-her-hands.html

   Grigg-Booth denied responsibility for any deaths, but relatives of the patients are relieved she died. As one said, "Why anyone would do such an evil and pointless thing is beyond me." Of course, that depends on whether she did. Is she a scapegoat? Did she feel remorse? Both? In any case, as a nurse she was presumably following orders. Indeed, much of the debate about this sorry case has been about whether the patients should have been prescribed opiates at all, as most were not in pain or terminally ill.

   It would be helpful for everyone to have an investigation, *with full awareness of digital risk*, and determine whether the Graseby syringe driver played a significant part, rather than automatically blaming the nurse at the sharp-end.

79. Page 86. **There's a good programming rule: if you can use a FSM, you should use a FSM. They are fast, efficient, easy to program, and — useful for safety-critical applications — they are easy to analyze to check they do what you want and have whatever properties you require. My book *Press On: Principles of Interaction Programming* (MIT Press) explains how using FSMs can help design high-quality user interfaces.**

80. Page 88. National Patient Safety Agency, *Rapid Response Report NPSA/2010/RRR019: Safer ambulatory syringe drivers*, 2010.

81. Page 88. The National Patient Safety Agency says milliliters is abbreviated as ml, but best practice is to abbreviate it as mL, to reduce the chance of confusing the letter l as the digit 1.

82. Page 89. Victoria Ward, "Gosport inquiry panel accused of 'NHS cover up' over faulty syringe drivers," *The Telegraph*, www.telegraph.co.uk/news/2018/06/23/gosport-inquiry-panel-accused-nhs-cover-faulty-syringe-drivers

83. Page 89. "UK's unsafe syringes found their way to Indian hospitals: Report," *The Times of India*, 8 July 2018. timesofindia.indiatimes.com/india/uks-unsafe-syringes-found-their-way-to-indian-hospitals-report/articleshow/64907985.cms

84. Page 89. www.apple.com/uk/shop/trade-in (accessed 2019).

85. Pages 90, 149, 477. The Principle of Dual Effect goes back to Thomas Aquinas, *Summa Theologica*, 1265–1274. A brief and very powerful discussion can be found in the page-turner by Rana Awdish, *In Shock: How Nearly Dying Made Me a Better Intensive Care Doctor*, Penguin, 2017.

      In Shock is a stunning and very human book documents some tragic healthcare suicides, where healthcare staff feel inadequate against the perfection standards they had been pressurized to live by.

86. Page 90. Graseby MS-16A advert by auctiontraderrsuk, who are no longer active.

87. Pages 93, 98, 134, 489, 557. The official report is Angela Hopkins, *Commissioned Review, June to September 2016. Review of the Blood Glucometry Investigations in Abertawe Bro Morgannwg University Health Board. Establishing lessons learned.* Abertawe Bro Morgannwg University Health Board, Wales, 2016.

      I've written a peer-reviewed paper about my own work as an expert witness in the case: Harold Thimbleby, "Misunderstanding IT: Hospital cybersecurity and IT problems reach the courts," *Digital Evidence and Electronic Signature Law Review*, **15**:11–32, 2018. DOI: 10.14296/deeslr.v15i0.4891

      In addition, the Judge has published his ruling on the case: R v Cahill; R v Pugh 14 October 2014, Crown Court at Cardiff, T20141094 and T20141061 before HHJ Crowther QC, *Digital Evidence and Electronic Signature Law Review*, **14**:67–71, 2017. DOI: 10.14296/deeslr.v14i0.2541

      The Princess of Wales Hospital at the time of the incident was in the Abertawe Bro Morgannwg University Health Board, which was renamed Swansea Bay University Health Board in 2019, but in the revision, the Princess of Wales Hospital was taken over by Cwm Taf University Health Board. Ironically for a book on digital health, their respective websites are not all correctly updated — which isn't helped by their helpful archived websites, which Google also finds, that predate the renamings and mergers.

88. Page 93. In the UK, expert witnesses work for the court, rather than for the defense or prosecution. An expert witness's job is to find out and tell the truth within their area of expertise. In the case described here, I was briefed by and worked closely with the defense team, since only they thought there was something wrong with the evidence.

89. Page 93. Reliable databases usually have auditing, so you know what operations have been performed on them. Or databases have checksums and other integrity checks, so you can tell if there's been any corruption. PrecisionWeb had absolutely nothing to audit, stop, detect, or recover from errors.

90. Page 96. XceedPro Good Design Award, www.g-mark.org/award/describe/36688/?locale=en

91. Page 96. Once the court found that the data used as evidence was rubbish, the case collapsed and the court didn't need to work out *why* the glucometer data was rubbish. I suspect it was corrupt long before Abbott was called in to fix it. I suspect that the Princess of Wales Hospital had all but ignored the state of the data in the PrecisionWeb database until the police asked for it. I read the hospital's extensive written evidence to the court on how they managed the database, and it showed considerable technical naïvety about managing clinical databases — but, of course, because of that very naïvety it didn't discuss what it didn't know!

92. Page 97. Incident and device reporting systems — in the US the FDA's MAUDE, and in the UK the MHRA's NRLS.

93. Page 97. Baystate Health System acknowledged their problems (rather than taking their nurses to court) and were able to improve their processes and managed to reduce the errors to just 3 per month — a twenty times improvement. See: Gaurav Alreja, Namrate Setia, James Nichols, and Liron Pantanowitz, "Reducing patient identification errors related to glucose point-of-care testing," *Journal of Pathology Informatics*, 2:22, 2011. DOI: 10.4103/2153-3539.80718 available at www.ncbi.nlm.nih.gov/pubmed/21633490

94. Page 97. I've just reported a bug to the UK's postal service, the Royal Mail. They replied to me, and asked me to provide a screenshot, a link to the URL (there's only one, so they should know what it is!), the browser I used, its version number, and a description of the device I was using. None of that is my job, and I still can't use their system!

95. Pages 97, 156, 171, 246, 532. Harold Thimbleby, "Three laws of paperlessness," *Digital Health*, 5:1-16, 2019. DOI: 10.1177/2055207619827722

96. Page 98. *PrecisionWeb Point of Care Data Management System User's Manual*, QC Manager 3.0, page 1-1, Abbott Diabetes Inc, ART12275 Rev.B04/09, 2009.

97. Pages 99, 100. One person's case in the Horizon scandal is discussed in detail in Paul Marshall, "The harm that judges do — misunderstanding computer evidence: Mr Castleton's story. An affront to the public conscience," *Digital Evidence and Electronic Signature Law Review*, **17**, 2020. DOI: 10.14296/deeslr.v17i0.5172

98. Pages 100, 101 twice, 103, 482. The profound nature of the legal problems is discussed in Peter B. Ladkin, Bev Littlewood, Harold Thimbleby, and Martyn Thomas, "The Law Commission presumption concerning the dependability of computer evidence," *Digital Evidence and Electronic Signature Law Review*, **17**, 2020. DOI: 10.14296/deeslr.v17i0.5143

99. Pages 100, 105. Stephen Mason, "Electronic evidence: A proposal to reform the presumption of reliability and hearsay," *Computer Law & Security Review*, **30**(1):80-84, 2014. DOI: 10.1016/j.clsr.2013.12.005

   Stephen has also edited the *the* reference book on digital evidence.[d]

100. Page 100. Chris Baynes, "Hundreds of Post Office workers 'vindicated' by High Court ruling over faulty IT system that left them bankrupt and in prison," *The Independent*, 17 December 2019. www.independent.co.uk/news/business/news/post-office-high-court-case-it-horizon-postmaster-prison-latest-a9249431.html

   See www.bbc.co.uk/news/video_and_audio/must_see/51120545/post-office-assisting-review-of-postmasters-convictions for a powerful video summary, and Stephen Mason, "Case Transcript: England & Wales – Regina v Seema Misra, T20090070 – Commentary and Index to the transcript by Stephen Mason," *Digital Evidence and Electronic Signature Law Review*, **12**, 2015. DOI: 10.14296/deeslr.v12i0.2217 for an overview of the cases.

   More recent details are here: Jonathan Ames and Andrew Ellson, "Call to prosecute bosses after postmasters cleared," and "Bankruptcy, imprisonment and suicide on the long journey to justice," *The Times*, (73454):10-12, 24 April 2021. www.thetimes.co.uk/article/postmasters-convictions-quashed-by-court-of-appeal-50pn7qm8v

101. Page 100. Horizon was originally developed by ICL, but ICL was taken over by Fujitsu in 2002.

102. Page 102. The Abbott XceedPro has many internal checks, but from the Princess of Wales Hospital case, it seems that there are very few if any checks on data reliability once patient data has left the device.

103. Page 103. The survey only looked at Picture Archiving and Communication Systems (PACS) using the Digital Imaging and Communications in Medicine (DICOM) protocol. Greenbone Networks GmbH, *Information Security Report: Confidential patient data freely accessible on the internet*, 2019. www.greenbone.net

104. Page 103. Ross Koppel and Craig Kuziemsky, "Healthcare Data Are Remarkably Vulnerable to Hacking: Connected Healthcare Delivery Increases the Risks," *Studies in Health Technology and Informatics*, **257**:218-222, IOS Press, 2019.

105. Page 106 twice. Rachel Krause, "Skill Mapping: A Digital Template for Remote Teams," 4 October 2020. www.nngroup.com/articles/skill-mapping — this helpful reference explains how to use skill maps and also provides a skill map template.

---

[d] See Chapter 33: Electronic Evidence, page 482 ←

9   The scale of the problem

106. Pages 109, 112, 243. Florence Nightingale's comment quoted at the beginning of the
      chapter — "The very first requirement in a hospital is that it should do the sick no
      harm" — comes from the preface of her *Notes on Hospitals* (Longman, Green,
      Longman, Roberts, and Green, 1863). This is clearly reminiscent of the famous
      Hippocratic Oath, "First do no harm." The problem is that this quote is usually sourced
      back to a Latin phrase, *primum non nocere*, but the big problem with that is
      Hippocrates was Greek, and he didn't speak Latin. The closest you can get to it is in
      his *Epidemics*, where he says (in Greek, obviously), "make a habit of two things — to
      help, or at least to do no harm." See more about Hippocrates in note 1.
          The interesting story is reviewed nicely in: Cedric M. Smith, "Origin and Uses of
      Primum Non Nocere — Above All, Do No Harm!" *The Journal of Clinical
      Pharmacology*, **45**(4):371–377, 2005. DOI: 10.1177/0091270004273680

107. Page 111. World Health Organization, *Family of International Classifications*, 2019.
      www.who.int/classifications/en

108. Page 111. US Centers for Disease Control and Prevention (CDC), *New ICD-10-CM
      code for the 2019 Novel Coronavirus (COVID-19)*, 1 April 2020. www.cdc.gov/
      nchs/data/icd/Announcement-New-ICD-code-for-coronavirus-3-18-2020.pdf

109. Page 112. Christina Jewett, "Hidden FDA Reports Detail Harm Caused By Scores Of
      Medical Devices," *Kaiser Health News*, 2019.
      khn.org/news/hidden-fda-database-medical-device-injuries-malfunctions

110. Pages 113 twice, 476. I've combined 2013 US Centers for Disease Control and
      Prevention (CDC) causes of death data with estimates of patient harm from a 2013
      paper by John T. James, "A new, evidence-based estimate of patient harms associated
      with hospital care," *Journal of Patient Safety*, **9**(3):122–128, 2013. DOI:
      10.1097/PTS.0b013e3182948a69
          James's methodology looked at hospital patient records, and if the patient records
      themselves were wrong thanks to (for instance) diagnostic errors, then this would not
      have been detected from the records alone. Estimates of fatalities in healthcare more
      generally — including primary care, pharmacies, dentists, nursing homes — would of
      course make the figures even higher.
          To draw the bar chart, I took the CDC fatality data, which ignores errors, and
      reduced each category by James's 16.9% (otherwise the preventable error bar would
      have been double-counting deaths classified under disease causes). However, I did not
      reduce suicides, as that category is not going to be much affected by preventable error.
          There have been studies sampling particular areas, such as infusions. See, for
      instance, the Eclipse project, www.eclipse.ac.uk

111. Page 113. **Lucian Leape's 1994 paper is a real classic on medical error. Lucian
      L. Leape, "Error in Medicine," *Journal of the American Medical Association*,
      272(23):1851–1857, 1994.**

112. Page 114. Facts taken from: World Health Organization, *Patient Safety Fact File*,
      2019, *10 facts on patient safety*, 2018, and *Patient Safety: Making Health Care Safer*,
      2017. www.who.int

113. Page 114. The air travel comparison is complicated. Many patients are very ill when
      they are admitted to hospital, and if you are very ill you are unlikely to go flying off on
      a trip from London to Brazil. So hospitals are going to have more deaths than aviation.
      However, the figures above were for *preventable* deaths, that is deaths that should not
      have happened in hospitals. Even if hospitals improved their safety by a factor of a
      thousand, they would still have a way to go to catch up with aviation safety.
          Airlines just have to get passengers and their baggage safely from A to B. Airline
      passengers are generally pretty well, whereas hospital patients start off being ill.
      Patients generally have all sorts of problems, lots of data (blood groups, drugs they are
      on, and more), and their blood pressure, heart rate, and other vital factors keep

changing. But just because patients are more complicated than plane passengers doesn't mean we should dismiss the aviation comparison! Hospitals have far more specialist staff and far more diagnostic equipment, and they need to have much better computer systems to keep track of everything.

Arguably, the biggest single difference between a hospital incident and a plane crash is the media coverage. When airplanes have problems, it's all over the news. When people die in hospital, for whatever reason, it's a private grief that very rarely gets reported. Only exceptional problems in hospitals reach the news, and the stories are usually about blaming doctors and nurses.

114. Page 114. A lot of people argue that the high preventable error estimates are wrong.

Surely it's implausible to have that huge a number of preventable errors? The numbers cited in this book (figure 9.1) are US numbers, and the US is different from other countries, so, arguably, the numbers are irrelevant for any other country, aren't they?

There is much discussion in the literature, including: Kaveh G. Shojania and Mary Dixon-Woods, "Estimating deaths due to medical error: the ongoing controversy and why it matters," *BMJ Quality & Safety*, **26**:423–428, 2017. DOI: 10.1136/bmjqs-2016-006144

A more recent systematic review and meta-analysis is Maria Panagioti, Kanza Khan, Richard N. Keers, Aseel Abuzour, Denham Phipps, Evangelos Kontopantelis, Peter Bower, Stephen Campbell, Razaan Haneef, Anthony J. Avery, and Darren M. Ashcroft, "Prevalence, severity, and nature of preventable patient harm across medical care settings: systematic review and meta-analysis," *BMJ*, **366**:l4185, 2019. DOI: 10.1136/bmj.l4185

Other surveys have specifically explored the role of computers in error: Farah Magrabi, Mei-Sing Ong, William Runciman, and Enrico Coiera, "An analysis of computer-related patient safety incidents to inform the development of a classification," *Journal of the American Medical Informatics Association*, **17**(6):663–670, 2010. DOI: 10.1136/jamia.2009.002444

For instance, they found 25% of medication errors were voluntarily reported as computer related — however, their survey of a voluntary incident reporting database used in one Australian state only found 0.2% of all reported incidents being computer-related. It's likely that the true figures are higher, since nobody in hospitals is trained to spot computer bugs, let alone go to the trouble of reporting them. Reporting bugs is tedious, as they usually have complicated symptoms, and by the time anyone has noticed a bug has caused problems, they have probably already focused on the workaround to get their job done. The details of the bug will be lost in history.

Finally, the simplest argument: estimated error numbers are higher than you expect because more often than not errors happen *because* we don't notice them happening. If we noticed errors, we'd stop them happening as they happen. The estimates are counting the extra errors we don't notice, so the rates seem high to us.

115. Page 114. Harms being 20 times worse than 16.9% sounds like an impossibly large estimate. No; 100% would be all the patients who die each year, but more people get harmed each year than die each year, so the harm rate can easily be 20 times higher than the death rate.

116. Page 115. Jessica Kim Cohen, "Physicians subpoenaed in Rhode Island, allegedly after reporting EHR risks," *Becker's Hospital Review*, 25 January 2019. www.beckershospitalreview.com/legal-regulatory-issues/physicians-subpoenaed-in-rhode-island-allegedly-after-reporting-ehr-risks.html

117. Page 115. Chitra Acharya, *Human-Computer Interaction and Patient Safety*, PhD Thesis, Swansea University, Wales, 2017.

118. Page 116. Samantha Poling, "Critical error: The Lisa Norris story," BBC Frontline, Scotland, 2007. news.bbc.co.uk/1/hi/scotland/6731117.stm

119. Pages 116, 556. Mark Davies, Paul Lee, Alan Chamberlain, and Harold Thimbleby, "Managing Gravity Infusion using a Mobile Application," *Proceedings BCS*

Conference on Human-Computer Interaction, 299–304, British Computer Society, 2014. DOI: 10.14236/ewic/HCI2014.48

120. Page 117. Jackie van Dael, Tom W. Reader, Alex Gillespie, Ana Luisa Neves, Ara Darzi, and Erik K. Mayer, "Learning from complaints in healthcare: a realist review of academic literature, policy evidence and front-line insights," *BMJ Quality & Safety*, epub ahead of print, 2020. DOI: 10.1136/bmjqs-2019-009704

121. Page 118. Here's a three-minute video of Peter Thimbleby's (my father's) death and what happened: www.harold.thimbleby.net/dad

10 Medical apps and bug blocking

122. Page 121. You can download the Mersey Burns app from merseyburns.com

123. Page 122. I checked and wrote up the Mersey Burns examples in September 2020; I was running the then most up-to-date iPhone version of Mersey Burns, version 1.6.4.

124. Page 123. Jamie Barnes, Annie Duffy, Nathan Hamnett, Jane McPhail, Chris Seaton, Kayvan Shokrollahi, M. Ian James, Paul McArthur and Rowan Pritchard Jones, "The Mersey Burns App: evolving a model of validation," *Emergency Medicine Journal*, **32**:637–641, 2015. DOI: 10.1136/emermed-2013-203416

125. Page 126. **Robert M. Wachter, *The Digital Doctor: Hope, Hype, and Harm at the Dawn of Medicine's Computer Age*, McGraw-Hill, 2015.**

126. Page 126. A single bed can produce 700 alarms in a day; and there is a very large literature on alarm fatigue and the hazards for patient safety. Quick places to get into the problems are Maria Cvach, "Monitor alarm fatigue: An integrative review," *Biomedical Instrumentation & Technology*, **46**(4):268–77, 2012. DOI: 10.2345/0899-8205-46.4.268 or Keith Ruskin and Dirk Hueske-Kraus, "Alarm fatigue: impacts on patient safety," *Current Opinion in Anaesthesiology*, **28**(6):685–690, 2015. DOI: 10.1097/ACO.0000000000000260

127. Page 126. Sue Sendelbach and Marjorie Funk, "Alarm Fatigue: A Patient Safety Concern," *American Association of Critical-Care Nurses (AACCN) Advanced Critical Care*, **24**(4):378–386, 2013. DOI: 10.1097/NCI.0b013e3182a903f9

128. Page 128. Chris Seaton, Mersey Burns, chrisseaton.com/merseyburns, 2018.

129. Page 129. For Wikipedia article on the Parkland formula, see en.wikipedia.org/wiki/Parkland_formula

   NICE, the UK National Institute for Health and Care Excellence, has a review of Mersey Burns at "Mersey Burns for calculating fluid resuscitation volume when managing burns," March 2016. www.nice.org.uk/advice/mib58

   The classic paper on the Parkland formula is: Charles R. Baxter and Tom Shires, "Physiological response to crystalloid resuscitation of severe burns," *Annals New York Academy of Science*, **150**:874–94, 1968. DOI: 10.1111/j.1749-6632.1968.tb14738.x

130. Page 129. There are some very nice ways to help humans calculate burn fluids reliably, but that's a different problem to getting apps bug-free. See David Williams and Ronald Doerfler, "Graphic Aids for Calculation of Fluid Resuscitation Requirements in Pediatric Burns," *Annals of Plastic Surgery*, **69**(3):260–264, 2012, DOI: 10.1097/SAP.0b013e3182586d4e

   — though of course if you're a burns patient, you'd far rather it was calculated correctly regardless of how it was done.

131. Page 129. The Mersey Burns app needs to know how long ago the burn happened, so the user can enter the time the burn happened (if they don't do this, a bug means that the previous patient's time of burn will be used instead). However, the clinician may enter an incorrect time, perhaps because the patient reported an incorrect burn time or or simply because of a use error.

   If the burn time is entered as up to 4 minutes ahead of the device's (say an iPhone) clock, the app simply takes the burn time as entered. However, if the time of burn is entered as 5 minutes ahead of the iPhone, without warning, the app will take the burn time to be 23 hours 55 minutes *in the past.*

The bug is that the app ignores time differences less than five minutes, which seems reasonable, as the user might take the time from their wrist watch or a wall clock, which could easily give a different time than the app's more accurate clock. Unfortunately, the app then makes a calculation error taking 5 minutes in the future to be in the past. Its time difference calculation has apparently ignored the hours in a day: if it is 8pm now, the app takes 8:04 to be 4 minutes *ahead* today, but it takes 8:05 as yesterday, so it takes it as 23 hours 55 minutes *earlier.*

There are lots of solutions ...

Solutions include that the user interface should validate the time entered correctly, and guard the internal assumption that time differences less than five minutes can be ignored.

Other cases in Mersey Burns of failing to validate user input occur in entering the patient weight (weights up to 4.5 tons are permitted on the iPhone); on the HTML version very large numbers can be entered, with so many digits, that they overflow the input field. Then, displaying fewer digits than are actually used, a very large number will look innocuous.

I pointed these and other bugs out to the app's authors in discussions in 2013, but these still remain. I am not particularly worried about these "extreme" bugs so much as the likelihood that such bugs getting through the development process implies other bugs will also have got through — and the other bugs may have greater practical significance. When a canary dies in a coal mine, you don't fix the canary, you fix the coal mine.

132. Page 130. Dimitris Bertsimas, Jack Dunn, George C. Velmahos, and Haytham M. A. Kaafarani, "Surgical Risk Is Not Linear: Derivation and Validation of a Novel, User-friendly, and Machine-learning-based Predictive OpTimal Trees in Emergency Surgery Risk (POTTER) Calculator," *Annals of Surgery*, **268**(4):574–583, 2018. DOI: 10.1097/SLA.0000000000002956

133. Page 133. The Ancient Egyptian pharaoh Rameses II was diagnosed with diffuse idiopathic skeletal hyperostosis using computed tomography in 2014. Rameses II is about 3,233 years old, so patients can legitimately have enormous ages! See Sahar N. Saleem and Zahi Hawass, "Brief Report: Ankylosing Spondylitis or Diffuse Idiopathic Skeletal Hyperostosis in Royal Egyptian Mummies of the 18th–20th Dynasties? Computed Tomography and Archæology Studies," *Arthritis & Rheumatology*, **66**(12):3311–3316, 2014. DOI: 10.1002/art.38864

134. Page 133. Tallal Hussain, Ian Braithwaite, and Stephen Hancock, "Errors and inaccuracies in internet medical calculator applications: an example using oxygenation index," *Archives of Disease in Childhood*, 2018. DOI: 10.1136/archdischild-2018-315323

   If you want to try out some oxygenation index calculations, you can google oxygenation calculations, or try this website: **www.medcalc.com/oxygen.html**

135. Page 134. Ben Shneiderman, *The new ABCs of research*, Oxford University Press, 2016.

136. Page 135. John Carreyrou, *Bad Blood — Secrets and Lies in a Silicon Valley Startup*, Picador, 2018.

137. Page 135. Hannah Wisniewski, Gang Liu, Philip Henson, Aditya Vaidyam, Narissa Karima Hajratalli, Jukka-Pekka Onnela, and John Torous, "Understanding the quality, effectiveness and attributes of top-rated smartphone health apps," *Evidence Based Mental Health*, **22**:4–9, 2019. DOI: 10.1136/ebmental-2018-300069

11 Cars are safer

138. Pages 140, 490. **Ralph Nader,** *Unsafe at Any Speed: The Designed-in Dangers of the American Automobile,* **Pocket Books, 1966.**

139. Page 141. George A. Akerlof, Nobel Prize speech, 2001. www.nobelprize.org/prizes/economic-sciences/2001/akerlof/article

140. Page 142. Jeanne Lenzer and ICIJ reporters, "Medical device industry: International investigation exposes lax regulation," *BMJ,* **363**:k4997, 2018. DOI: 10.1136/bmj.k4997

12 Safety Two

141. Page 146. Sidney Dekker, *Foundations of Safety Science: A Century of Understanding Accidents and Disasters,* CRC Press, 2019. This is an excellent textbook covering the history of safety.

142. Page 146. An excellent website with lots of resources on civility is www.civilitysaveslives.com

    There is plenty of research on civility in healthcare, including the following:

    Arieh Riskin, Amir Erez, Trevor A. Foulk, Amir Kugelman, Ayala Gover, Irit Shoris, Kinneret S. Riskin, and Peter A. Bamberger, "The Impact of Rudeness on Medical Team Performance: A Randomized Trial," *Pediatrics,* **136**(3):487–495, 2015. DOI: 10.1542/peds.2015-1385

    Joy Longo, "Combating Disruptive Behaviors: Strategies to Promote a Healthy Work Environment," *The Online Journal of Issues in Nursing,* **15**(1), 2010. ojin. nursingworld.org/MainMenuCategories/ANAMarketplace/ANAPeriodicals/OJIN/ TableofContents/Vol152010/No1Jan2010/Combating-Disruptive-Behaviors.html

143. Page 147. What I call Safety One and Safety Two are usually called Safety I and Safety II, that is using Roman numerals, but I think this can cause unnecessary problems, as I (meaning me) and I (meaning the Roman numeral one) are readily confusable. Moreover, Safety II can look like Safety 11 (thus confusing Roman two and Arabic eleven) when written in some fonts.

    The English words "One" and "Two" don't have these problem, and since we are all for improving safety, let's make a good example out of our terminology.

144. Pages 148, 462. Liam Donaldson, "When will health care pass the orange-wire test?" *The Lancet,* **364**(9445):1567–1568, 2004. DOI: 10.1016/S0140-6736(04)17330-3

145. Page 149. Retractable Technologies Inc., www.retractable.com/Products#Injectiondevices

146. Page 149. Steven Shorrock, "Learning Teams, Learning from Communities," *Humanistic Systems,* 13 January 2019. humanisticsystems.com/2019/01/13/learning-teams-learning-from-communities

13 Computational Thinking

147. Page 151. I stressed *digital* computer, as so far as I am aware, the first serious analog computer was the Antikythera mechanism, built around 100BC. Prior to Babbage there were of course various simple digital devices, such as Blaise Pascal's calculator, which Pascal made in 1645 when he was still a teenager, but these devices (like the Antikythera mechanism) were not programmable.

148. Page 151 twice. Luigi Federico Menabrea, "Sketch of the analytical engine invented by Charles Babbage, Esq," *Article XXIX, Scientific memoirs,* translated into English with

notes by Ada King, Countess of Lovelace, daughter of Byron, **3**:694, 1843. A facsimile of the original can be found at
repository.ou.edu/uuid/6235e086-c11a-56f6-b50d-1b1f5aaa3f5e

149. Page 152. The story about building the replica Difference Engine will have you on the edge of your seat: Doron Swade, *The Difference Engine: Charles Babbage and the Quest to Build the First Computer*, Penguin, 2002.

150. Page 152. There's a fascinating video of a wooden Turing Machine working: www.youtube.com/watch?v=vo8izCKHiF0 made by Richard J. Ridel in 2015. One of the comments on the video is somebody who wants to hook up their hamster wheel so their hamster could run it, thus getting close to proving that hamsters are Turing Complete too.

151. Page 155. A great place to start is with Alan Turing's own writings, and so I very strongly recommend Charles Petzold, *The Annotated Turing*, Wiley Publishing Inc, 2008, which is a very readable tour through Turing's ground-breaking work, along with lots of fascinating and helpful explanations. Alternatively, why not relax and read a gripping, well-told story about the real drama of building computers, like Tracy Kidder's Pulitzer Prize winning *The Soul of a New Machine*, Back Bay Books, 2000. But if you want to follow up on the deep ideas stemming from Turing, the general topic is called **computability**, and there is lots on it to read, though a lot of it is very mathematical and quite hard work. The best advice is recursive: use a computer — a search engine like Google — to help you find the sort of book or websites you want.

152. Page 155. And who bothers to prove that their ideas are computable? It turns out to be very hard, unless your problem is very simple. Instead, we just hope that we're asking computers to do things that are possible, rather than nearly possible. Where they aren't quite possible, they'll *have* to go wrong in some way.

153. Page 156. The early history of computing is quite controversial, as so many things happened so fast. The legacy of World War II computers was kept secret until the 1970s, so most of the histories of computing are unaware of much earlier work, such as the Colossus, which was already running in 1943 during the war.
    Turing had a leading role in the wartime computing, and he went on to develop the Automatic Computing Engine, the ACE, in 1945. The British Manchester Baby was the first "fully modern computer" — however you define that — and was running in 1948. See en.wikipedia.org/wiki/Colossus_computer for more on this fascinating story.

154. Page 157. www.historicsimulations.com/edsac.html

155. Page 157. There's a good description of the story of Apollo 13 in the Wikipedia description of the film at en.wikipedia.org/wiki/Apollo_13_(film)

156. Page 158. David Harel and Yishai Feldman, *Algorithmics: The Spirit of Computing*, third edition, Addison-Wesley, 2004.

157. Page 158. Jeannette Wing has written a lot on Computational Thinking; this article is probably her most accessible: Jeannette Marie Wing, "Computational Thinking," *Communications of the ACM*, **49**(3):33–35, 2006. DOI: 10.1145/1118178.1118215
    Also, do read this: Enrico Nardelli, "Do We Really Need Computational Thinking?" *Communications of the ACM*, **62**(2):32–35, 2019. DOI: 10.1145/3231587 It's an article written over a decade later that provides (arguably!) more mature ideas.
    This book's further reading chapter[e] suggests more things to read on Computational Thinking.[f]

158. Page 158. "Without error" needs caveats. Maybe our program is calculating numbers and we'd be happy with answers that are close enough. The answers may not be

---

[e] See Chapter 33: Good reading, page 471 ←

[f] See Chapter 33: Magic and Computational Thinking reading, page 484 ←

exactly correct, but they are good enough for the purpose. So "error" doesn't just mean being wrong; it means being *too* wrong, for some numerical, statistical, or other meaning of that.

159. Page 161. A good — and brief — introduction to reproducibility is Shannon Palus, "Make Research Reproducible," *Scientific American*, **319**(4):48–51, 2018.

My own early foray into reproducibility was: Harold Thimbleby, "Give your computer's IQ a boost," *Journal of Machine Learning Research, Times Higher Education Supplement*, 9 May 2004.
www.timeshighereducation.co.uk/story.asp?sectioncode=26&storycode=176549

160. Page 161. Here's one way to increase reproducibility in Computer Science: Harold Thimbleby and David Williams, "A tool for publishing reproducible algorithms & A reproducible, elegant algorithm for sequential experiments," *Science of Computer Programming*, **156**:45–67, 2018. DOI: 10.1016/j.scico.2017.12.010

A recent article about the reproducibility crisis in digital healthcare is Enrico Coiera, Elske Ammenwerth, Andrew Georgiou, and Farah Magrabi, "Does health informatics have a replication crisis?" *Journal of the American Medical Informatics Association*, **25**(8):963–968, 2018. DOI: 10.1093/jamia/ocy028

161. Page 162. Sendhil Mullainathan, *Scarcity: The True Cost of Not Having Enough*, Penguin, 2014.

162. Page 163. Claude E. Shannon, "Programming a Computer for Playing Chess," *Philosophical Magazine*, series 7, **41**(314), 1950. This paper created the field of computer chess, which in turn was one of the main drivers that developed AI — chess is too hard for a computer to play well without using AI.

163. Page 163. If you have come across the term **API**, you've already heard something about **modules**. A module interacts with the rest of the world *only* through its API. This eliminates the combinatorial explosion.

Parnas's original paper is still a wonderful read, and should be on all programmers' reading lists: David Lorge Parnas, "On the Criteria to Be Used in Decomposing Systems into Modules," *Communications of the ACM*, **15**(12):1053–1058, 1972. DOI: 10.1145/361598.361623

164. Page 163. Mersey Burns does include some internal double-checking to confirm that its key calculations are correct. This is very good so far as it goes. However, Mersey Burns has no checking to confirm whether what the user does is correctly interpreted by the program. Are the numbers used in the calculation correct? Are the results displayed correctly? And so on.

165. Pages 164, 377. C. A. R. Hoare, "The Emperor's Old Clothes," *Communications of the ACM*, **24**(2):75–83, 1981. DOI: 10.1145/358549.358561

166. Page 166. Melissa Cunningham, "He died alone after his medical test results were faxed to wrong number," *The Age*, 10 May 2018.
www.theage.com.au/national/victoria/he-died-alone-after-his-medical-test-results-were-faxed-to-wrong-number-20180510-p4zeia.html

167. Page 166. Carl Macrae, "When no news is bad news: communication failures and the hidden assumptions that threaten safety," *Journal of the Royal Society of Medicine*, **111**(1):5–7, 2018. DOI: 10.1177/0141076817738503

168. Page 168. Colin Runciman and Harold Thimbleby, "Equal Opportunity Interactive Systems," *International Journal of Man-Machine Studies*, **25**(4):439–451, 1986. DOI: 10.1016/S0020-7373(86)80070-0

169. Page 168. Here's an old book, but it's all the more readable for that: R. D. Tennent, *Principles of Programming Languages*, Prentice Hall International Series in Computing Science, 1981.

170. Page 169. We should log everything to understand errors, and other problems to analyze how things are used — and to learn how to improve things. This seems so obvious! Indeed, logging was clearly described way back in 1975 by Brian R. Gaines and Peter V. Facey, "Some Experience in Interactive Systems Development and

Application," *Proceedings IEEE*, **63**(6):894–911, 1975. DOI: 10.1109/PROC.1975.9854

171. Page 171. See the insightful foreword Don Knuth wrote for Marko Petkovsek, Herbert S. Wilf, and Doron Zeilberger, *A=B*, A K Peters, 1996.

172. Page 172. Brett Kelman, "Vanderbilt ex-nurse indicted on reckless homicide charge after deadly medication swap," *Nashville Tennessean*, 6 February 2019. eu.tennessean.com/story/news/health/2019/02/04/vanderbilt-nurse-reckless-homicide-charge-vecuronium-versed-drug-error/2772648002

173. Page 173. Adolphe Quetelet (1796–1874) was a fascinating chap. He found that as people grow, for most of their lives their weight is closely proportional to their height squared. Hence his index, which divides one by the other, is therefore is a good indicator of excess weight for age. It was about a century later that people started to notice that his index was related to life expectancy, and hence led to calls to reduce obesity, which could be measured by his index. See Garabed Eknoyan, "Adolphe Quetelet (1796–1874) — the average man and indices of obesity," *Nephrology Dialysis Transplantation*, **23**(1):47–51, 2008. DOI: 10.1093/ndt/gfm517

174. Page 173. Liam Thorp, "I was invited for a covid vaccine because the NHS thought I was 6cm tall — Hilarious mix-up may have highlighted a potential issue with the vaccine roll-out," *Liverpool Echo*, 17 February 2021. www.liverpoolecho.co.uk/news/liverpool-news/invited-covid-vaccine-because-nhs-19857990

175. Page 174. Institute for Safe Medication Practices, "Another Round of the Blame Game: A Paralyzing Criminal Indictment that Recklessly 'Overrides' Just Culture," 14 February 2019. www.ismp.org/resources/another-round-blame-game-paralyzing-criminal-indictment-recklessly-overrides-just-culture

    Here's one insightful quote from that article: "[The criminal charges] may also prompt organizations to inappropriately forbid any ADC overrides, inevitably leading to unauthorized stashes of medications. The detrimental effects of criminal prosecution on reporting, learning, culture, and safety strategies far outweigh its negligible impact on improving individual performance."

14 Risky calculations

176. Page 177. Carol M. Ostrom, "Nurse's suicide follows tragedy," *The Seattle Times*, 20 April 2011. www.seattletimes.com/seattle-news/nurses-suicide-follows-tragedy

177. Page 177. According to David Bundy, Elizabeth Mack, Sheila Scarbrough, and Danielle Scheurer, "Building a Culture of Safety," www.scha.org/files/cultureofsafety\bunderline panel.pot\bunderline .pdf

178. Page 178. G. M. Souza, M. F. A. Jesus, M. V. S. Ferreira, V. P. Cataneli, and L. K. W. Eller, "Dissemination of Methicillin-Resistant Staphylococcus aureus (MRSA) by University Student's Cell Phones," *ASM Microbe 2019 Conference*, 2019. www.abstractsonline.com/pp8/##!/7859/presentation/15327 See media report: Molly Walker, "Resistant Bacteria Abundant on Nursing Students' Cell Phones Small study raises possibility of nosocomial infections, transfer to patients," *MedPage Today*, 22 June 2019. www.medpagetoday.com/meetingcoverage/asmmicrobe/80657

179. Page 178. Clare Gerada, "Preventing suicide in medical staff," *BMJ*, **366**:l5231, 2019. DOI: 10.1136/bmj.l5231

180. Page 179. If the iPhone is used in landscape, the displayed number can be much longer, so the population of the world will be handled correctly. The iPhone's answer to the problem will end up being right.

    If the calculator is immediately turned from landscape into portrait after entering the world's population, it'll be displayed correctly as 7.1e9 (that is 7.1×10^9) in portrait. But it won't do this if the number is entered directly in portrait mode.

    Why can't it automatically handle big numbers this way without having to turn it in and out of landscape? Surely, even in portrait, the iPhone could have gone from displaying 710,000,000 to displaying 7.1e9 when the next digit was pressed — it's clearly able to display numbers this way if it wants to. Doing so would have fixed the bug.

Finally, I think it's worth pointing out that the iPhone has a very high-resolution display, and it has no reason to display large numbers obscurely, like 7.1e9, when it's perfectly able to display numbers conventionally like 7.1×10^9 directly.

181. Page 180. On the iPhone, deletion is done by swiping your finger left or right across the number displayed. Other calculators, when they provide a delete function, usually have a special button for it.

182. Page 181. Harold Thimbleby and Andy Gimblett, "Applying Theorem Discovery to Automatically Find and Check Usability Heuristics," *Proceedings ACM Conference on Engineering Interactive Computer Systems*, 101–106, ACM, 2013. DOI: 10.1145/2494603.2480320

183. Page 181. Almost all countries give you the same problems as with the UK, but if you try doing the sums with the population of India (about 1.339 billion) or the population of China (about 1.386 billion), curiously you will get the right answers.

The problem is that the calculators secretly don't handle numbers in the billions or larger correctly — they silently lose the extra digits after their screens have filled up with however many digits they can cope with. They make a mistake with the world population (about 7.6 billion people) and *the same* mistake with the populations of India or China, so the errors coincidentally cancel out, and you'll get the right answer to the question. Here, two wrongs really do make a right!

184. Page 181. The 2000 paper explaining conventional calculator problems was cited earlier, in note 47.

A vastly superior approach to calculator design that reduces errors is introduced in a 2005 paper: Will Thimbleby and Harold Thimbleby, "A Novel Gesture-Based Calculator and Its Design Principles," *Proceedings 19th British Computer Society HCI Conference*, **2**:27–32, British Computer Society, 2005. I must add that Will did all the creative hard work here. I strongly recommend you go to Will Thimbleby's website for more details: see will.thimbleby.net

185. Page 185. Toby Helm, "Austerity cuts are blamed for 130,000 preventable deaths," *The Observer*, 16, 2 June 2019. (Note the title of 130,000 deaths refers to 2012 to date.)

An alarming report is Philip Alston, "Statement on Visit to the United Kingdom," United Nations, London, 16 November 2018. www.ohchr.org/Documents/Issues/Poverty/EOM_GB_16Nov2018.pdf. The medical profession's view of this is summarized in the BMJ: Sophie Arie, "UK's 'austerity experiment' has forced millions into poverty and homelessness, say UN rapporteur," *BMJ*, **365**:l2321, 2019. DOI: 10.1136/bmj.l2321

186. Page 185. Growth in a time of debt, en.wikipedia.org/wiki/Growth_in_a_Time_of_Debt

187. Page 185. Thomas Herndon, Michael Ash, and Robert Pollin, "Does high public debt consistently stifle economic growth? A critique of Reinhart and Rogoff," *Cambridge Journal of Economics*, **38**(2):257–279, 2014. DOI: 10.1093/cje/bet075

188. Page 185. John Cassidy, "The Reinhart and Rogoff Controversy: A Summing Up," *The New Yorker*, 26 April 2013. www.newyorker.com/news/john-cassidy/the-reinhart-and-rogoff-controversy-a-summing-up, or if you prefer a Nobel Prize winner, try Paul Krugman, "The Excel Depression," *The New York Times*, 18 April 2013. www.nytimes.com/2013/04/19/opinion/krugman-the-excel-depression.html?_r=0

189. Page 185. Programmers will be able to think of many sensible approaches to help Excel be more reliable, though all such approaches have trade-offs, because the safety checks they introduce have possible bugs themselves due to the obvious problems of implementing the techniques correctly (especially as Excel provides no help in

following the new spreadsheet use conventions that most such techniques would rely on).

Instead of blindly hoping that SUM gives the right answer, a safer approach is to double-check every cell being added up. One way to do this is to use =ISNUMBER(A1:A100), which seems to work (by which I mean that for every SUM that goes wrong that I've tried, ISNUMBER is FALSE, but I don't *know* whether this can be relied on in every case). Unfortunately, lots of Excel users are not professional programmers, so they probably won't think defensively like this.

The problem is, once you start putting ISNUMBERs in a spreadsheet, your spreadsheet starts getting more complicated: protecting yourself from errors *itself* becomes a likely source of even more complicated errors. Worse, each additional ISNUMBER makes sense and doesn't seem to make things too complicated — so each one has a good reason to be added, and you add another, and another and another — but a while later, the spreadsheet will be an unmanageable mess. Excel has no way to help you now.

190. Page 187. Patrick Oladimeji, Harold Thimbleby, and Anna L. Cox, "A Performance Review of Number Entry Interfaces," *Proceedings IFIP Conference on Human-Computer Interaction — Interact 2013, Designing for Diversity*, Lecture Notes in Computer Science, **8117**:365–382, Springer-Verlag, 2013. DOI: 10.1007/978-3-642-40483-2_26

191. Page 188. Harold Thimbleby, Jeremy Gow, and Paul Cairns, "Misleading Behaviour in Interactive Systems," in *Proceedings British Computer Society HCI Conference*, **2**:33–36, Research Press International, 2004.

15   Who's accountable?

192. Page 193. The Mersey Burns (version 1.6.2) warranty quoted was found at merseyburns.com/manual/v1.6.2/disclaimer.html, 2019.

193. Page 193. "You must check the disclaimer page of the App prior to each use of the App" — in fact, you can't do this, as you can only see the disclaimer page when the app is downloaded and used for the first time. Either the disclaimer is incorrect or the code has a bug.

194. Page 194. Medical Calculators Algorithms, version 2.9, 2019. Available from Apple app store.

195. Page 194. 2019 iOS Software License Agreement, www.apple.com/legal/sla/docs/iOS12.pdf

196. Page 195. David J. DeWitt and his fight to publish research about commercial computer systems is described in en.wikipedia.org/wiki/David_DeWitt

A new update on the issues for researchers was written in the *Scientific American*, "Universities Should Encourage Scientists to Speak Out about Public Issues," 1 February 2018. www.scientificamerican.com/article/universities-should-encourage-scientists-to-speak-out-about-public-issues

197. Page 196. My book *Press On: Principles of Interaction Programming* (MIT Press)[g] has some ideas for programmers to generate user manuals automatically, which ensures they are correct, and — because it is automatic and easy — encourages the designers to modify the designs to make the manuals easier to understand. A complex user manual is a symptom of a poor design.

198. Page 197. Kieran Beattie, "NHS Grampian patients locked into controversial bedside TV service until 2027, while contract with NHS Highland runs out next week," *Press and Journal*, 9 January 2020. www.pressandjournal.co.uk/fp/news/aberdeenshire/1941149/nhs-grampian-patients-locked-into-controversial-bedside-tv-service-

---

[g] See Chapter 33: *Press On: Principles of Interaction Programming*, the book, page 483 ←

until-2027-while-contract-with-nhs-highland-runs-out-next-week

199. Page 197. Anna W. Mathews, "Behind Your Rising Health-Care Bills: Secret Hospital
      Deals That Squelch Competition," *Wall Street Journal*, 18 September 2018.
      www.wsj.com/articles/behind-your-rising-health-care-bills-secret-hospital-
      deals-that-squelch-competition-1537281963

200. Page 198. The Architects Registration Board's website is www.arb.org.uk

16   Regulation needs fixing

201. Page 201. At the time of writing, Brexit may or may not happen to the UK. Whatever
      happens, something equivalent to CE marking will have to be implemented, otherwise
      there will be no trade on medical devices with the EU.

202. Page 201. Christopher Hodges, "The regulation of medical products and medical
      devices," Chapter 17 in Judith M. Laing and Jean V. McHale, editors, *Principles of
      Medical Law*, 4th edition, Oxford University Press, 2017, especially section 17.122
      onward.

203. Page 202. The terms Class I, Class II, etc, mean different things around the world
      which adds to the complexity. Goodness knows what will happen during or after
      Brexit, which is certainly a growing problem for UK manufacturers.

204. Page 202. Simon Bowers and Deborah Cohen, "How lobbying blocked European
      safety checks for dangerous medical implants," *BMJ*, **363**:k4999, 2018. DOI:
      10.1136/bmj.k4999

205. Page 203. Checking program equivalence is non-computable. For example, two
      programs might *seem* to be the same, but one has bugs that you haven't yet noticed, so
      in fact they are not the same. Unfortunately bugs can hide themselves indefinitely, so
      you will never know whether two programs are equivalent. (I used "bugs" as an
      example difference; of course, bugs may not be the only difference.)

206. Page 204. Over a million emails were sent to NHS staff, and email was delayed for
      hours. News reports say Accenture, the developers, still hadn't provided safeguards to
      stop this basic sort of error, despite it being an NHS requirement. Gareth Corfield,
      "NHS reply-all meltdown swamped system with half a billion emails: Accenture
      blamed for system swamp," *The Register*, 31 January 2017. https://www.theregister.
      com/2017/01/31/nhs_reply_all_email_fail_half_billion_messages

          More details can be found in James Temperton, "NHS email blunder catches 1.2
      million staff in 'reply all' chaos," *Wired*, 14 November 2016.
      www.wired.co.uk/article/nhs-email-reply-all-down

          Wikipedia has various entries on email problems, like these **email storms** —
      en.wikipedia.org/wiki/Email_storm

207. Page 204. Denis Campbell, "NHS gender identity clinic discloses email contacts of
      2,000 patients," *The Guardian*, 6 September 2019. www.theguardian.com/society/
      2019/sep/06/nhs-gender-identity-clinic-discloses-email-contacts-data-breach

208. Page 205. Cardinal Health, "Alaris GP Volumetric Pump," Instructions for Use,
      1000DF00009 Issue 3, 2005–2006.

209. Page 206. National Institute for Health and Care Excellence, *SINGLE TECHNOLOGY
      APPRAISAL Lumacaftor and ivacaftor combination therapy for treating cystic fibrosis
      homozygous for the F508del mutation [ID786]*, February 2016.
      www.nice.org.uk/guidance/ta398/documents/committee-papers

210. Page 206. National databases to register clinical studies (or any other kind of research)
      help reduce **cherry picking**. If you do an experiment, after you've got all the data,
      you might hunt for more interesting results to get something worth publishing — with
      enough data there is *always* something or other interesting to find, but it may just be a
      coincidence.

          By registering, you state your objectives, and then report on what you found out about them. Of course you can report serendipitous discoveries, but you can't manipulate your results.

The database used for registering the cystic fibrosis experiment is clinicalTrials.gov — where the trial can be found under number NCT01931839. DOI: 10.1016/S2213-2600(16)30427-1

211. Page 206. IOM (Institute of Medicine), *Medical devices and the public's health: The FDA's 510(k) clearance process at 35 years*, US National Academies of Science, The National Academies Press, 2011. www.nap.edu/read/13150

212. Page 207. REGULATION (EU) 2017/745 OF THE EUROPEAN PARLIAMENT AND OF THE COUNCIL of 5 April 2017 on medical devices, amending Directive 2001/83/EC, Regulation (EC) No 178/2002 and Regulation (EC) No 1223/2009 and repealing Council Directives 90/385/EEC and 93/42/EEC, eur-lex.europa.eu/legal-content/EN/ALL/?uri=CELEX:32017R0745

213. Pages 207, 327. Here's the story of Aaron Davidson's jail sentence, which is reported in several places: "Jail for illegal gas fitter who put his customers' lives at risk," *The Gas Engineer*, 4 August 2020. registeredgasengineer.co.uk/jail-for-illegal-gas-fitter-who-put-his-customers-lives-at-risk and "Plumber jailed for illegal gas work," Health and Safety Executive, 9 July 2020. press.hse.gov.uk/2020/07/09/plumber-jailed-for-illegal-gas-work

214. Pages 207, 491. Kirby Dick and Amy Ziering, *The Bleeding Edge*, Netflix, 27 July 2018.

215. Page 207. www.hse.gov.uk/work-equipment-machinery/uk-law-design-supply-products.htm

17   Safe and secure

216. Page 212. Jessica Davis, "Australian hospitals fighting system failure after botched WannaCry patch," *Healthcare IT News*, 26 May 2017. www.healthcareitnews.com/news/australian-hospitals-fighting-system-failure-after-botched-wannacry-patch

217. Page 213. Patricia Mazzei, "Hit by Ransomware Attack, Florida City Agrees to Pay Hackers $600,000," *New York Times*, 19 June 2019.

218. Page 213. Your national cybersecurity center is the best place to start learning about cyberattacks and defenses, and their websites will stay up-to-date. The Wikipedia article on multi-factor authentication is another good place to go to: en.wikipedia.org/wiki/Multi-factor_authentication

219. Page 213. National Cybersecurity and Communications Integration Center report ICSMA-18-037-02, 2018: see ics-cert.us-cert.gov/advisories/ICSMA-18-037-02

220. Page 214 twice. Chris Baraniuk, "Anaesthetic devices 'vulnerable to hackers'," BBC News, 10 July 2019. www.bbc.co.uk/news/technology-48935111

221. Page 214. Zoe Kleinman, "Therapy patients blackmailed for cash after clinic data breach," BBC News, 26 October 2020. www.bbc.co.uk/news/technology-54692120
    And see the English reports from the Finnish agency UUTISET which has several articles on the topic, including this one: "Psychotherapy centre's database hacked, patient info held ransom," 21 October 2020. yle.fi/uutiset/osasto/news/psychotherapy_centres_database_hacked_patient_info_held_ransom/11605460

222. Page 215. "Irish health service hit by cyber attack," BBC News, 14 May 2021. www.bbc.co.uk/news/world-europe-57111615

223. Page 216. Office of the Information and Privacy Commissioner, Ontario, "Statement from the Office of the Information and Privacy Commissioner of Ontario and the Office of the Information and Privacy Commissioner for British Columbia on LifeLabs Privacy Breach," 17 December 2019. It has a very long URL, so you may be better off searching for it instead! www.newswire.ca/news-releases/statement-from-the-

office-of-the-information-and-privacy-commissioner-of-ontario-and-the-office-of-the-information-and-privacy-commissioner-for-british-columbia-on-lifelabs-privacy-breach-821489025.html

In addition, there are many popular news reports, such as this: Charlie Smith, "LifeLabs CEO Charles Brown says he doesn't know if hacked test-result data was encrypted," *The Georgia Straight*, 18 December 2019. www.straight.com/life/1338251/lifelabs-ceo-charles-brown-says-he-doesnt-know-if-hacked-test-result-data-was-encrypted

224. Page 217. Backing up data is an essential precaution against digital problems, including cyberattacks. However, remember that you may have backed up something *already* attacked, and your backup systems may also be attacked directly. It's not sufficient just to back up; can you tell when your data is corrupted or deleted?

Cybersecurity is a huge problem! You must get up-to-date external expert advice — nobody on their own can keep up with the developments. Start with your national cybersecurity center's advice; the UK Centre, for instance, provides lots of helpful and up-to-date guidance.

For more information, see www.ncsc.gov.uk/guidance

225. Page 220. To explain short selling (of which there are many types), let's use car hire as a simple, concrete analogy.

I hire a new car for a week, paying the rental company, let's say, $100 to cover comprehensive insurance and the week's rent. However, I sell the car to a friend of mine for $10,000.

At this stage, I've made a profit of $9,900 — though I still have the contract that I must return the car by the end of the week.

Let's say that my friend has a crash and wrecks the hired car. The car is now only worth $100 as scrap, so I buy it back. I've still made a profit of $9,800.

I now return the damaged car back to the rental company.

Thanks to the insurance I bought, I've nothing further to pay.

Effectively, I've got an insurance scam that makes $9,800 easy money out of an accident covered by the garage's car insurance (which I paid the premium for). My profit of $9,800 is based on me betting the value of the car will go down — it needed my friend to have a crash after buying the car off me — so that I can buy it back for a pittance at the end of the week.

You could do the same, borrowing St Jude shares instead of a car, betting that they would decrease in value. As with the car, just sell the shares on — but unlike selling a hire car, this is perfectly legal to do. Instead of needing a car accident, we disclose the St Jude cybersecurity vulnerabilities, and the shares crash in value. We then buy them back very cheaply at their crashed market value, then return them to the trader we originally borrowed them from. The shares are back where they started. We've made a nice profit.

226. Page 221. www.accessdata.fda.gov/scripts/cdrh/cfdocs/cfmaude/search.cfm

227. Pages 221, 463. For an example of a quite typical free, open, publicly available aviation report after a serious incident, see: ATSB (Australian Transport Safety Bureau) Transport Safety Report, Aviation Occurrence Investigation AO-2010-089, Final - 27 June 2013: "In-flight uncontained engine failure Airbus A380-842, VH-OQA, overhead Batam Island, Indonesia, 4 November 2010," www.atsb.gov.au/media/4173625/ao-2010-089_final.pdf

18 Who profits?

228. Page 225. Seth Shulman, "Patent absurdities," *The Sciences*, **39**(1):30–33, January–February 1999. DOI: 10.1002/j.2326-1951.1999.tb03410.x

229. Page 225. Madhumita Murgia and Max Harlow, "How top health websites are sharing sensitive data with advertisers," *Financial Times*, 13 November 2019. www.ft.com/content/0fbf4d8e-022b-11ea-be59-e49b2a136b8d

230. Page 226. Tom Knowles, "Facebook uses iPhones to track users' movements," *The Times*, 18 September 2019.

231. Pages 226, 328. Sidney Fussell, "The Sneaky Genius of Facebook's New Preventive Health Tool – The feature looks likely to fill gaps in care — and to further draw users into Facebook's ecosystem," *The Atlantic*, 8 January 2020. www.theatlantic.com/technology/archive/2020/01/facebook-launches-new-preventative-health-tool/604567

232. Page 226. A very nice article reviewing GP changes in prescribing practices using prescription data from 8,078 GP practices, covering a population of 55 million is Alex J. Walker, Felix Pretis, Anna Powell-Smith, and Ben Goldacre, "Variation in responsiveness to warranted behavior change among NHS clinicians: novel implementation of change detection methods in longitudinal prescribing data," *BMJ*, **367**:l5205, 2019. DOI: 10.1136/bmj.l5205

   The paper has lots of ideas on open science and using computers for analyzing health data. Also, do have a look at the great Twitter thread by one of the authors, Ben Goldacre, @bengoldacre, at
   threadreaderapp.com/thread/1181231445265850369.html

233. Page 226. Toby Helm, "Revealed: how drugs giants can access your health records — Experts say information sold on by Department of Health and Social Care can be traced back to individual medical records," *The Observer*, 8 February 2020. www.theguardian.com/technology/2020/feb/08/fears-over-sale-anonymous-nhs-patient-data

   An authoritative blog on health privacy, and many related issues, is run by Prof Ross Anderson's Security Group at the University of Cambridge. Start here: www.lightbluetouchpaper.org — he's also got a good book on security, I recommend in Good reading.[h]

234. Page 227. Sam Shead, "Google DeepMind is funding NHS research at Moorfields Eye Hospital," *Business Insider*, 3 August 2017. uk.businessinsider.com/deepmind-is-funding-nhs-research-2017-7

235. Page 228. Gary Finnegan, "Google's DeepMind Health told to explain how it will make money," *Science | Business*, 19 June 2018. sciencebusiness.net/healthy-measures/news/googles-deepmind-health-told-explain-how-it-will-make-money

236. Page 228. Although the report seems to have disappeared, a brief summary is available here: understandingpatientdata.org.uk/news/deepmind-health-independent-review-panel-second-annual-report

237. Page 228. Andrew Orlowski, "Google swallows up DeepMind Health and abolishes 'independent board'," *The Register*, 14 November 2018. www.theregister.co.uk/2018/11/14/google_swallows_up_deepmind_health_and_abolishes_independent_board

238. Page 230. Santiago Romero-Brufau, Kim Gaines, Clara T. Nicolas, Matthew G. Johnson, Joel Hickman, and Jeanne M. Huddleston, "The fifth vital sign? Nurse worry predicts inpatient deterioration within 24 hours," *JAMIA Open*, **2**(4):465–470, 2019. DOI: 10.1093/jamiaopen/ooz033

239. Page 230. "Covid Symptom Study regrets Samantha Cameron mask ad," BBC News, 20 October 2020. www.bbc.co.uk/news/technology-54621308 Interestingly, the BBC

---

[h] See Chapter 33: Good reading, page 471 ←

News report also advertises the same range of COVID masks as the app did. ZOE's website for the COVID Symptom Study is covid.joinzoe.com

240. Page 231. Steven A. Julious and Mark A. Mullee, "Confounding and Simpson's paradox," *BMJ*, **309**:1480, 1994. DOI: 10.1136/bmj.309.6967.1480

241. Page 231. Tom Chivers, "We should be very wary of the R value: A rise in the Covid-19 infection rate actually means that lockdown is working," *UnHerd blog*, 12 May 2020. unherd.com/2020/05/what-the-headline-covid-figures-dont-tell-you

242. Page 231. Skin color is an obvious potential bias. A more subtle one is **length time bias**. If the AI is trained on patients, then patients who have diseases (such as skin cancers) that last a long time are going to be over-represented in the data.

    As a rule, slow cancers are less likely to be fatal, so it'll appear that the diagnostic system is reducing the severity of cancer. That is, on average the patients whose cancers are detected by the AI do better than the patients whose cancers are missed, because it is preferentially detecting cancers that are typically less malignant.

243. Pages 232, 233. A popular article on racial bias is Shraddha Chakradhar, "Widely used algorithm for follow-up care in hospitals is racially biased, study finds," *STAT*, 24 October 2019.
    www.statnews.com/2019/10/24/widely-used-algorithm-hospitals-racial-bias. The article interviewed the authors of this more academic article: Ziad Obermeyer, Brian Powers, Christine Vogeli, and Sendhil Mullainathan, "Dissecting racial bias in an algorithm used to manage the health of populations," *Science*, **366**(6464):447–453, 2019. DOI: 10.1126/science.aax2342

244. Page 233. Blood hemoglobin concentration is estimated and measured in grams per liter. Worryingly, many publications measure concentration using g/l, which can easily be misread as g divided by one (since l looks like 1) — which encourages unnecessary human error. For details, see L. F. Miles, T. Larsen, M. J. Bailey, K. L. Burbury, D. A. Story, and R. Bellomo, "Borderline anaemia and postoperative outcome in women undergoing major abdominal surgery: a retrospective cohort study," *Anaesthesia*, **75**(2):210–217, 2019. DOI: 10.1111/anae.14870

245. Page 233. **This amazing book won the 2019 Royal Society Science Book Prize: Caroline Criado Perez, *Invisible Women: Exposing Data Bias in a World Designed for Men*, Chatto & Windus, 2019.**

246. Page 233. An interesting insight is the two way synergy between digital and ethics: as ethics helps digital (AI or whatever), digital also helps ethics because digital brings with it a precision that a lot of ethics lacks.

    Two of my PhD students have done good research on digital trust and ethics:
    Stephen Marsh, *Formalising Trust as a Computational Concept*, PhD Thesis, Stirling University, Scotland, 1994.
    Penny Duquenoy, *The internet: A framework for understanding ethical issues*, PhD Thesis, Middlesex University, London, 2001.
    A more recent, and more accessible, book on ethics is Michael Kearns and Aaron Roth, *The Ethical Algorithm: The Science of Socially Aware Algorithm Design*, Oxford University Press, 2020.

247. Page 234. Biplav Srivastava and Francesca Rossi, "Towards Composable Bias Rating of AI Services," *Proceedings AAAI/ACM Conference on AI, Ethics, and Society*, 284–289, ACM, 2018. DOI: 10.1145/3278721.3278744

    A thought-provoking book on sexism is Criado Perez, *Invisible Women: Exposing Data Bias in a World Designed for Men*, Chatto & Windus, 2019. A good popular article is Katyanna Quach, "Q. If machine learning is so smart, how come AI models are such racist, sexist homophobes? A. Humans really suck. Our prejudices rub off on our computer pals, sadly," *The Register*, 5 September 2019.
    www.theregister.co.uk/2019/09/05/ai_racist_sexist Like many things in digital healthcare, the field is moving very rapidly, and the best thing to do is to run an internet search to find out what's up-to-date.

248. Page 234. Shneiderman gives an excellent overview of the algorithmic bias problem: Ben Shneiderman, "Opinion: The dangers of faulty, biased, or malicious algorithms requires independent oversight," *Proceedings National Academy of Sciences*, **113**(48):13538–13540, 2016. DOI: 10.1073/pnas.1618211113

249. Page 235. Andre Esteva, Brett Kuprel, Roberto A. Novoa, Justin Ko, Susan M. Swetter, Helen M. Blau, and Sebastian Thrun, "Dermatologist-level classification of skin cancer with deep neural networks," *Nature*, **542**:115–118, 2 February 2017. DOI: 10.1038/nature21056

250. Page 235. Lisette Hilton, "The Artificial Brain as Doctor," *Dermatology Times*, 15 January 2018. www.medpagetoday.com/dermatology/generaldermatology/70513

251. Page 235. Will Douglas Heaven, "Hundreds of AI tools have been built to catch covid. None of them helped." *MIT Technology Review*, 30 July 2021. technologyreview.com/2021/07/30/1030329/machine-learning-ai-failed-covid-hospital-diagnosis-pandemic
    A very readable article on AI biases is Ramya Srinivasan and Ajay Chander, "Biases in AI Systems: A survey for practitioners," *ACM Queue*, **19**(2):45–64, March-April 2021. DOI: 10.1145/3466132.3466134

252. Page 236. Dave Lee, "Why Big Tech pays poor Kenyans to teach self-driving cars," BBC News, 3 November 2018. www.bbc.co.uk/news/technology-46055595
    A good analysis of how algorithmic bias affects all of us who use the internet is Safiya Umoja Noble, *Algorithms of Oppression: How Search Engines Reinforce Racism*, NYU Press, 2018.

253. Page 237. Rana Awdish, twitter.com/RanaAwdish/status/1072333983898316800, 11 December 2018.

254. Page 237. Kenneth H. Lai, Maxim Topaz, Foster R. Goss, and Li Zhou, "Automated misspelling detection and correction in clinical free-text records," *Journal of Biomedical Informatics*, **55**:188–195, 2015. DOI: 10.1016/j.jbi.2015.04.008

255. Page 237. Ivan Evtimov, Kevin Eykholt, Earlence Fernandes, Tadayoshi Kohno, Bo Li, Atul Prakash, Amir Rahmati, and Dawn Song, "Robust Physical-World Attacks on Machine Learning Models," *Computing Research Repository* (CoRR), **abs/1707.08945**, 2017. arxiv.org/abs/1707.08945

256. Page 238. Tom Knowles, "Tape trick fools Tesla into speeding 50mph over limit," *The Times*, 20 February 2020.

257. Page 238. Andrew Ilyas, Shibani Santurkar, Dimitris Tsipras, Logan Engstrom, Brandon Tran, and Aleksander Madry, "Adversarial Examples Are Not Bugs, They Are Features," arxiv.org/abs/1905.02175, 2019.

258. Page 239. Marshall Allen, "You Snooze, You Lose: Insurers Make The Old Adage Literally True," *ProPublica*, 21 November 2018. www.propublica.org/article/you-snooze-you-lose-insurers-make-the-old-adage-literally-true

259. Page 239. Privacy International, "Alexa, what is hidden behind your contract with the NHS?," 6 December 2019. privacyinternational.org/long-read/3298/alexa-what-hidden-behind-your-contract-nhs

260. Page 240. Shanti Das and Andrew Gregory, "Amazon ready to cash in on free access to NHS data," *Sunday Times*, page 4, 8 December 2019.

261. Page 240. A good review of blockchain, available as a lecture and as transcript, is Martyn Thomas, "Will Bitcoin and the Blockchain Change the Way we Live and Work?" Gresham College Lecture, 9 January 2018. www.gresham.ac.uk/lectures-and-events/will-bitcoin-and-the-block-chain-change-the-way-we-live-and-work

262. Page 241. John Burg, Christine Murphy, and Jean Paul Petraud, "Blockchain for International Development: Using a Learning Agenda to Address Knowledge Gaps," 2018. merltech.org/blockchain-for-international-development-using-a-learning-agenda-to-address-knowledge-gaps

263. Page 242. Jane Feinmann, "How volunteer doctors help the world's most vulnerable patients, from Yemen to Ukraine, Bangladesh to Bethnal Green," *BMJ*, **363**:k4993, 2018. DOI: 10.1136/bmj.k4993

264. Page 242. The UK Government funds doctors primarily on the basis of the size of local population they serve. Matt Burgess and Nicole Kobie, "The messy, cautionary tale of how Babylon disrupted the NHS," *Wired*, Monday 18 March 2019. www.wired.co.uk/article/babylon-health-nhs and Matt Burgess and Nicole Kobie, "Major concerns are being raised about Babylon's impact on the NHS," *Wired*, 26 April 2019. www.wired.co.uk/article/babylon-health-gp-at-hand-nhs-inquiry-andy-slaughter

265. Page 243. Ellen L. Idler, editor, *Religion as a Social Determinant of Health*, Oxford University Press, 2014.

    A typical rigorous case study of religion as a social determinant of health is reviewed here: Tyler J. VanderWeele, Shanshan Li, Alexander C. Tsai, and Ichiro Kawachi, "Association Between Religious Service Attendance and Lower Suicide Rates Among US Women," *Journal of the American Medical Association Psychiatry*, **73**(8):845–851, 2016. DOI: 10.1001/jamapsychiatry.2016.1243

19   Interoperability

266. Page 245. David W. Bates and Lipika Samal, "Interoperability: What Is It, How Can We Make It Work for Clinicians, and How Should We Measure It in the Future?" *Health Services Research*, **53**(5):3270–3277, 2018. DOI: 10.1111/1475-6773.12852

267. Page 247. Some RFID technologies (especially NFCs) don't work very well near to liquids, so a good solution to ensuring the prescription/bag/infusion pump/patient all pair up safely is not just a matter of throwing technology at the problem.

268. Page 247. Peter J. Pronovost, "Here's a Crucial Technological Fix to Rising Health-Care Costs," *The Wall Street Journal*, 30 October 2016. blogs.wsj.com/experts/2016/10/30/heres-a-crucial-technological-fix-to-rising-health-care-costs/

269. Page 247. Leigh R. Warren, Jonathan Clarke, Sonal Arora, and Ara Darzi, "Improving data sharing between acute hospitals in England: an overview of health record system distribution and retrospective observational analysis of inter-hospital transitions of care," *BMJ Open*, **9**:e031637, 2019. DOI: 10.1136/bmjopen-2019-031637

270. Page 248. When a cosmic ray interferes with a computer's memory, bits can get flipped.

    In Marie Moe's pacemaker, flipping a bit was detected and caused it to enter a "safe mode." However, it's possible to make pacemakers — and any other devices — resistant to bit flips. You could, for example, use three bits instead of one. The pacemaker hardware then takes a majority of two bits, so — even with this simple method — it would be resistant to any single bit being flipped. Failing from a bit flip is a bug, or at least a financial decision that safety is not worth the added cost of redundancy.

    There are, of course, far more sophisticated ways to add redundancy than a simple "majority of two" algorithm. This Wikipedia article is a good place to find out more: "Error detection and correction," en.wikipedia.org/wiki/Error_detection_and_correction Note that error correction is also very powerful in user interfaces, not just inside computers and networks.

271. Page 251. John Seddon, *Systems Thinking in the Public Sector: The Failure of the Reform Regime and a Manifesto for a Better Way*, Triarchy Press Ltd, 2008.

272. Page 254. Kim Thomas, "Wanted: a WhatsApp alternative for clinicians," *BMJ*, **360**, 2018. DOI: 10.1136/bmj.k622

273. Page 255. WhatsApp bugs are regularly in the news. A recent case is Dave Lee,

"WhatsApp flaw 'puts words in your mouth'," BBC News, 8 August 2019. www.bbc.co.uk/news/technology-49273606

Full details of the bug, as found by Checkpoint Research, and how it can be exploited, are described here: Dikla Barda, Roman Zaikin, and Oded Vanunu, "Black Hat 2019 — WhatsApp Protocol Decryption for Chat Manipulation and More," 7 August 2019. research.checkpoint.com/fakesapp-a-vulnerability-in-whatsapp

274. Page 256. "Royal Cornwall Hospitals NHS Trust reduces medication errors in pharmacy dispensing,"
healthcare.gs1uk.org/cases/royal-cornwall-hospitals-nhs-trust-medication-errors

20   Human Factors

275. Page 259. Caroline E. Preston and Stanley Harris, "Psychology of drivers in traffic accidents," *Journal of Applied Psychology*, **49**(4):284–288, 1965. DOI: 10.1037/h0022453

In this paper, Preston and Harris show that most car drivers think they are better than average, even when they have a record of bad driving and, when they were interviewed for the study, are recovering in hospital from a car crash they'd caused!

276. Page 262. There are some terrific books on how stage magic works, and how we are systematically seduced by psychologically based subterfuge. The point is, if entertainers can do it deliberately, in a hospital it can certainly happen unintentionally — and everybody should know what the "tricks" (or poor design features in digital systems) are that force us to make mistakes again and again.

I strongly recommend these two books: Gustav Kuhn, *Experiencing the impossible: The science of magic*, MIT Press, 2019; and Stephen Macknik, Susana Martinez-Conde, and Sandra Blakeslee, *Sleights of Mind*, Profile Books, 2011.

277. Page 263. **This is the moving account of a hero who turned a catastrophe into a movement to improve patient safety for everyone. Martin Bromiley, "The husband's story: from tragedy to learning and action," BMJ Quality & Safety, 24:425–427, 2015. DOI: 10.1136/bmjqs-2015-004129**

A summary of Elaine Bromiley's surgery is "The Case of Elaine Bromiley," which can be found under chfg.org/chfg-history

278. Page 263. Cricothyrotomy means cutting a hole in the neck through which the patient can breathe.

279. Page 264. What I call near mistakes are usually, inaccurately, called near misses, which is a strange phrase. A "near miss" is a miss; I think a near miss itself would be better called a near hit.

280. Page 264. The contrast between healthcare and aviation safety cultures is brilliantly discussed in Matt Syed's book *Black Box Thinking*. Matt puts Elaine and Martin's stories side-by-side with aviation accidents, and contrasts the responses. I'll discuss Matt's book more in Good reading.[i]

281. Page 264. It sounds unhelpfully negative to say healthcare doesn't want to know about failure, but healthcare is full of gag clauses that restrict people, both staff and patients, from talking openly about incidents. You can easily Google lots, but here's just one high-profile example: Andrew Hosken, "NHS chief 'stopped from speaking on patient safety'," BBC News, 14 February 2013. www.bbc.co.uk/news/health-21444058

Or read Dr David Hilfiker's honest, searing article about his own mistakes and the pervasive healthcare culture within which he worked: "Facing Our Mistakes," *New England Journal of Medicine*, **310**:118–122, 1984. DOI: 10.1056/NEJM198401123100211

Dr Hilfiker says,

---

[i] See Chapter 33: Good reading, page 471 ←

We are not prepared for our mistakes, and we don't know how to cope with them when they occur. [...] Doctors hide their mistakes from patients, from other doctors, even from themselves. Open discussion of mistakes is banished from the consultation room, from the operating room, from physicians' meetings. [...] We either deny the misfortune altogether or blame the patient, the nurse, the laboratory, other physicians, the system, fate — anything to avoid our own guilt. The medical profession seems to have no place for its mistakes.

282. Page 265. Helen Jones, "Why I ... garden," *BMJ*, **367**:l6647, 2019. DOI: 10.1136/bmj.l6647

283. Page 266. Details of the WHO Surgical Checklist are available on the WHO website. See www.who.int/patientsafety/safesurgery/checklist/en

284. Page 266. Cleve Bryan, "EXCLUSIVE: Lourdes Hospital Transplant Center Admits Giving Wrong Person Kidney Transplant," *CBS Philly*, 26 November 2019. philadelphia.cbslocal.com/2019/11/26/exclusive-lourdes-hospital-transplant-center-admits-giving-wrong-person-kidney-transplant

285. Page 266. Liam Donaldson, "An organisation with a memory," *Clinical Medicine*, **2**:452–457, 2002.

286. Page 266. Danielle Ofri, "The Business of Health Care Depends on Exploiting Doctors and Nurses — One resource seems infinite and free: the professionalism of caregivers," *New York Times*, 8 June 2019. www.nytimes.com/2019/06/08/opinion/sunday/hospitals-doctors-nurses-burnout.html

287. Page 268. An edited collection of personal resilience ideas is Peter Lees and Myra Malik, editors, *Building resilience: A practical resource for healthcare professionals*, CRC Press, 2018. A recommended, powerful personal story is re-humanising.co.uk/2019/03/29/resilience-lets-treat-the-cause-not-the-symptoms, 29 March 2019. Finally, a rather academic review of resilience is Siri Wiig, Karina Aase, Stephen Billett, Carolyn Canfield, Olav Røise, Ove Njå, Veslemøy Guise, Cecilie Haraldseid-Driftland, Eline Ree, Janet E. Anderson, and Carl Macrae, "Defining the boundaries and operational concepts of resilience in the resilience in healthcare research program," *BMC Health Services Research*, **20**:330, 2020. DOI: 10.1186/s12913-020-05224-3

288. Page 270. Walter Quattrociocchi, Antonio Scala, and Cass R. Sunstein, "Echo Chambers on Facebook," draft, 2019. www.researchgate.net/publication/331936299_Echo_Chambers_on_Facebook

289. Page 270. The NHS has a brief *Just Culture Guide*. See improvement.nhs.uk/resources/just-culture-guide

290. Page 271. Saif S. Khairat, Cameron Coleman, Paige Ottmar, Thomas Bice, Ross Koppel, and Shannon S. Carson, "Physicians' gender and their use of electronic health records: findings from a mixed-methods usability study," *Journal of the American Medical Informatics Association*, DOI: 10.1093/jamia/ocz126

291. Page 272. The 2019 Stack Overflow survey covers many details as well as gender. See *Developer Survey Results*, 2019. insights.stackoverflow.com/survey/2019

292. Page 273. "TUI plane in 'serious incident' after every 'Miss' on board was assigned child's weight," *The Guardian*, 9 April 2021. www.theguardian.com/world/2021/apr/09/tui-plane-serious-incident-every-miss-on-board-child-weight-birmingham-majorca?CMP=Share_AndroidApp_Other More technical details at: assets.publishing.service.gov.uk/media/604f423be90e077fdf88493f/Boeing_737-8K5_G-TAWG_04-21.pdf

293. Page 274. Hugh Dubberly, *How do You Design: A Compendium of Design Models*, Dubberly Design Office, 2004. www.dubberly.com/wp-content/uploads/2008/06/ddo_designprocess.pdf

294. Page 274. John Ziman, *Reliable knowledge: An exploration of the grounds for belief in science*, Cambridge University Press, revised edition 2008.

295. Page 274. Daniel M. Wegner, "How to Think, Say, or Do Precisely the Worst Thing for Any Occasion," *Science*, **325**(5936):48–50, 2009. DOI: 10.1126/science.1167346

296. Page 275. This quote on personal change has been attributed to many people, and my attempts to find the source weren't helped by Jacob Braude himself being an avid collector of quotes. If in doubt, attributing a wise saying to Benjamin Franklin always sounds respectable.

297. Page 275. Chip Heath and Dan Heath *Switch: How to change things when change is hard*, Random House Business 2011.

21   Computer Factors

298. Page 277. Dean Buonomano, *Brain Bugs: How the Brain's Flaws Shape Our Lives*, W. W. Norton & Company, 2012.

299. Page 278. See the facsimile of Edison's letter at the Thomas Edison Papers repository: 11/13/1878 Edison, Thomas Alva to Puskas, Theodore (Morgan (J.S.) & Co; Drexel Morgan & Co; Fabbri and Chauncey; Fabbri, Egisto Paolo; Serrell, Lemuel Wright; Griffin, Stockton L) Sales and service; Inventions and creativity; Electric light and power [LB003] Letterbook Series — General Letterbooks: LB-003 (1876–1878) [LB003487; TAEM 28:913] edison.rutgers.edu/NamesSearch/SingleDoc.php?DocId=LB003487, cited in Alexander B. Magoun and Paul Israel, "Did You Know? Edison Coined the Term 'Bug'," *IEEE Spectrum*, August 2013. spectrum.ieee.org/the-institute/ieee-history/did-you-know-edison-coined-the-term-bug

300. Page 278. Patterns have a long history in Computer Science, having being inspired by Chris Alexander's work in architecture, most notably his inspiring book *Notes on the Synthesis of Form*, Harvard University Press, 1974. A maintained and up-to-date list of computing patterns can be found at en.wikipedia.org/wiki/Software_design_pattern

301. Page 282. Like many popular programming languages used in healthcare, JavaScript has unsafe types. For example, the expression "1"+1 is equal to 11 and not equal to 2, as you'd probably expect. The second 1, which is a number, is silently converted — that is, its type is silently changed — to a string, then appended to the string "1" which results in the string "11". Having what you think is 1+1 being equal to 11 is rarely what anyone expects or wants.

    Confusingly, if you did "1"-1 instead, you'd get zero. In other words, + converts 1 to a string then joins the strings, but - converts "1" to a number, then subtracts the numbers!

    These examples may make some sort of sense, but imagine what happens in a program when you write a+b, as the result will depend in very strange ways on the types of the values that the variables a and b have. Weirdly, in general, it means that a+b isn't equal to b+a.

    Bugs happen when this sort of quirky behavior occurs by accident. Every JavaScript program is just a typo away from chaos. Somebody else may have written the code that gives your variables values, but your code has to work correctly whatever the types that come in to it. That's not at all easy to do. Using better programming languages than JavaScript — strongly typed languages — avoids such problems.

302. Page 283. Wikipedia doesn't discuss Computer Factors, but it does give an up-to-date list of bugs. "Wikipedia: Software bug," en.wikipedia.org/wiki/Software_bug

303. Page 283. The Curiosity Mars Rover is a car-sized roving vehicle designed to explore Mars. It was launched in 2011 and is still operational years later. The main reason for its success is that its software and hardware are redundant. A good article on it is Gerard J. Holzmann, "Mars Code," *Communications of the ACM*, **57**(2):64–73, 2014. DOI: 10.1145/2560217.2560218

304. Page 284. Another reason not to program in Javascript: the test if(a < 10) succeeds without error when the variable a is either true or false! In decent programming languages, it'd be a compile time error to compare a Boolean variable with an integer.

305. Page 284. C. Jeya K. Henry, "The biology of human starvation: some new insights," *Nutrition Bulletin*, **26**:205–211, 2008. DOI: 10.1046/j.1467-3010.2001.00164.x

306. Page 286. See Daniel Keane, "Health boss unsure how many patients impacted by dosage bungle blamed on Windows upgrade," *ABC News*, 7 May 2021. http://www.abc.net.au/news/2021-05-07/sa-health-unsure-of-patient-impact-of-medication-dosage-bungle/100122958

    Emily Cosenza, "SA nurses on high alert after computer glitch adds extra digit to medicine dosages: A computer glitch has caused an extra digit to be incorrectly added to some medicine dosages at several hospitals in one Australian state," NCA NewsWire, 6 May 2021. www.news.com.au/national/south-australia/sa-nurses-on-high-alert-after-computer-glitch-adds-extra-digit-to-medicine-dosages/news-story/9ff9959cd12f634e30195db405df0dab

    According to Emily Cosenza's report, "Technology experts are working to determine the cause of the glitch." Well, the cause of the "glitch" (really, you can call a ten-times drug overdose just a *glitch*?) is easy: bad programming, then buying and using poor quality programs — and, ultimately, the poor regulation and lack of professional oversight that lets any of that happen.

307. Page 288. A good programming language will check that guards cover all possible cases, and, if there's any logical overlap between guards, that the code still does the same thing under all cases.

    Although 1976 now seems a long time ago, Edsger Dijkstra has an excellent discussion of this philosophy and how it improves program quality: Edsger Wybe Dijkstra, *A Discipline of Programming*, Prentice Hall, 1976.

308. Pages 291, 441. Alan Mathison Turing, Lecture to the London Mathematical Society on the Design of the Automatic Computing Engine, 20 February 1949. Turing Digital Archive AMT/B/1. www.turingarchive.org/browse.php/B/1

309. Page 290. Nunjucks is an open source template language primarily intended for rapid development of websites: it generates HTML and JavaScript. Nunjucks is available on Github at mozilla.github.io/nunjucks

310. Page 290. The ACM Digital Library is at dl.acm.org and the IEEE Xplore Library is at ieeexplore.ieee.org

311. Page 298. Jon Loeliger and Matthew McCullough, *Version Control with Git: Powerful tools and techniques for collaborative software development*, O'Reilly Media, 2012. (Make sure you get the latest edition!)

312. Page 299. I'm always baffled that we need any special term like **Formal Methods**. When you design an airplane or a sports car, you don't just throw it together and see if it works; you don't leave it to special occasions to use "Formal Methods." No; engineers use hard mathematics *all the time*. For some reason, programmers typically throw software together, and only very rarely use any explicit mathematics at all.

    Unlike conventional engineering, as used in aviation and cars, few programs have any rigorous reasoning in them at all. It's a shame Formal Methods has become an arcane specialty. Needing such a term at all is really an acknowledgment that almost all software development is seat-of-the-pants and pretty sloppy.

313. Page 299. Daniel Jackson, *The Essence of Software: Why Concepts Matter for Great Design*, Princeton University Press, 2021.

314. Page 299. Edsger Wybe Dijkstra, *Selected Writings on Computing: A Personal Perspective*, Springer-Verlag, 1982.

315. Page 299. The quote is from Dijkstra's Turing Award Lecture: Edsger Wybe Dijkstra "The Humble Programmer," in *ACM Turing Award Lectures: The First Twenty Years*, pages 17–32, Addison-Wesley Publishing Company, 1987.

    The ACM Turing Awards are the Computer Science equivalent of the Nobel Prize;

the Turing Award Lectures, written by the Award winners, are without exception brilliant and well worth reading.

316. Pages 299, 362. E. W. Dijkstra in O.-J. Dahl, E. W. Dijkstra, and C. A. R. Hoare, *Notes on Structured Programming*, Academic Press, 1972.

22   User Centered Design

317. Page 302. "Test your idea with real users in real situations" — you need to test your ideas with a representative sample of *real* users. Testing with a few users is not sufficient; your tests have to be statistically valid. Testing using people from a group of "test users" you always use because they're convenient is also not good enough — they've already got used to your designs. If you are making a product for national use, say, then testing with users from nearby is not sufficient either. There are likely to be variations across the country that a local sample of users will not represent.

318. Page 302. Jeffrey Braithwaite, Robert L. Wears, and Erik Hollnagel, *Resilient Health Care, Volume 3: Reconciling Work-as-Imagined and Work-as-Done*, CRC Press, 2016.

319. Page 302. Ross Koppel, Sean Smith, Jim Blythe, and Vijay Kothari, "Workarounds to Computer Access in Healthcare Organizations: You Want My Password or a Dead Patient?" *Studies in Health Technology and Informatics*, **208**:215–220, 2015. DOI: 10.3233/978-1-61499-488-6-215

320. Page 303. There are many books and papers on task analysis. My advice is to read up from a chapter in a book on user interface design — task analysis, like UCD itself, is only one of many great ideas for improving systems. The chapter Good reading[j] has many ideas.

321. Page 303. An entire issue of *HindSight*, **25** (European Organisation for Safety of Air Navigation), Summer 2017, is devoted to Work as Imagined and Work as Done. www.eurocontrol.int/sites/default/files/publication/files/hindsight25.pdf

     The editor-in-chief is Steven Shorrock, who is well worth Googling for all things Human Factors, including his extensive work on WAD-WAI. The special issue also has articles by names you'll recognize from elsewhere in this book: Sidney Dekker, Erik Hollnagel, Martin Bromiley, and others.

322. Page 304. Jakob Nielsen and Thomas K. Landauer, "A mathematical model of the finding of usability problems," *Proceedings ACM INTERCHI'93 Conference*, 206–213, ACM, 1993. DOI: 10.1145/169059.169166

     More recent discussions can be found at Jakob Nielsen, "Why You Only Need to Test with 5 Users," www.nngroup.com/articles/why-you-only-need-to-test-with-5-users

     Note that most of the discussion is about *usability* problems for generic systems (websites and so on). Problems certainly need fixing, but in healthcare we have patients and trained professionals. Digital healthcare usability is a different issue than for general users; we are more concerned about *safety*, which these conventional usability studies say nothing about.

323. Pages 304, 319. Sketching is a technical term in design; it doesn't mean using a rough drawing, but a sketch could be a mock-up made out of wood even. Probably the best book on sketching is Saul Greenberg, Sheelagh Carpendale, Nicolai Marquardt, and Bill Buxton, *Sketching User Experiences*, Morgan Kaufmann, 2012.

     There is a whole world on good practice in UCD (such as sketching and expert heuristic evaluation), and while it's fascinating and essential to use, it'd take us too far beyond the core of this book. The point of my discussion on how many users is enough for UCD is to make clear that, at least in healthcare contexts, five users is

---

[j] See Chapter 33: Good reading, page 471 ←

nothing like enough to ensure safety or effectiveness — in fact, safety is a formal property that requires solid software engineering (certainly supported by UCD), but UCD alone is not sufficient, however many users are tested.

324. Page 305. The first person who seemed to have noticed this critical question — who are the users? — was Wilfred J. Hansen, "User Engineering Principles for Interactive Systems," *Proceedings Fall Joint Computer Conference, AFIPS'71*, 523–532, AFIPS, 1971. DOI: 10.1145/1479064.1479159

    This classic 1971 article has the great advantage that Hansen's insights into how to design better interactive systems are not obscured by lots of modern technology distractions.

325. Page 306. Denis Campbell, "NHS faces £24m bill after glue injected into girl's brain at Great Ormond Street," *The Guardian*, 27 January 2014. www.theguardian.com/society/2014/jan/27/nhs-24m-bill-glue-injected-girls-brain-great-ormond-street

326. Page 306. R. Evley, J. Russell, D. Mathew, R. Hall, L. Gemmell, and R. P. Mahajan, "Confirming the drugs administered during anæsthesia: a feasibility study in the pilot National Health Service sites, UK," *British Journal of Anæsthesia*, **105**(3):289–296, 2010. DOI: 10.1093/bja/aeq194

327. Page 307. Daphna Stroumsa, Elizabeth F. S. Roberts, Hadrian Kinnear, and Lisa H. Harris, "The Power and Limits of Classification – A 32-Year-Old Man with Abdominal Pain," *New England Journal of Medicine*, **380**(20):1885–1888, 16 May 2019. DOI: 10.1056/NEJMp1811491

    A more popular newspaper article is here: Marilynn Marchione, "Nurse mistakes pregnant transgender man as obese. Then, the man births a stillborn baby," *USA Today*, 16 May 2019. www.usatoday.com/story/news/health/2019/05/16/pregnant-transgender-man-births-stillborn-baby-hospital-missed-labor-signs/3692201002

328. Page 307. Rhiannon Williams, "Facebook's 71 gender options come to UK users," *The Telegraph*, 27 June 2014. www.telegraph.co.uk/technology/facebook/10930654/Facebooks-71-gender-options-come-to-UK-users.html

329. Page 308. Prue Thimbleby, Sarah Wright, and Rhian Solomon, "'Reconstructing Ourselves" — An arts and research project improving patient experience," *Journal of Applied Arts & Health*, **9**(1):113–124, 2018. DOI: 10.1386/jaah.9.1.113_1

330. Page 310. E. Michael Canham and Michael J. Weaver, "Copy, Paste, and Cloned Electronic Records," *Chest*, **146**(3):e101, 2014. DOI: 10.1378/chest.14-0759

331. Page 310. Ross Koppel, "Illusions and delusions of cut, pasted, and cloned notes," *Chest*, **145**(3):444–445, 2014. DOI: 10.1378/chest.13-1846 — see also the comments on Ross Koppel's paper: Justin M. Weis and Paul G. Levy, "Copy, paste, and cloned notes in health records," *Chest*, **145**(3):632–638, 2014. DOI: 10.1378/chest.13-0886

332. Page 311. Patrick Vlaskovits, "Henry Ford, Innovation, and That 'Faster Horse' Quote," *Harvard Business Review*, 29 August 2011. hbr.org/2011/08/henry-ford-never-said-the-fast

23 Iterative Design

333. Page 314. A company was using a simple web form, which, unknown to them, was putting customers off — it was only two buttons and two fields; how could that possibly go wrong? But they didn't know what they didn't know. The customers who were giving up never crossed their radar.

    UCD experts ran focus groups, and identified some serious design problems with the form. Fixing the design problems increased the income of the company by $300 *million* a year!

    This famous UCD story is described here: Luke Wroblewski, *Web Form Design: Filling in the Blanks*, Rosenfeld Media, 2008.

334. Page 319. Design Council, *What is the framework for innovation? Design Council's evolved Double Diamond*, 2019. www.designcouncil.org.uk/news-opinion/what-framework-innovation-design-councils-evolved-double-diamond

335. Page 319. More precisely, *we* — me and Mandy — might both be idiosyncratic, but that is much less likely than one user is idiosyncratic. More to the point, I'll admit to being idiosyncratic in some ways — I'm very interested in UCD, for a start — but Mandy is different to me, so it's reassuring and a good check to see the UCD problems I discussed at the beginning of the chapter being experienced by somebody who isn't into UCD at all.

336. Page 320. Clinipad's website is softwareofexcellence.co.uk/solutions/clinipad

337. Page 320. One problem is that Clinipad has made the iPads visually very faithfully represent the old paper forms, but apparently overlooked providing any digital advantages. There's no apparent Computational Thinking — the forms are harder for the user to fill in than paper was (but they keep a record, even if errors happen, for the manager). Many of the useful features of paper forms are gone too: you can't cross out a section, for instance. Clinipad have created new problems too; for instance, in the "old days," lots of patients waiting could fill in their paper forms; now, the queue behind the receptionist gets longer and longer, as the two expensive iPads are devoted to just one patient. See note 95 for more discussion on the paperless revolution.

24 Wedge Thinking

338. Page 328. I could wire up a socket with low current wire. The socket will seem to work fine when I check it, but if, say, a high power heater is plugged in, my thin wiring will get hot. This could cause a fire.

    Outdoor wiring and wiring near water pose additional risks that amateur electricians may ignore and not provide the appropriate protections for. When the wiring is dry, it'll seem to work just fine, but when it's wet, it can kill.

339. Page 329. For more on the Enigma and its Human Factors chaos, see Harold Thimbleby, "Human Factors and missed solutions to Enigma design weaknesses," *Cryptologia*, **40**(2):177–202, 2016. DOI: 10.1080/01611194.2015.1028680

340. Page 329. A lot of very interesting research has been done on how we are unconsciously over-confident when we communicate — what we say seems obvious to us, but it's less obvious to others.

    (I think my jokes are very good — I already know why they are funny — but unfortunately other people don't always get them. That's the same problem!)

    When it comes to programming, that means what we program seems more obvious to us than it does to users later, and the research shows that we do not realize how critical this difference really is.

    This article has some nice stories and pointers to the wider literature: Boaz Keysar and Anne S. Henly, "Speakers' Overestimation of Their Effectiveness," *Psychological Science*, **13**(3):207–212, 2002.

341. Page 330. Peter J. Pronovost and Eric Vohr, *Safe Patients, Smart Hospitals*, Penguin, 2011. This book is so powerful, it's also discussed in Good reading.

342. Page 331. One of the problems in industry is that it sort of makes sense to have separate technical authors to write instructions, and they can't write instructions until the design is finished. But this is so wrong! Once the instructions are written, they should be checked and tested and the design improved iteratively to help make the instructions clearer and clearer.

343. Page 331. A good place to start on technical debt is the Wikipedia article on it: en.wikipedia.org/wiki/Technical_debt

344. Page 331. For more on User Centered Design and Human Computer Interaction, please see the Good reading chapter for more information.[k]

345. Page 333. Here is the classic — eye-opening — paper on *N* version programming. The authors compared 15 independently-developed programs for seismic data analysis. The programs (which had been used professionally) had numerous previously unknown bugs revealed by the *N* version programming. Les Hatton and Andy Roberts, "How accurate is scientific software?" *IEEE Transactions on Software Engineering*, **20**(10):785–797, 1994, DOI: 10.1109/32.328993

346. Page 334. **Atul Gawande, *The Checklist Manifesto: How to Get Things Right*, Profile Books, 2011. Programming and healthcare are both complex activities, and it's easy to forget or overlook important ideas — checklists are your way out. Gawande has written a very readable and fascinating account of these under-rated checklists and how they are used in all successful, complex activities. The World Health Organization's surgical checklist is one example, but checklists are used in aviation, fire fighting, large building construction, and more.**

347. Page 334. The National Cancer Research Institute (NCRI), *Cancer research in the UK 2002–2011: An overview of the research funded by NCRI Partners*, 2013.

25   Attention to detail

348. Page 338. Paul B. Batalden and Frank Davidoff, "What is 'quality improvement' and how can it transform healthcare?" *BMJ Quality & Safety*, **16**:2–3, 2007. DOI: 10.1136/qshc.2006.022046

349. Page 340. There is a discrepancy between the printed units (mL/h) and the displayed units (mg/h). Is this a programming bug or a hardware bug? Which was designed first? Did the programmer not use the hardware specification, or did the hardware designer not use the program specification? Why didn't the programmer update the software after the discrepancy occurred? I think it's pointless worrying whether bugs are hardware or software, or even where they come from. Computers are both hardware and software.

350. Pages 340, 345. Watch the video at youtu.be/eK3oIYU060g or read Harold Thimbleby, "Reasons to Question Seven Segment Displays," *Proceedings ACM Conference on Computer-Human Interaction, ACM CHI*, 1431–1440, ACM, 2013. DOI: 10.1145/2470654.2466190

     Although the Alaris PC suffers from the problems I pointed out that are common with seven-segment displays, the Alaris PC actually uses a 12-segment display, but it shares the same problems. It's pointless to question whether the problems with the Alaris PC arise from a segment display or from recessing the display too much; the point is, it can be misread.

351. Page 341. Matt Burgess and Nicole Kobie, "The messy, cautionary tale of how Babylon disrupted the NHS," *Wired*, 18 March 2019. www.wired.co.uk/article/babylon-health-nhs

352. Page 341. Aliya Ram and Sarah Neville, "High-profile health app under scrutiny after doctors' complaints," *Financial Times*, 13 July 2018. www.ft.com/content/19dc6b7e-8529-11e8-96dd-fa565ec55929

353. Page 341. Leo Kelion, "Babylon Health admits GP app suffered a data breach," BBC News, 10 June 2020. www.bbc.co.uk/news/technology-52986629

354. Page 341. Rory Glover's Twitter handle is @Rory_Glover

355. Page 342. Laura Lovett, "Chatbot Babylon fires back at Twitter critic by publicly analyzing his search data. The company's move has come under fire for privacy

[k] See Chapter 33: User Centered Design reading recommendations, page 482 ←

concerns," *mobihealthnews*, 25 February 2020. mobihealthnews.com/news/
chatbot-babylon-fires-back-twitter-critic-publicly-analyzing-his-search-data

Natasha Lomas, "AI chatbot maker Babylon Health attacks clinician in PR stunt
after he goes public with safety concerns," *TechCrunch*, 26 February 2020.
techcrunch.com/2020/02/25/first-do-no-harm

356. Pages 342 twice, 343. press@babylonhealth.com, "Babylon results published after
2400 Twitter troll tests," assets.babylonhealth.com/pdfs/Babylon-results-
published-after-2400-Twitter-troll-tests.pdf, 24 February 2020.

357. Page 342. My harsh assessment of Babylon and the regulators is an increasingly
common perspective. For an independent summary of the issues, see Gareth
Iacobucci, "Row over Babylon's chatbot shows lack of regulation," *BMJ*, **368**:m815,
2020. DOI: 10.1136/bmj.m815

358. Page 342. Katherine Middleton, Mobasher Butt, Nils Hammerla, Steven Hamblin,
Karan Mehta, and Ali Parsa, "Sorting out symptoms: design and evaluation of the
'babylon check' automated triage system," *ArXiv*, abs/1606.02041, 2016.

359. Page 342. This article is well-researched and includes further references: "Babylon
Health," *Best Practice Artificial Intelligence*,
bestpractice.ai/studies/babylon_health_claims_82_accuracy_for_video_medical_
diagnosis_based_on_machine_learning_and_natural_language_processing,
undated, but viewed 26 February 2020.

360. Pages 344, 534. Interestingly, this book *is* a program. I wrote it in LaTeX, which not
only did the typesetting but is also a complete, if rather quirky, programming system.

For example, this note 360 you're reading right now, refers back to the page
numbers of the pages where it was referred to — and you can see it's been referenced
on two pages, one of which is this one. The book *as a program* works out (hopefully)
the correct numbers to use for notes and their pages.

The word "Pages," above, however, is not "in" the book but is in the program that
runs the book. The same program also generates details like the index and the table of
contents, and many other features, like the note numbers themselves.

From an internationalization perspective, this means that if the book is translated
to another language, then all English words like "Page" in the program will also have to
be translated — otherwise the notes will go wrong. Even worse, the word "English" in
the previous sentence, but probably nowhere else, will need, not translating, but
changing to the name of the new language the book is translated into.
Internationalization isn't easy!

361. Page 345. David Shepardson, "GM recalls 4.3 million vehicles over air bag-related
defect," Reuters, 9 September 2016.
www.reuters.com/article/us-gm-recall-idUSKCN11F2AH

26   Planes are safer

362. Page 347. Kathy McGrath, "The LASCAD Project: A Failed Implementation or a Way
of Understanding the Present?" *Journal of Intelligent Systems*, **10**(5–6):509–538,
2011. DOI: 10.1515/JISYS.2000.10.5-6.509

363. Page 347. BBC News, "London ambulance service hit by New Year fault," 1 January
2017. www.bbc.co.uk/news/uk-38482746

364. Page 350. My figures combine data from the World Bank at
data.worldbank.org/indicator/IS.AIR.PSGR?end=2017&start=1970&view=chart and
from Boeing, via Wikipedia at
en.wikipedia.org/wiki/Aviation_accidents_and_incidents##Statistics

The industry standard data is from Boeing, and is fascinating and well presented;
see *Statistical Summary of Commercial Jet Airplane Accidents Worldwide Operations,
1959–2016*,

www.boeing.com/resources/boeingdotcom/company/about_bca/pdf/statsum.pdf

365. Page 351. I compared the risk of dying on a plane with the risk of sitting in an armchair — arguing that flying is safer — because it helps you to think about statistics and sampling (what population of people are we measuring?). Most people flying walk onto the plane, so almost all passengers are healthy, and certainly they are mobile. In contrast, a lot of people sitting in armchairs are, as a whole, more likely to be less mobile than passengers. Many people sitting in armchairs are old or ill people; certainly there are more old and ill people sitting in armchairs right now than there are sitting in planes. In short, on *average* people sitting in armchairs are more likely to die. This doesn't mean that *you* can lengthen your life by going off flying instead of collapsing in an armchair!

366. Page 351. Sully Sullenberger, "We must not forget," *Blog*, www.sullysullenberger.com/we-must-not-forget

367. Page 352. "US Airways Flight 1549", Wikipedia, en.wikipedia.org/wiki/US_Airways_Flight_1549

368. Pages 352, 354. The software Boeing put in the 737 MAX was called the Maneuvering Characteristics Augmentation System, or MCAS. Gregory Travis, "How the Boeing 737 Max Disaster Looks to a Software Developer," *IEEE Spectrum*, 18 April 2019. spectrum.ieee.org/aerospace/aviation/how-the-boeing-737-max-disaster-looks-to-a-software-developer
    The 737 MAX story is complex, investigations are ongoing, and the report by Travis is not without controversy. A more recent, and very readable, summary of the story is available on the BBC: Theo Leggett, "What went wrong inside Boeing's cockpit," 17 December 2019. bbc.in/2HoGKrx

369. Page 353. FDA, "MDR Data Files," 21 June 2019. www.fda.gov/medical-devices/medical-device-reporting-mdr-how-report-medical-device-problems/mdr-data-files

370. Page 353. Ben Hallman, "FDA Releases Vast Trove Of Hidden Medical Device Injury And Malfunction Reports," The International Consortium of Investigative Journalists, 24 June 2019. www.icij.org/investigations/implant-files/fda-releases-vast-trove-of-hidden-medical-device-injury-and-malfunction-reports and Christina Jewett, "FDA To End Program That Hid Millions Of Reports On Faulty Medical Devices," *Kaiser Health News*, KHN, 3 May 2019. khn.org/news/fda-to-end-program-that-hid-millions-of-reports-on-faulty-medical-devices

371. Page 353. "Kaiser Health News Wins Feddie Award," 1 November 2019. nationalpress.org/newsfeed/kaiser-health-news-wins-feddie-award

372. Page 353. The Indonesian investigation into the accident, *KNKT.18.10.35.04, Aircraft Accident Investigation Report, PT. Lion Mentari Airlines, Boeing 737-8 (MAX); PK-LQP*, can be found here: knkt.dephub.go.id/knkt/ntsc_aviation/baru/2018%20-%20035%20-%20PK-LQP%20Final%20Report.pdf
    A more accessible BBC News report on it is here: Theo Leggett, "Boeing 737 Max Lion Air crash caused by series of failures," BBC, 25 October 2019. www.bbc.co.uk/news/business-50177788

373. Page 354. See James Dean, "US aircraft watchdog staff 'afraid to challenge Boeing'," *The Times*, 30 July 2019. www.thetimes.co.uk/article/us-aircraft-watchdog-staff-afraid-to-challenge-boeing-vrrrkps0r

374. Page 355. This comparison of pilot and surgeon skill was made by Jeremy Hunt, the then UK Secretary of State for Health, in the 2017 World Health Organization's Global Ministerial Summit in Bonn, Germany.

375. Page 355 twice. Stephanie Nebehay, "Going into hospital far riskier than flying: WHO," *Health News*, 21 July 2011. www.reuters.com/article/us-safety-idUSTRE76K45R20110721

376. Page 356. "Software and IT systems." Some people want to make distinctions between algorithms, software, programs, electronics, and so on. There are useful

professional distinctions between the terms, but in Computer Science, all are formally equivalent: anything you can do in software you can do in hardware, and there are no hard-and-fast distinctions.

377. Page 356. James Rodger, "Stephen Pettitt's heartbroken family speak out after he died following robotic heart surgery," *Birmingham Live*, 8 November 2018. www.birminghammail.co.uk/news/uk-news/stephen-pettitts-heartbroken-family-speak-15390579

378. Page 358. Justin Kruger and David Dunning, "Unskilled and Unaware of It: How Difficulties in Recognizing One's Own Incompetence Lead to Inflated Self Assessments," *Journal of Personality and Social Psychology*, **77**(6):1121–1134, 1999. DOI: 10.1037/0022-3514.77.6.1121

    It's a great paper which is well worth reading. It even won the authors the Ig Nobel Prize.

379. Page 358. Meta-skills are skills about skills. When you are programming, you obviously think about the programming you are doing, but if you have meta-skills you also think about *how* you are programming, how you are solving problems, how you can get better, and so on.

    Everyone makes mistakes, but people with meta-skills think about the mistakes they may have made but haven't noticed yet — people trained with meta-skills are not only much better programmers, but they continue to get better and better. People rarely learn to practice meta-skills effectively without coaching.

380. Page 358. Nicola Woolcock, "Firms hold hacking contests to recruit teenage IT experts," *The Times*, 29 May 2017. www.thetimes.co.uk/article/firms-hold-hacking-contests-to-recruit-teenage-it-experts-bb0s5g0vm

381. Page 359. Walter Loeb, "Amazon Is The Biggest Investor In The Future, Spends $22.6 Billion On R&D," *Forbes*, 1 November 2018. www.forbes.com/sites/walterloeb/2018/11/01/amazon-is-biggest-investor-for-the-future/#7f7a4c961f1d

382. Page 360. A very few things, like transplants and blood transfusions, are amazingly fungible, provided you do enough homework first to avoid rejection.

383. Page 363. Sophie Borland, "Up to 300,000 heart patients may have been given wrong drugs or advice due to major NHS IT blunder," *Daily Mail*, 12 May 2016. www.dailymail.co.uk/health/article-3585149/Up-300-000-heart-patients-given-wrong-drugs-advice-major-NHS-blunder.html or Alex Matthews-King, "GPs to review 260,000 patients as full scale of CV risk calculator error revealed," *PULSE*, 9 June 2016. www.pulsetoday.co.uk/clinical/clinical-specialties/cardiovascular/gps-to-review-260000-patients-as-full-scale-of-cv-risk-calculator-error-revealed/20032035.article

384. Page 363. Many clinical programs use codes (such as SNOMED-CT) for systematically classifying medical terms. The bugs with SystmOne/QRISK arose because some clinical codes were accidentally omitted and some codes were incorrectly mapped between two different coding schemes. So, while the basic calculator QRISK was "correct," the data (based on the code mapping it was using) was incorrect. See Ben Heather, "QRisk2 in TPP "fixed" but up to 270,000 patients affected," *Digitalhealth*, 10 June 2016. www.digitalhealth.net/2016/06/qrisk2-in-tpp-fixed-but-up-to-270000-patients-affected

385. Page 363. Chris Smyth, "Medical records of 150,000 patients shared by mistake," *The Times*, 3 July 2018. See also: BBC News, "NHS data breach affects 150,000 patients in England," 2 July 2018. www.bbc.co.uk/news/technology-44682369

386. Page 363. Kath Moser, Sarah Sellars, Margot Wheaton, Julie Cooke, Alison Duncan, Anthony Maxwell, Michael Michell, Mary Wilson, Valerie Beral, Richard Peto, Mike Richards, and Julietta Patnick, "Extending the Age Range for Breast Screening in England: Pilot Study to Assess the Feasibility, Acceptability of Randomization," *Journal of Medical Screening*, **18**(2):96–102, 2011. DOI: 10.1258/jms.2011.011065

387. Page 363. Laura Donnelly, "Breast screening scandal deepens as IT firm says senior health officials ignored its warnings," *Daily Telegraph*, 4 May 2018. www.telegraph.co.uk/news/2018/05/04/breast-screening-scandal-deepens-firm-says-senior-health-officials

388. Page 363. *Independent Breast Screening Review*, Her Majesty's Stationery Office, 2018.

27   Stories for developers

389. Page 367. For simplicity, I wrote "say("*")" in the code, as I think it's a clear way to show what I mean. If you want to run this code in a browser, you'll need to write something like "document.write("*");" (or define the function say(s) yourself), but these easy details aren't what the question is about.

390. Page 368. It's fairly obvious that f(n) prints lots of stars — but *exactly* how many stars does it print?

    It's easy enough to work out in your head that for $n < 0$, $n = 0$, $n = 1$ or $n = 2$ then f(n) prints 1 star; if n is 3, it prints 2 stars. Then it starts to get a bit harder! If n is 4, it prints 3 stars. Then it probably gets too hard to do reliably in your head. Instead, you could try running the code f(n) to check things, but that doesn't really help you understand *exactly* what f(n) does in general.

    In general, f(n) prints as many stars as f(n−1) and f(n−2) combined. This is reminiscent of the Fibonacci series; indeed, for $n > 0$, f(n) prints F_n stars, where F_n is the nth Fibonacci number. You could work this out by trying out the program to see what it does — you could just recognize the pattern, as it prints 1, 1, 2, 3, 5, 8, 13, 21... stars — which are the first few Fibonacci numbers.

    However, to *prove* it is the Fibonacci series is a bit harder, but it's essential to do so, because you don't really know what any piece of program does until it's proven.

    Usually we are not so lucky to get a problem with a form, here Fibonacci numbers, that we recognize. In most cases, then, we need to use sophisticated tools, such as symbolic mathematics systems, such as Mathematica. To use them effectively, we need to first learn the sort of material found in *Concrete Mathematics: A Foundation for Computer Science* by Ronald L. Graham, Donald E. Knuth, and Oren Patashnik, second edition, Addison-Wesley, 1994, which tells you pretty much everything.

391. Page 369. Heartbleed, en.wikipedia.org/wiki/Heartbleed

392. Page 369. Farhad Manjoo, "Users' Stark Reminder: As Web Grows, It Grows Less Secure," *New York Times*, 9 April 2104. www.nytimes.com/2014/04/10/technology/users-stark-reminder-as-web-grows-it-grows-less-secure.html?ref=farhadmanjoo&_r=0

393. Page 369. A revelation of the Boeing 737 MAX story was that a lot of the safety-critical programming was out-sourced to other countries, and almost certainly had less oversight.

394. Page 370. BBC News, "Health records 'put at risk by security bugs'," 7 August 2018. www.bbc.co.uk/news/technology-45083778

395. Page 370. In PHP, if you misspell a name, the name is taken to be a constant. So typing **tem** incorrectly instead of **temp** is not a recognized error, but gives you the value **tem** (a string) rather than the value of the variable, **temp**, you wanted. Your program won't work, and PHP won't help you find the problem. In JavaScript, misspelling a name is an error, and the system will help you track it down.

396. Page 371. Kevin C. O'Kane, *The Mumps Programming Language*, CreateSpace Independent Publishing Platform, 2008.

397. Page 371. Ross Koppel and Christoph U. Lehmann, "Implications of an emerging EHR monoculture for hospitals and healthcare systems," *Journal of the American Medical Informatics Association*, **22**:465–471, 2015. DOI: 10.1136/amiajnl-2014-003023

398. Page 373 twice. Sydney Lupkin, "Like clockwork: How daylight saving time stumps hospital record keeping," *USA Today*, 3 November 2018. eu.usatoday.com/story/news/health/2018/11/03/daylight-saving-time-hospital-electronic-medical-records-emergency-fall-back/1864579002

399. Page 373. Harold Thimbleby, "Can Anyone Work the Video?," *New Scientist*, **129**(1757):48-51, 1991.

400. Page 373. The Y2K problem arose because programmers were tempted to store the year using only two digits, a seemingly nice plan to cover the years from 1900 to 1999. Unfortunately, this idea meant that the next year after 99 would be 0, so instead of 1999 becoming 2000 with the turn of the new millennium, it would turn into 1900 instead.

401. Page 373. Harold Thimbleby, "Heedless Programming: Ignoring Detectable Error is a Widespread Hazard," *Software — Practice & Experience*, **42**(11):1393-1407, 2012. DOI: 10.1002/spe.1141

402. Page 374. I've made the analogy that English is a type, and I want my book to make sense in the specific type of English. So if I write words that are from another language, that would be reported as an error.
    Serious programming languages go a step further with **polymorphic types**, which, as it were, means I'd be able to say I want the book to make sense in *any* language, which I don't have to specify explicitly, say French or German, so long as the book makes consistent sense throughout in *that* language. (Does anyone want to translate my book, please?)

403. Page 375. There has been a lot of research on what we *think* are dependable programming languages, but surprisingly little research on how safe programming languages are when they are *actually* used, and — surprise, surprise! — even less research on what is safe and effective for digital healthcare.
    Here is a very interesting bit of research that has a very useful discussion on its limitations: Emery D. Berger, Celeste Hollenbeck, Petr Maj, Olga Vitek, and Jan Vitek, "On the Impact of Programming Languages on Code Quality," arXiv:1901.10220 [cs.SE], 2019.

404. Page 375. Ralf Jung, Jacques-Henri Jourdan, Robbert Krebbers, and Derek Dreyer, "Safe Systems Programming in Rust," *Communications of the ACM*, **64**(4):144-152, 2021. DOI: 10.1145/3418295

405. Pages 375, 485. Good reading[1] has more ideas, but a short paper that is easy to access on Alloy is Daniel Jackson, "Alloy: A lightweight Object Modelling Notation," *ACM Transactions on Software Engineering and Methodology*, **11**(2):256-290, 2002. DOI: 10.1145/505145.505149

406. Page 375. One of the problems writing a book like this is everything is changing. On MISRA C, for instance, there's a 2018 paper describing the next version, which is called MISRA C:2012 — even it's struggling to catch up! See Frank van den Beuken, "The Future MISRA C under the Spotlight," *Proceedings Twenty-sixth Safety Critical Systems Symposium*, 155-164, SCSC Publications, 2018.
    There is of course much more about safe programming that *Fix IT* cannot cover; the point is to be aware that there are many resources, and then find out what's best practice at the time it's needed.

407. Page 376. For discussion of Formal Methods and benefits, such as reducing bugs per thousand lines of code, see these classics:
    John A. McDermid and Tim P. Kelly, "Software in Safety Critical Systems: Achievement and Prediction," *Nuclear Future*, **2**(3):34-40, 2006. DOI: 10.1680/nuen.2006.2.3.140
        and
    Jean-Louis Boulanger, editor, *Industrial Use of Formal Methods: Formal Verification*, John Wiley & Sons, 2012.

---

[1] See Chapter 33: Good reading, page 471 ←

Counting bugs can be used to improve the quality of code, regardless of Formal Methods. For example, count bugs found per kLoC every week, and fit the data to a distribution (a Poisson distribution will do). Now you can calculate how much effort to put into getting whatever target level of defects per kLoC you want before the software is released for use.

408. Page 377. MISRA C forbids recursion, since you do not want to run out of stack space in a safety-critical system. The example code at the beginning of this chapter is recursive, so would be banned by MISRA C on those grounds alone. (So if you use MISRA C, you don't need to answer the question!)

409. Pages 378, 390. There is a lot of popular excitement on Agile methods. Far and away the best — though more academic than practical — resource on Agile is Bertrand Meyer, *Agile! The Good, the Hype and the Ugly*, Springer, 2014.

410. Page 378. Facebook's now historic slogan has been discussed widely, and it isn't just a problem for healthcare. See Jonathan Taplin, *Move Fast and Break Things: How Facebook, Google and Amazon Have Cornered Culture and Undermined Democracy*, Pan, 2018.

28   Finding bugs

411. Page 383. Bank account numbers have check digits. I didn't use Grete Fossbakk's actual account number, and I used a very simple check digit scheme to make it easy to understand what happened. In my example, the eleventh digit is the sum of all other digits, and then take the remainder when divided by 10. This very simple scheme does not detect transposing digits, something real check digit schemes can easily cope with. See Kai A. Olsen, "The $100,000 Keying Error," *IEEE Computer*, **41**(4):106–108, 2008. DOI: 10.1109/MC.2008.135

The *IEEE Computer* journal's citation (available at the DOI) for this article was given as pages 108–107 [sic], which piqued my copy editor's interest! In fact, the article's first page is 108, then it jumps backward to page 106, then it finishes part way down page 107. So the computer-generated citation looks backwards, and it certainly misses out page 106. It's a bug.

The programmer didn't expect articles to jump around a journal non-sequentially — despite it being quite common for the final paragraphs of an article to continue elsewhere, so that the page layout can be made neat. Given that *IEEE Computer* is a flagship journal, it's surprising that such an elementary bug wasn't noticed during testing — but, as we know, detailed tests are often skimped.

412. Page 384. Patrick Collinson, "I lost my £193,000 inheritance – with one wrong digit on my sort code. When Peter Teich's money went to another Barclays customer, the bank offered £25 as a token gesture," *The Guardian*, 7 December 2019. www.theguardian.com/money/2019/dec/07/i-lost-my-193000-inheritance-with-one-wrong-digit-on-my-sort-code

413. Page 385. The code in the body of the book is the most deeply indented line in the HTML shown below; the rest of the HTML is needed to tell your browser that you want the JavaScript code to be run and not just treated as more HTML.

Type this into a word processor (the indentation isn't important):

```
<!DOCTYPE html>
    <html>
        <body>
            <script>
                alert(parseFloat("40.5"));
            </script>
        </body>
    </html>
```

and save it as a file called t.html (it need not be t.html; it can be any name ending in .html to ensure it is an HTML file), then open the HTML file in any web browser to see what it does.

It should just pop up a dialog box, the alert, and say 40.5.

Now change the "40.5" in the code to, say, "40.5 mcg", save the file again and refresh your browser. You'll see that the code completely ignores the critical mcg bit (which means a millionth of a gram) — the number now means 0.0000405 grams. The standard JavaScript code neither recognizes mcg as a unit, nor does it warn the user that it is completely ignoring it.

414. Page 387. Here's a paper that explains the method in more detail with infusion pumps as the example. Paolo Masci, Rimvydas Rukšėnas, Patrick Oladimeji, Abigail Cauchi, Andy Gimblett, Yunqiu (Karen) Li, Paul Curzon, and Harold Thimbleby, "The Benefits of Formalising Design Guidelines: A Case Study on the Predictability of Drug Infusion Pumps," *Innovations in Systems and Software Engineering*, **11**(2):73–93, 2015. DOI: 10.1007/s11334-013-0200-4

415. Page 388. Paolo Masci, Anaheed Ayoub, Paul Curzon, Michael Harrison, Insup Lee, and Harold Thimbleby, "Verification of interactive software for medical devices: PCA infusion pumps and FDA regulation as an example," *Proceedings SIGCHI Symposium on Engineering Interactive Computing Systems*, 81–90, ACM, 2013. DOI: 10.1145/2494603.2480302

See www.pvsioweb.org for up-to-date information.

416. Page 390. There is lots of advice on fuzzing. My book, Harold Thimbleby, *Press On: Principles of Interaction Programming* (MIT Press) has lots of ideas — and unlike most of the guidance on fuzzing, *Press On: Principles of Interaction Programming* is full of practical ideas to help evaluate and improve user interface design. *Press On: Principles of Interaction Programming* is also a recommended book in the Good reading.[m]

The Wikipedia page on fuzzing is en.wikipedia.org/wiki/Fuzzing and is also recommended. (Wikipedia is always recommended, as it'll be kept up-to-date.)

417. Pages 390, 391, 392. This paper explains the details of the user interfaces that were fuzzed, along with full details of the techniques for evaluating the safety of the interface designs: Harold Thimbleby, Paul Cairns, and Patrick Oladimeji, "Unreliable numbers: Error and harm induced by bad design can be reduced by better design," *Journal Royal Society Interface*, **12**(110):20150685, 2015. DOI: 10.1098/rsif.2015.0685 — the Royal Society paper includes working code that can be copied.

The original ISMP rules (described in the paper above) were designed for making handwritten numbers more reliable; for instance, writing .5 might be misread as 5, so ISMP requires numbers less than 1 to always start with a zero, in this case by writing 0.5 instead of .5

That's fine, and easy to require in a digital system, except that as you enter a number interactively into a device, you may go through intermediate stages that ISMP does not recommend. For instance, to enter 0.5, you'd first have to enter 0. (which isn't permitted by ISMP rules) at some point. So what do you do?

We discussed a safe solution to this problem in Harold Thimbleby and Andy Gimblett, "Dependable Keyed Data Entry for Interactive Systems," *FMIS 2011, 4th International Workshop on Formal Methods for Interactive Systems*, in *Electronic Communications of the EASST*, **45**:1/16–16/16, 2011. DOI: 10.1145/1996461.1996497

A working implementation, including several demos, is at harold.thimbleby.net/regex

418. Page 392. Jane Wakefield, "Artificial intelligence-created medicine to be used on humans for first time," BBC, 30 January 2020. www.bbc.co.uk/news/technology-51315462

---

[m] See Chapter 33: *Press On: Principles of Interaction Programming*, the book, page 483 ←

419. Page 393. One of the best no-nonsense explanations of RCTs can be found in David Spiegelhalter, *The Art of Statistics: Learning from Data*, Pelican Books, 2020. It's also a fantastic book if you want to get a very readable introduction to statistics or if you want to get new insights from a world leader.
420. Page 394. Robert W. Yeh, Linda R. Valsdottir, Michael W. Yeh, Changyu Shen, Daniel B. Kramer, Jordan B. Strom, Eric A. Secemsky, Joanne L. Healy, Robert M. Domeier, Dhruv S. Kazi, and Brahmajee K. Nallamothu, "Parachute use to prevent death and major trauma when jumping from aircraft: randomized controlled trial," *BMJ*, **363**:k5094, 2018. DOI: 10.1136/bmj.k5094

    Note that there is a correction in *BMJ* **363**:k5343, 2018.
421. Page 395. Tarveen Jandoo, "WHO Guidance for Digital Health: What It Means for Researchers," *Digital Health*, **6**:1–4, 2020. DOI: 10.1177/2055207619898984
422. Page 395. The best critique of RCTs and discussion of powerful alternatives — in fact, a whole new approach to clearer thinking — is Judea Pearl and Dana Mackenzie, *The Book of Why: The New Science of Cause and Effect*, Penguin, 2018. Everyone working in computing, especially AI, will have heard of Judea Pearl, and I think this is his best and most accessible book by a long way.

    Here's an excellent article on the way RCTs and the quest for strong evidence undermines responding effectively with the time pressures driven by a pandemic: Trisha Greenhalgh, "Thinking in a pandemic," *Boston Review*, 29 May 2020. bostonreview.net/science-nature/trisha-greenhalgh-will-evidence-based-medicine-survive-covid-19

    Greenhalgh also wrote a more academic paper: "Evidence based medicine: a movement in crisis?," *BMJ*, **348**:g3725, 2014. DOI: 10.1136/bmj.g3725
423. Page 396. Andrew J. Copas, James J. Lewis, Jennifer A. Thompson, Calum Davey, Gianluca Baio, and James R. Hargreaves, "Designing a stepped wedge trial: three main designs, carry-over effects and randomisation approaches," *Trials*, **16**:352, 2015. DOI: 10.1186/s13063-015-0842-7

    A broader review of other choices can be found at Alain Bernard, Michel Vaneau, Isabelle Fournel, Hubert Galmiche, Patrice Nony, and Jean Michel Dubernard, "Methodological choices for the clinical development of medical devices," *Medical Devices: Evidence and Research*, **7**:325–334, 2014. DOI: 10.2147/MDER.S63869
424. Page 396. Billy Kenber and Chris Smyth, "Test and Trace: Where did it all go wrong?" *The Times*, 11 November 2020. www.thetimes.co.uk/article/test-and-trace-where-did-it-all-go-wrong-66kfkg3wm
425. Page 399. Editorial, "Is digital medicine different?" *The Lancet*, **392**:95, 14 July 2018. DOI: 10.1016/S0140-6736(18)31562-9
426. Page 399. See: Joseph M. Smith, "Digital health startups may not want to do randomized trials, but they need to," *STAT*, 15 October 2018. www.statnews.com/2018/10/15/digital-health-startups-randomized-trials, and Reflexion Health, "Reflexion Health and Duke Clinical Research Institute Announce Results of the First Randomized Controlled Trial Demonstrating Virtual Physical Therapy Outperforms Traditional Approach," reflexionhealth.com/virtual-physical-therapy-news/veritas-study-results-announcement, 15 October 2018.

29 Choose safety

427. Page 403. Leapfrog uses letter grades A, B, C, D, E, and F — A being best. Each year the group re-evaluates hospitals, and the thresholds for each grade are adjusted. (In contrast the EU energy rating retains the same gradings, but adds more A+, A++ grades at the top.) The end result is the same: a clear way to be able to compare safety and effectiveness. Leapfrog's safety rating website is at www.hospitalsafetygrade.org. There is also an interesting paper on it: J. Matthew Austin, Guy D'Andrea, John D.

Birkmeyer, Lucian L. Leape, Arnold Milstein, Peter J. Pronovost, Patrick S. Romano, Sara J. Singer, Timothy J. Vogus, and Robert M. Wachter, "Safety in Numbers: The Development of Leapfrog's Composite Patient Safety Score for U.S. Hospitals," *Journal of Patient Safety*, **10**(1):64–71. 2013. DOI: 10.1097/PTS.0b013e3182952644

428. Page 404. An RFID tag would mean just getting your mobile phone (running the right app, or, better, configured by your hospital to do this automatically) close to the label would transfer the information across.

429. Page 405. The full summary of our work was published here: Patrick Oladimeji and Harold Thimbleby, "Open Metrics for Evaluating and Designing Safer Interactive Health Systems: A Case Study in Procuring Infusion Pumps," *2015 USENIX Summit on Information Technologies for Health, HealthTech*, Washington DC, USA, 2015.

430. Page 407. Thomas Sullivan, "A Tough Road: Cost To Develop One New Drug Is $2.6 Billion; Approval Rate for Drugs Entering Clinical Development is Less Than 12%," *Policy & Medicine*, 21 March 2019.
www.policymed.com/2014/12/a-tough-road-cost-to-develop-one-new-drug-is-26-billion-approval-rate-for-drugs-entering-clinical-de.html

431. Page 408. Levels and tiers are often used in designing complex computer systems, such as the **OSI Levels** (e.g., data layer, network layer, application layer) — or the **Three-Tier Architecture** (i.e., user interface, business logic, and data storage layers). Unfortunately, issues such as safety interact across the layers; if one layer is unsafe, they all potentially become unsafe. The user interface layer (the main concern of this book) can say things that mislead the user about the capability of the other layers, and then things start to go wrong.

432. Page 409. See Institute for Safe Medication Practices, www.ismp.org

433. Page 409. Patrick Oladimeji, Harold Thimbleby, and Anna L. Cox, "Number entry interfaces and their effects on error detection," *Proceedings 13th IFIP TC13 Conference on Human-Computer Interaction*, **IV**:178–185, Springer-Verlag, 2011. DOI: 10.1007/978-3-642-23768-3_15

434. Page 409. Abigail Cauchi, Patrick Oladimeji, Gerrit Niezen, and Harold Thimbleby, "Triangulating Empirical and Analytic Techniques for Improving Number Entry User Interfaces," *Proceedings ACM SIGCHI Symposium on Engineering Interactive Computing Systems*, **EICS'14**:243–252, ACM, 2014. DOI: 10.1145/2607023.2607025

435. Pages 410, 411. Patrick Oladimeji, Anna L. Cox, and Harold Thimbleby, "A Performance Review of Number Entry Interfaces," *Proceedings IFIP Conference on Human-Computer Interaction, Designing for Diversity, Lecture Notes in Computer Science*, **8117**:365–382, Springer-Verlag, 2013. DOI: 10.1007/978-3-642-40483-2_26

436. Pages 411, 557. In my autoimmune disease, B cells are destroying the myelin sheaths on my nerves, which gives me chronic inflammatory demyelinating polyneuropathy.

     Rituximab is a monoclonal antibody that kills B cells (white blood cells), and thus gives my nerve sheaths a chance to grow back. It's working so far, although it has side effects that need managing. I have the dilemma that rituximab makes me more susceptible to COVID-19, but that's not the concern here ...

     It's a worrying contrast that full details of rituximab (like its chemical formula, $C_{6416}H_{9874}N_{1688}O_{1987}S_{44}$) and *lots* of detailed research on it are quite routinely available — including its effectiveness on my own disease. Yet the design of the Alaris GP infusion pump that is infusing me with it, and how safe it is, is "commercially confidential."

437. Page 411. Participants in this number experiment were not nurses. We used university students, 22 females, 11 males, average age 23.5, $\sigma = 4.86$.

438. Page 413. People often want to reduce the number of mouse clicks as well as the number of keystrokes; indeed, what is widely regarded as the first book on the science of human computer interaction focused almost exclusively on ways to estimate and

reduce times. See: Stuart K. Card, Thomas P. Moran, and Allen Newell, *The Psychology of Human-Computer Interaction*, CRC Press, 1986.

439. Page 413. Melinda Ashton, "Getting Rid of Stupid Stuff," *New England Journal of Medicine*, **379**:1789–1791, 2018. DOI: 10.1056/NEJMp1809698

30 Signs of life

440. Page 417. Medal describe their app and development approach at blog.medicalalgorithms.com/clinical-algorithm-development, and their website is www.medicalalgorithms.com

441. Page 418. Patient Safety Alert, "Risk of death and severe harm from failure to obtain and continue flow from oxygen cylinders," NHS/PSA/W/2018/001, 2018. improvement.nhs.uk/documents/2206/Patient_Safety_Alert_-_Failure_to_open_ oxygen_cylinders.pdf

442. Page 419. Zoë Norris, @dr_zo, 10 September 2018. twitter.com/dr_zo/status/1039116040981110785?s=20 and replied to by Matt Hancock, @MattHancock, 10 September 2018. twitter.com/MattHancock/status/1039126578163339264?s=20

443. Page 420. Andy Hertzfeld, "Steve wants to make the Macintosh boot faster," *Folklore*, August 1983. www.folklore.org/StoryView.py?story=Saving_Lives.txt

444. Page 420. Here's a small systematic review of eICUs: Sajeesh Kumar, Shezana Merchant, and Rebecca Reynolds, "Tele-ICU: Efficacy and Cost-Effectiveness of Remotely Managing Critical Care," *Perspectives in Health Information Management*, Spring:1–13, 2013.

445. Page 421. Ben Goldacre, *Bad Pharma* is excellent on these sorts of issue. His book is discussed in Good reading.[n]

446. Page 421. Tom J. Pollard, Alistair E. W. Johnson, Jesse D. Raffa, Leo A. Celi, Roger G. Mark, and Omar Badawi, "The eICU Collaborative Research Database, a freely available multi-center database for critical care research," *Scientific Data*, **5**:180178 EP, 2018. DOI: 10.1038/sdata.2018.178

447. Pages 423, 555. My wife, Prue Thimbleby, runs an accredited training course on Digital Storytelling at the University of South Wales. Contact her by email at prue@thimbleby.net

The first job preparing a Digital Story is to get the **story shape** right.

The story itself may be prepared as a written script of about 250 words, but it will sound much better, more spontaneous, and authentic, if it is done conversationally *without* reading it. Quite a bit of editing may need to be done to the voice recording to help the storyteller communicate well — knowing the recording will be edited allows the teller to have a few goes at getting their words sorted out. Then the images can be added.

There are many Digital Storytelling tools available which run on PCs and mobiles — hackastory.com is one place to start looking for them. There are also lots of expensive professional editing tools. But in healthcare, it's very important that the digital hurdles to start storytelling are minimized. In fact, the more "professional" the storytelling process is made, the more everyone's expectations of production quality increase, which soon intrude on the process, which takes attention away from the listening and communicating power of simple, direct storytelling.

The story images can be animated by slowly zooming in on areas of interest, or panning from one face or point of interest to another. These techniques date from rostrum cameras, but are often called Ken Burns effects. These techniques work very well with Digital Stories, grabbing attention, perhaps focusing on a photograph of the

---

[n] See Chapter 33: Good reading, page 471 ←

patient or a family member or what they are doing. Very often people have plenty of photographs to work from, and the effects enliven the images without introducing the production problems of video. Simple photographs, particularly ones taken in the past giving context to the story (like ordinary family photographs of the patient before an incident), are very effective, and have a powerful authenticity. Sometimes drawings work better, they are easy to anonymize if that's required.

In contrast to still photos with simple zooming and panning, video raises expectations and makes it much harder to do a good job. So much video we watch, like in movies, is produced professionally and sets very high standards. Videos are very much harder to record and edit, too, especially editing the video to synchronize with the voice-over. So, for Digital Stories, use still photographs or simple drawings.

Finally, thought must be given to consent and permissions, especially if the stories are going to be put on the internet. Digital Stories are very personal, and they must be used with respect.

448. Page 423. Wikipedia gives a summary of Digital Stories: en.wikipedia.org/wiki/Digital_storytelling and the Berkeley storytelling center, StoryCenter, is at www.storycenter.org

449. Page 423. Arts in Health Wales does a huge amount of digital patient storytelling. www.artsinhealth.wales/patient-experience.html

450. Page 424. Christopher Richard Evans and J. Wilson, "A program to allow computer based history-taking in cases of suspected gastric ulcer," *National Physical Laboratory Report*, Com 49, 1971. For more context, see S. S. Somerville, J. S. Stewart, and G. E. T. Raine, "Mickie: Experiences of Interviewing Patients by Micro," in J. P. Paul, M. M. Jordan, M. W. Ferguson-Pell, and B. J. Andrews (eds) *Computing in Medicine*, Strathclyde Bioengineering Seminars, Palgrave, London, 1982. DOI: 10.1007/978-1-349-06077-1_5
   An interesting and technically more detailed article is: Nigel Bevan, Peter Pobgee and Shirley Somerville, "MICKIE — A microcomputer for medical interviewing," *International Journal of Man-Machine Studies*, **14**:39–47, 1981.

451. Page 424. Chris Evans was way ahead of his time. His *The Mighty Micro* is amazingly prescient — and still very interesting to read — considering it was written in 1980: see Christopher Richard Evans, *The Mighty Micro*, Coronet Books, 1980.

452. Page 425. If you don't know about pulmonary hypertension, Bella's lovely story might be balanced in the non-digital scales of the heart-breaking loss of Elaine Pagels's young child Mark to pulmonary hypertension. See Elaine Pagels, "Finding the heart," *The New Yorker*, 4 November 2018. www.newyorker.com/culture/personal-history/finding-the-heart?mbid=social_twitter&utm_source=twitter&utm_brand=tny&utm_social-type=owned&utm_medium=social

453. Page 427. Marie Elisabeth Gaup Moe, "Go Ahead Hackers. Break My Heart," *Wired*, www.wired.com/2016/03/go-ahead-hackers-break-heart

454. Page 430. Signs of Safety's website is www.signsofsafety.net

455. Page 430. See www.signsofsafety.net/signs-of-safety-practice-it-alignment-learning-lab-exceeds-expectations-of-north-tyneside-council

456. Page 431. Isabel Healthcare Ltd. See www.isabelhealthcare.com
   Although the Isabel website has lots of information, an interesting open-access review of 23 digital symptom checkers, including Isabel, which discusses benefits and challenges of the technology, is: Hannah L. Semigran, Jeffrey A. Linder, Courtney Gidengil, and Ateev Mehrotra, "Evaluation of symptom checkers for self diagnosis and triage: Audit study," *BMJ*, **351**(h3480), 2015. DOI: 10.1136/bmj.h3480

457. Page 432. J. Luis Zabala-Genovez, Edwarda Golden, and Farah Ciftci, "Isabel to the Rescue!" Abstract 1085 at Conference on Hospital Medicine, *Journal of Hospital Medicine*, 2019. www.isabelhealthcare.com/pdf/SHM_poster_PDF_version.pdf

458. Page 433. Julia Cumberlege, *First Do No Harm. The report of the Independent Medicines and Medical Devices Safety Review*, July 2020. Available at www.gov.uk/official-documents

459. Page 434. I recommend starting with the Patient Experience Library's *Inadmissible Evidence: The double standard in evidence-based practice, and how it harms patients*, 2020. Find it at www.patientlibrary.net

31 The pivotal pandemic?

460. Page 437. Chris Pleasance, *Daily Mail*, 19 March 2020. www.dailymail.co.uk/news/article-8130379/First-person-die-coronavirus-Indiana-say-goodbye-partner-iPad.html

461. Page 437. Jimmy McCloskey, "Man with Down syndrome died lonely coronavirus death on his 30th – 7 days after it killed his mom," *MetroUK*, 10 April 2020. metro.co.uk/2020/04/10/man-syndrome-died-lonely-coronavirus-death-30th-birthday-12541023
      Some reports of Thomas Martins call him Thomas Martins-Reitz. I sincerely apologize if I've made a mistake.

462. Page 437. Paul Lynch and Daniel Wainwright, "Coronavirus: How GPs have stopped seeing most patients in person," BBC, 11 April 2020. www.bbc.co.uk/news/uk-england-52216222

463. Page 438. There are some interesting trade-offs: the patients sent home with oxygenation meters need to know how to use them and what to do. That requires some sort of assessment and training (however simple), which is more work for already overloaded hospitals.
      On the other hand, that extra work needs to be traded off against the hopefully huge saving of workload because the patients have gone home. See Ingrid Torjesen, "Covid-19: Patients to use pulse oximetry at home to spot deterioration," *BMJ*, **371**:m4151, 2020. DOI: 10.1136/bmj.m4151

464. Page 438. Perhaps the quickest way to get into wearable computing is to buy an Arduino and an oxygenation sensor. There are numerous suppliers of such kit, and it's worth spending a while searching for the stuff that best suits your needs. Even better, go to a hacker club and chat to people who are already doing this.

465. Page 439. Luca Ferretti, Chris Wymant, Michelle Kendall, Lele Zhao, Anel Nurtay, Lucie Abeler-Dörner, Michael Parker, David Bonsall, and Christophe Fraser, "Quantifying SARS-CoV-2 transmission suggests epidemic control with digital contact tracing," *Science*, published online, 2020. DOI: 10.1126/science.abb6936

466. Page 439. Tim Biggs, "COVIDSafe may interfere with diabetes-monitoring apps," *Sydney Morning Herald*, 1 May 2020. www.smh.com.au/technology/covidsafe-may-interfere-with-diabetes-monitoring-apps-20200501-p54oyd.html

467. Page 439. Paresh Dave and Stephen Nellis, "Colombia had to abandon contact tracing from its coronavirus app because it didn't work properly," *Business Insider*, 7 May 2020. www.businessinsider.com/colombia-contact-tracing-apple-google-coronavirus-app-2020-5?r=US&IR=T

468. Page 440. Rebecca Smithers, "Fraudsters use bogus NHS contact-tracing app in phishing scam," *The Guardian*, 13 May 2020. www.theguardian.com/world/2020/may/13/fraudsters-use-bogus-nhs-contact-tracing-app-in-phishing-scam?CMP=share_btn_tw

469. Page 440. The cost of testing and tracing in the UK to July 2020 has been widely criticized. See Andrew Woodcock, "Coronavirus: Government has set aside £10bn for Test and Trace system for England," *The Independent*, 8 July 2020. www.independent.co.uk/news/uk/politics/coronavirus-test-and-trace-system-england-government-budget-a9608656.html

470. Pages 440, 442. Harriet Brewis, "Failed test-and-trace app cost more than £11 million, Government figures show," *Evening Standard*, 19 June 2020. www.standard.co.uk/news/uk/test-and-trace-app-cost-uk-government-11million-a4474386.html

471. Page 440. *The Guardian* of 6 October 2020 has several good articles about the Test and Trace problem. The leading front cover article was: Josh Halliday, Peter Walker, and Denis Campbell, "Race to warn 50,000 people of virus risks after 'catastrophic' IT blunder," *The Guardian*, 6 October 2020. Or see Elisabeth Mahase, "Covid-19: Only half of 16,000 patients missed from England's official figures have been contacted," *BMJ*, **371**, 6 October 2020. DOI: 10.1136/bmj.m3891

472. Page 441. At the time of writing, nobody seems very clear what happened. The journalists reporting the problems are not technical or don't have access to accurate technical information, and the politicians discussing it seem to want to down-play any problems. My understanding, from reading inconsistent reports and listening to parliamentary discussions, is that large quantities of data were probably emailed in CSV formats to central handling centers. For some reason, possibly because their software couldn't import CSV directly or the CSV files weren't all in the same format, the CSV files were converted to XLS, probably by using Excel, as that would be the easiest way to do it, and certainly the easiest way to make simple corrections to varying data.

Here's one of many reports: Leo Kelion, "Excel: Why using Microsoft's tool caused Covid-19 results to be lost," *BBC News*, 5 October 2020. www.bbc.co.uk/news/technology-54423988

A bit later I published a short letter about the atrocious design of the system in the *British Medical Journal*: Harold Thimbleby, "The problem isn't Excel, it's unprofessional software engineering," *BMJ*, **371**:m4181, 2020. DOI: 10.1136/bmj.m4181

473. Page 443. David Adam, "A guide to *R* — the pandemic's misunderstood metric: What the reproduction number can and can't tell us about managing COVID-19," *Nature*, **583**:346–348, 3 July 2020. www.nature.com/articles/d41586-020-02009-w, DOI: 10.1038/d41586-020-02009-w

474. Page 444. Laura Spinney, *Pale Rider: The Spanish Flu of 1918 and how it changed the world*, Vintage, 2017.

Despite its being pre-digital (and even pre-knowing about viruses) the book *Pale Rider* has many lessons for today, but the modern story of the COVID-19 pandemic is brilliantly covered in Michael Lewis, *The Premonition: A Pandemic Story* (Allen Lane, 2021) — I review this engrossing book in the Good reading chapter.[°]

475. Page 444. Nick Carding, "Hancock grants GCHQ powers over NHS IT systems," *HSJ*, 29 April 2020. www.hsj.co.uk/free-for-non-subscribers/nhs-developing-coronavirus-contact-tracking-app/7027163.article

476. Pages 445, 446, 447. The SIR model's documentation is at www.harold.thimbleby.net/sir, which contains a link to the model itself at www.harold.thimbleby.net/sir/sir.html

When you run the model, you should get the graph shown in the book (figure 31.1). You may need to adjust its size to make it easier to read, and you may want to change the fonts because I wanted the diagram to use the fonts used in the rest of this book.

° See Chapter 33: *The Premonition*, page 477 ←

477. Page 446. The SIR model is based on the number of susceptible people, S, the number of people infected, I, and the number of people who have recovered, R (this is a different R from the reproduction number).

Mathematically, SIR involves some simple differential equations, and a program to understand SIR solves these equations with the given parameters. However, it's much easier to write a program to run a SIR model by taking small time steps, like one day, and simply iterating the basic equations for updating the S, I, and R parameters.

478. Page 447. David Adam, "Modelling the pandemic: The simulations driving the world's response to COVID-19," *Nature*, **580**:316–318, 2020. DOI: 10.1038/d41586-020-01003-6

479. Pages 447, 449. There have been many very strong criticisms of Ferguson's code. For example, David Richards and Konstantin Boudnik, "Neil Ferguson's Imperial model could be the most devastating software mistake of all time," *The Telegraph*, 16 May 2020, www.telegraph.co.uk/technology/2020/05/16/neil-fergusons-imperial-model-could-devastating-software-mistake

See also: Jonathan Leake, "Neil Ferguson interview: No 10's infection guru recruits game developers to build coronavirus pandemic model," *The Sunday Times*, 29 March 2020. www.thetimes.co.uk/article/neil-ferguson-interview-no-10s-infection-guru-recruits-game-developers-to-build-coronavirus-pandemic-model-zl5rdtjq5

480. Page 447. Harold Thimbleby, "A proposal to achieve professional software engineering in scientific research." Preprint available at www.harold.thimbleby.net/reliable-models.pdf

481. Pages 448, 556. Neil M. Ferguson, @neil_ferguson, 22 March 2020. twitter.com/neil_ferguson/status/1241835454707699713

Ferguson's tweet is also accessible and discussed in Hector Drummond, "Anon IT Professional: Can we trust Neil Ferguson's flu pandemic model?" *Hector Drummond Magazine*, 24 April 2020. hectordrummond.com/2020/04/24/guest-post-can-we-trust-neil-fergusons-flu-pandemic-model and in Mike Jackson, "Better software, better COVID-19 research," Software Sustainability Institute, 7 May 2020. www.software.ac.uk/blog/2020-05-07-better-software-better-covid-19-research

482. Page 449. Sarah Boseley, "Neil Ferguson: coronavirus expert who is working on despite symptoms — Epidemiologist is taking on a marathon of mathematical modelling at sprint speed," *The Guardian*, 18 March 2020. www.theguardian.com/world/2020/mar/18/neil-ferguson-coronavirus-expert-who-is-working-on-despite-symptoms

483. Page 449. A nice brief article describing the benefits and uses of lab notebooks is Santiago Schnell, "Ten Simple Rules for a Computational Biologist's Laboratory Notebook," *PLoS Computational Biology*, **11**(9):e1004385, 2015. DOI: 10.1371/journal.pcbi.1004385

484. Page 449. There are *lots* of automatic and semi-automatic documentation generators. The Wikipedia article is an up-to-date source of information: en.wikipedia.org/wiki/Comparison_of_documentation_generators

I've developed a tool to help document program code: Harold Thimbleby and Dave Williams, "A tool for publishing reproducible algorithms & A reproducible, elegant algorithm for sequential experiments," *Science of Computer Programming*, **156**:45–67, 2018. DOI: 10.1016/j.scico.2017.12.010 All the code is available online too at github.com/haroldthimbleby/relit

485. Page 450. Imperial College, COVID-19 Emergency Ventilator, 2020. www.imperial-consultants.co.uk/areasofexpertise/emergency-ventilator

486. Page 450. Tom Dare, "'Creepy' plan to spy on mobile phones of Birmingham patients including your calls and daily movements," *BirminghamLive*, 18 February 2020. www.birminghammail.co.uk/news/midlands-news/creepy-plan-spy-mobile-phones-17767137

487. Page 450. House of Commons, House of Lords, Joint Committee on Human Rights, *Human Rights and the Government's Response to Covid-19: Digital Contact Tracing*, 6 May 2020. publications.parliament.uk/pa/jt5801/jtselect/jtrights/343/343.pdf

488. Page 451. The Declaration of Helsinki makes a salutary case study. It started in 1964 as a tight document on medical ethics principles (responding to numerous outrages), but it has since grown and become more prescriptive. For instance, it now mentions animal experiments and impact on the environment.

    As the Declaration added more and more issues, it inevitably became more controversial — it is no longer followed by, for instance, the US FDA, which inevitably creates a "pick and choose" approach to ethical principles and makes any principled approach *harder* to follow. The Declaration is likely to continue growing in complexity when it faces up to digital health interventions, especially as the huge commercial opportunities in digital rarely align with individual interests.

    We don't want Software Engineering Boards to fall into the same trap as the Declaration of Helsinki.

    World Medical Association, "World Medical Association Declaration of Helsinki Ethical Principles for Medical Research Involving Human Subjects," *Journal of the American Medical Association*, **310**(20):2191–2194, 2013. DOI: 10.1001/jama.2013.281053

489. Page 452. Sunil S. Bhopal, Jayshree Bagaria, Bayanne Olabi, and Raj Bhopal, "Children and young people remain at low risk of COVID-19 mortality," *The Lancet Child & Adolescent Health*, 10 March 2021. DOI: 10.1016/S2352-4642(21)00066-3

    The Spanish Government responded, as reported in this newspaper article a week later: Beatriz García and Ariadna Reina García, "Sanidad admite un error en la mortalidad infantil por covid: 'Cuentan centenarios como menores'" *NIUS*, 17 March 2021. www.niusdiario.es/sociedad/sanidad/sanidad-reconoce-datos-muertes-ninos-covid-erroneos-contabilizaban-centenarios-como-menores_18_3107220241.html

    The story about bugs is worrying — what public health policies in Spain were misdirected? — but the really important point the data begs is: what can we learn from South Korea, who have had *zero* child deaths (according to the paper's data) from COVID-19?

490. Page 453. David M. Cutler and Lawrence H. Summers, "The COVID-19 Pandemic and the $16 Trillion Virus," *Journal of the American Medical Association*, published online 12 October 2020. DOI: 10.1001/jama.2020.19759

32   Living happily ever after

491. Page 457. Frank Bajak, "FBI warns ransomware assault threatens US healthcare system," 29 October 2020. apnews.com/article/fbi-warns-ransomware-healthcare-system-548634f03e71a830811d291401651610 See also for more technical background and lots of useful advice and pointers to many resources: US National Cyber Awareness System, Alert (AA20-302A): "Ransomware Activity Targeting the Healthcare and Public Health Sector," 28 October 2020. us-cert.cisa.gov/ncas/alerts/aa20-302a

492. Page 458. Here's a story of a large Indian diagnostic lab's cybersecurity problems: "After Dr Lal PathLabs here's the Rx on healthcare data security: Scan, test, and treat immediately," see: economictimes.indiatimes.com/prime/technology-and-startups/after-dr-lal-pathlabs-heres-the-rx-on-healthcare-data-security-scan-test-and-treat-immediately/primearticleshow/78628718.cms

493. Page 458. Lizzie Dearden, "Coronavirus: UK vaccine programs face ongoing threat of cyber attacks by hostile states: National Cyber Security Centre says a quarter of record recorded incidents in the past year were coronavirus-related," *The Independent*, 3

November 2020. www.independent.co.uk/news/uk/home-news/covid-19-vaccine-uk-cyberattacks-oxford-b1536171.html

494. Page 459. Co-regulation is described in many places, and is a method employed by the EU. Here's an interesting US chapter on it: Ira Rubinstein, "The Future of Self-Regulation is Co-Regulation," *The Cambridge Handbook of Consumer Privacy*, Cambridge University Press, 2016.

495. Page 460. IEC 61508 is an international standard. Lots has been written about it and about the various derived standards (such as for MISRA-C we've talked about in this book).

The standard IEC 61508 is covered well in many books, such as David J. Smith and Kenneth G. L. Simpson, *Functional Safety: A straightforward guide to applying IEC 61508 and related standards*, second edition, Elsevier, 2004.

The 61508 Association has a useful website which has lots of information and pointers to lots of resources: www.61508.org

496. Page 461. The website for the National Association of Medical Device Educators & Trainers (NAMDET) is namdet.org

497. Page 461. Eirini Oikonomou, Jane Carthey, Carl Macrae, and Charles Vincent, "Patient safety regulation in the NHS: Mapping the regulatory landscape of healthcare," *BMJ Open*, **9**(7):e028663, 2019. DOI: 10.1136/bmjopen-2018-028663

498. Page 463. HSIB, the Healthcare Safety Investigation Branch's website is www.hsib.org.uk

499. Page 464. The World Health Organization (WHO): see www.who.int

500. Page 464. The International Medical Device Regulators Forum is a group of regulators working together to harmonize device regulation. As of 2019, its members include representatives from Australian regulators (Therapeutic Goods Administration), Chinese ones (National Medical Products Administration), the EU, Japan, ... US, and more (but not the UK).

More details are on their web site, www.imdrf.org

501. Page 464. Institute for Healthcare Improvement: see www.ihi.org

502. Page 466. Edward R. Melnick, Christine A. Sinsky, and Harlan M. Krumholz, "Implementing Measurement Science for Electronic Health Record Use," *JAMA*, 2021. DOI: 10.1001/jama.2021.5487

503. Page 466. Bug bounties are provided by many companies, including Google. Bounties can reach $1.5 million, so they are a strong motivation to find and report bugs. www.bbc.co.uk/news/technology-50515647

504. Page 466. As an expert witness, I've repeatedly seen how manufacturers don't want to disclose information, they really don't want to appear in court, and even when they do, they don't want a cup of coffee.

505. Page 467. Global NCAP, the Global New Car Assessment Program; see www.globalncap.org

506. Page 469. The World Medical Association's Declaration of Geneva can be found at www.wma.net/what-we-do/medical-ethics/declaration-of-geneva

33   Good reading

507. Page 471. The detailed reasons why the NHS COVID-19 app failed are of course complicated, but the underlying reason is Cat Thinking leading to over-confidence in rapidly developing complex digital healthcare solutions on the whims of politicians who aren't at all grounded in what is technologically feasible to deliver.

For a quick UK-centered summary, see: Rory Cellan-Jones, "Coronavirus: What went wrong with the UK's contact tracing app?" BBC, 20 June 2020. www.bbc.co.uk/news/technology-53114251

A more insightful report is this: James Ball, "The UK's contact tracing app fiasco is a master class in mismanagement," *MIT Technology Review*, 19 June 2020. **www.technologyreview.com/2020/06/19/1004190/uk-covid-contact-tracing-app-fiasco**

508. Page 471. RIPPLE20 is the catchy name given to a whole range of bugs in internet connectivity software used in many digital health devices, as well as in many IoT (Internet of Things) products, from domestic fridges to hospital blood banks.

All internet connections require software to sort out the internet packets, using a **TCP/IP Stack** (more briefly, the IP Stack).

Treck Inc (**treck.com**) is one of many companies that make TCP/IP stack solutions, but Trek's has serious bugs, which were identified in June 2020 by JSOF, a small cybersecurity company. Some of Trek's bugs are basic coding errors, like not checking there is enough memory before starting an operation.

Treck's buggy — and vulnerable — software is often embedded in small electronic components, typically little boxes as small as 2 cm by 4 cm (about 0.75 by 1.5 inches). These components are hidden inside medical devices and in many other connected devices. A serious problem is that people have pretty much lost track of where they are, and even whether their medical devices have affected components.

For full details, see JSOF's website, which has details and reports at **www.jsof-tech.com/ripple20**, June 2020.

Like most cybersecurity stuff, just do an internet search for RIPPLE20 to make sure you get the most up-to-date information.

509. Page 471. Brandon Vigliarolo, "IBM finds vulnerability in IoT chips present in billions of devices," *TechRepublic*, 19 August 2020. **www.techrepublic.com/article/ibm-finds-vulnerability-in-iot-chips-present-in-billions-of-devices**

510. Page 472. Benjamin Mazer, "Are medical errors a huge problem that's simple to fix?" *BMJ Online*, 9 November 2018. **blogs.bmj.com/bmj/2018/11/09/benjamin-mazer-are-medical-errors-a-huge-problem-thats-simple-to-fix**

511. Page 474. Ronald M. Davis, "BMJ bans 'accidents'," *BMJ*, **322**:1320, 2001. DOI: 10.1136/bmj.322.7298.1320

512. Page 480. Karl R. Popper, *Conjectures and Refutations: The Growth of Scientific Knowledge*, Routledge and Kegan Paul, 1963.

513. Page 480. Karl R. Popper and Neil McIntyre, "The critical attitude in medicine: The need for a new ethics," *BMJ*, **287**:1919–1923, 1983.

514. Page 490. Robert L. Wears, "Using information technology to reduce rates of medication errors in hospitals," *BMJ*, **320**:788–791, 2000. DOI: 10.1136/bmj.320.7237.788

515. Page 492. Civica Rx: see civicarx.org

516. Page 493. Beth Griffith's story is told on her twitter account, @bethangriffith

34   Notes

517. Page 497. DOIs illustrate a typical example of digital ambiguity and risks being ignored in international standards (in this case, ISO 26324, 2010).

The DOI standard permits any printable characters in a DOI, which means DOIs can include ordinary punctuation. Curiously, that means their use in text, such as in a bibliography — as they are used throughout these notes — can cause serious ambiguities.

Here's an example of the DOI problem. Does this DOI, DOI: 10.1098/rsif.2010.0112, include the final comma? According to the international standard, yes, according to common sense, no.

Hence, throughout these notes, DOIs have, so far as possible, always been written at the end of a line or paragraph so there should be no ambiguity.

In short, DOIs are a parable for this book: all the work that goes into an international standard, and yet the DOI standards team completely overlooked Work

As Done, reliability, and human error. They had not thought about all the uses of DOIs. Ironically, overlooking human error is *itself* a common human error.

My writing a blank after each DOI is a **workaround** that ensures we can get a badly designed computer standard to work in the real world (as represented by this book anyway). Another, more effective workaround, would be for all programmers to agree that they program their computers to ignore any trailing punctuation when reading a DOI. This workaround would fix the international standard, and, even better, requires no further work from us users. As always, fixing problems at the thick end of the wedge has a much wider impact, and in this case, simplifies use and reduces error.

35   Healthcare openness and acknowledgments

518. Page 553. VW's "dieselgate" emission trick, which affected over 11 million vehicles, is well known. VW diesel cars were programmed to detect when they were being tested for emissions, and they reduced their emissions to pass the test. However when they detect they are on the open road, not being tested, they switch to better performance by incurring worse emissions. See: Guilbert Gates, Jack Ewing, Karl Russell, and Derek Watkins, "How Volkswagen's 'Defeat Devices' Worked," *The New York Times*, 16 March 2017. www.nytimes.com/interactive/2015/business/international/vw-diesel-emissions-scandal-explained.html

519. Page 554. The approach to identifying patients, staff, hospitals, and systems taken in this book is consistent with the *British Medical Journal's* (BMJ's) consent policies. Peter A. Singer and the BMJ Ethics Committee, "Consent to the publication of patient information," *BMJ*, **329**:566–8, 2004. DOI: 10.1136/bmj.329.7465.566

In addition to a wider-ranging and thoughtful discussion, this paper says, "Publications about error should be encouraged as they are core to improvements in patient safety in both relation to analysis of root causes and engendering a culture of openness about error."

I and Raden Norfiqri, this book's artist, have redrawn screenshots and other pictures where there may otherwise have been copyright issues, or issues where bystanders could have been identified. The details that are shown explicitly in the pictures are necessary to explain and understand the issues.

520. Page 555. See the CHI-MED website, www.chi-med.ac.uk for lots of details of this very productive research project, "Computer-Human Interaction for Medical Devices."

Traditional healthcare views of confidentiality are challenged by digital healthcare. This chapter also includes heartfelt thanks to all the patients and healthcare staff and others who've told their stories and brought this book to life.

35

Healthcare openness and acknowledgments

This book explored and told the stories of people who have been injured or who have died in healthcare, and it told the stories of clinicians who have been affected by those incidents. Their names are highlighted in **bold** in the index at the end of this book. I want to particularly acknowledge and thank all of them and their families.

Some readers, especially those with traditional healthcare or clinical backgrounds, may be uncomfortable about the open approach to discussing problems, devices, staff and patient details that I took in this book.

Let me explain why it is important to be open in digital healthcare.

Legislation and regulation drives improvements in safety. Today, for instance, most countries are tightening pollution legislation, because car emissions harm people and cars can be made safer. There are occasional glitches when manufacturers have kept their problems secret,[518] but these scandals prove the rule. Being open helps everyone to improve. Openness helps people see how design affects safety. Openness creates a virtuous circle: now we know cars can be safer, we want to buy the safer cars, and therefore manufacturers want to make safer cars. And car manufacturers certainly want us to know which cars are which, so we buy *their* cars!

That is the culture of an industry that wants to make safer products.[a] Today, very little about car safety is kept secret. If there is an accident, news stories will mention the make of car, especially if it is new or innovative in any way — like, if it is driverless.

In contrast, healthcare has a long tradition of respecting confidentiality and privacy. Patient confidentiality is foundational in healthcare, but healthcare isn't only about patients. In modern healthcare, there are many devices

[a] See Chapter 11: Cars are safer, page 137 ←

Fix It: See and solve the problems of digital healthcare. Harold Thimbleby,
Oxford University Press. © Harold Thimbleby 2021.
DOI: 10.1093/oso/9780198861270.003.0035

and systems — almost all digital or embedded digital — that are used widely. Unlike patients, though, it really matters *which* devices we are using. What are their identities? In contrast to personal patient details, it really matters, and it profoundly affects care, which devices and systems are involved in the incident. Even the version number of an infusion pump may be the difference between life and death for a patient being treated by it.

This book told the stories of digital healthcare systems. All the stories were about common, typical digital products. It'd be bizarre if a book about drugs discussed problems like side effects but didn't name any drugs; likewise, it's obvious that it wouldn't have been possible to discuss digital systems properly and honestly in this book without naming them and exploring them in some detail. Moreover, naming and clearly identifying these things enables anyone to check the details of what I said.

One reason we are happy discussing drugs by name is that it's obvious that different drugs are different from each other — they do different things — and therefore it obviously matters which drugs are used. Therefore they need naming.

I hope, by now, this book has made it very clear, too, that infusion pumps, medical accelerators, patient record systems — every digital device or system in healthcare, even calculators and beds — are different from each other. It really matters which ones are being used. They must be named. Besides, it's just good science to be clear.

Some of the systems I discussed have won awards. The systems that illustrate this book's stories weren't picked on because they're terrible; they're here because they are some of the best — indeed, many have saved lives. Many of the stories in this book vividly illustrate how hard it is to make digital safe, and how hard it is for healthcare (and politicians and others) to recognize that we urgently need to improve digital healthcare. It's harder than winning prizes.

Manufacturers and hospitals may point out that the specific systems or versions of systems that have caused problems are obsolete models, and there are new versions or completely different systems that are now in use. That's good, but the critical issue is whether their *thinking* has changed too. If we don't improve our thinking, we'll get more of the same old problems. We have to learn the lessons, and that starts by being clear what the problems are, and that in turn requires being explicit about all the specific digital system identities.

Many stories in this book first appeared in the public domain, in newspapers, on television, and in social media. In this book, all use of public domain material has been fully cited; all other identifiable material used has had consent from the people concerned. This is standard practice.[519]

Personal acknowledgments

I am very grateful to See Change (R&MA-P, Scotland) who very generously fund all my work. My work was previously funded by the UK Engineering and Physical Sciences Research Council (EPSRC), in particular through a grant called "Computer-Human Interaction for Medical Devices" (CHI-MED), which involved a wonderful multi-university team.[520]

Many individuals have helped me enormously. I particularly want to thank the people who told their personal stories in chapter 30, *Signs of Life*, and I want to mention a few very important people who have sustained me beyond the call of duty: Chitra Acharya, Aidan Byrne, Nick Fine, Ross Koppel, Peter Ladkin, Paolo Masci, Patrick Oladimeji, Robin and Marianne Anker-Petersen, Martyn Thomas, Dave Williams, John Williams, and my OUP editor, Jamie Oates. Many thanks to the entire next generation of my family — Deborah, Em, Isaac, Jemima, Oi, Sam, and Will — who have read it and given me detailed comments too. But above all, this book would not exist without the encouragement and support and tremendously thoughtful input of my wife, Prue Thimbleby.[447]

All of the book's weaknesses or errors are entirely my fault, despite all my friends' best efforts to help me. I thank my reading group — in addition to those I named above — who waded through the many drafts of this book, for their fantastic, detailed comments, and encouragements:

Stuart Anderson	Kevin Fu	Rosie Plummer
Ann Blandford	Bod Goddard	Rowan Pritchard Jones
Angela Branston	Julie Greenall	Philip Scott
Simon Braybrook	Carolyn Greig	Martin Sheldon
Carol Butler	Beth Griffith	Ben Shneiderman
Paul Cairns	Rob Griffiths	Mike Smith
Abigail Cauchi	Michael Harrison	Deborah Symmons
Rod Chapman	Sue Heatherington	Joel Telles
Bella Cheham	Jan Hoogewerf	Lisa Thomas
Alan Cox	Daniel Jackson	Sian Thomas
Peter Croft	Michael Jackson	Sarah Tombs
Paul Curzon	Dagmar Lüttel	David Watkins
Jelle Damhuis	Paul Marshall	David Whitaker
Jim Dawton	Stephen Mason	Dan White
Paul DeMuro	Jason Maude	Graham White
Hanan Edrees	Marie Moe	David Widdows
Daniel Feldman	Rhian Morris	Suzette Woodward
Karen Francis	Martin Newby	Xixi Yao
Emma Friesen	Josh Pike	Alex Yeates

Picture and other credits

All the line drawings in this book are by Raden Norfiqri; please do see his website link radenoactive.com for more of his excellent work. However, I did all the graphs and charts, which were drawn in *Mathematica*.

More specific acknowledgements are as follows:

❶ Front cover photographer Johan B. Skre ❶ Page 2: Drawing based on a fragment of the Hippocratic Oath written on the third century Papyrus Oxyrhynchus 2547; Wellcome L0034090. Wellcome Trust, CC BY 4.0. ❶ Page 28: CAT scan drawings based on ChumpusRex, en.wikipedia.org/wiki/File:Ct-workstation-neck.jpg, CC BY-SA 3.0. ❶ Page 40: Drawing based on a photo by Carlos Monroy, cmonroya@gmail.com, used with permission. ❶ Page 50: Photograph of drug bag label by Institute for Safe Medication Practices Canada, used with permission. ❶ Page 82: X-ray of Anna Bertha Röntgen's hand. Wilhelm Röntgen, who took the X-ray in 1895, died in 1923: this work is now in the public domain. ❶ Page 83: Clarence Dally taking an X-ray, from *New York World*, 1, 3 August 1903. CC BY-NC 3.0. ❶ Page 116: Artist drawing based on screenshots from an app I helped build.[119] ❶ Page 249: Drawing based on a photo of Dr Marie Moe, used with permission. ❶ Page 252: Drawing based on a photo by Prof Ross Koppel, used with permission. ❶ Page 253: Drawing of Swiss Gornergrat Bahn just below the top station Gornergrat, based on a photo by David Gubler, 2013, www.bahnbilder.ch CC BY-SA 3.0. ❶ Page 278: Photograph of Rear Admiral Grace Murray Hopper's notebook, where she'd taped the first bug, a moth caught up in the machinery; from the US Naval History and Heritage Command collection, catalog number NH 96566-KN, 1945. www.history.navy.mil/our-collections/photography/numerical-list-of-images/nhhc-series/nh-series/NH-96000/NH-96566-KN.html ❶ Page 342: Tweet by Dr David Watkins, used with permission. ❶ Page 419: Tweet by Dr Zoë Norris, used with permission. ❶ Page 429: Artist drawing based on the Untire app, by Jelle Damhuis, used with permission. ❶ Page 448: Tweet by Prof Neil Ferguson, in public domain.[481]

Good-faith efforts have been made to contact copyright holders of material used in this book, but in a few instances the author has been unable to locate or get a response from the sources. Copyright holders are invited to contact Oxford University Press. Over time, internet resources move around, so if there are any "link rot" problems with this book's links, URLs, or DOIs — or problems with any other information, for that matter — please email me at harold@thimbleby.net

Prof Harold Thimbleby
harold@thimbleby.net – @haroldthimbleby
See Change Fellow in Digital Health
Wales

August 11, 2021

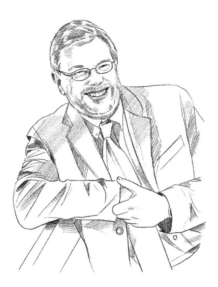

Prof Harold Thimbleby is See Change Fellow in Digital Health, based at Swansea University, Wales. Harold is a popular speaker, and has been invited to talk in over 30 countries.

Harold has been an expert witness in NHS criminal cases; his work exposing problems in digital healthcare has stopped nurses going to prison — a little of this story is mentioned in this book.[87]

Harold won the British Computer Society's Wilkes Medal, and his last book, *Press On: Principles of Interaction Programming* (MIT Press), won several international awards.

Although a professor of Computer Science, he is an Honorary Fellow of the Royal College of Physicians, the Edinburgh Royal College of Physicians, and the Royal Society of Arts; he's also a Fellow of the Learned Society of Wales and a fellow of the Royal Society of Medicine. He has been a Royal Society Wolfson Research Merit Award holder and a Leverhulme Trust Senior Research Fellow, and he is 28th Gresham Professor of Geometry. Harold is Expert Advisor on IT to the Royal College of Physicians, a member of WHO's Patient Safety Network, Patient Safety Council Member of the Royal Society of Medicine, and an advisor to the Clinical Human Factors Group and the UK Medicines & Healthcare products Regulatory Agency (MHRA).

Harold is also a patient. He has peripheral neuropathy,[436] which makes everyday activities like walking and writing painful and increasingly difficult.

More details, including offprints of hundreds of articles and videos, are available from Harold's website, **www.harold.thimbleby.net**

Harold's twitter handle is @haroldthimbleby

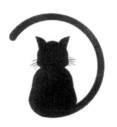

Fonts for cancer

Buy Fonts Save Lives (BFSL) is a generous project that was founded by the designer Paul Harpin after his niece Laura died of cancer when she was only 26. BFSL sells typefaces to raise money in support of Cancer Research UK and Macmillan Cancer Support. See typespec.co.uk for details of BFSL, to buy fonts, or to donate more fonts.

Nick Cooke designed the Organon fonts, and donated them to BFSL. The body text for this book is set in Organon Serif, and his complementary font Organon Sans Serif is used to make quotes and figure captions stand out. Both I and Oxford University Press, this book's publisher, have made donations to BFSL for the use of the fonts.

The modern Organon fonts have been subtly complemented with Roboto Slab for "computer text," which is used in this book mainly for URLs and program source code — the techy stuff.

Monospaced fonts, like Roboto Slab, hark back to the days of old typewriters, when a font having a constant width made the early mechanical typewriters considerably simpler to build. Today, monospaced fonts have been taken up by programmers because their constant-width characters make laying out program source code with neat indentations much easier. Consistent indentation in turn makes programs easier to check, which itself is an important contribution to reducing bugs.

Roboto Slab was designed by Christian Robertson. Visually, it's a typical "computer" font, which is one reason I liked it for this book. Roboto Slab is an Open (free) font, and encourages other people to contribute to it, for instance to provide more styles, such as letters for more languages. See fonts.google.com/specimen/Roboto+Slab for more details.

Fix IT was typeset with these fonts using LATEX (a powerful typesetting system) with my own macros. One of LATEX's many jobs was to generate a *slanted Organon font* by using PostScript transformations.

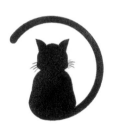

Index

🛈 All abbreviations used in this book can be found in the index.

🛈 **Names in bold** are in recognition of the fact that people have been harmed or adversely affected as victims or as second victims.[67]

🛈 Normal page numbers — 2, 3, 4 — refer to concepts and ideas in passing. For instance, if there is a patient incident at a hospital, the hospital name can be found in the index, but the index entry isn't *about* the hospital, it's just a detail of the story.

🛈 Page numbers in bold — **2, 3, 4** — are entries discussing topics in greater depth.

🛈 Page numbers in italics — *2, 3, 4* — are for authors of articles, papers, or reports. These mostly refer to authors appearing in the Notes.[a]

---

[a] See Chapter 34: Notes, page 497 ←

The problem is not so much to see what nobody has yet seen, as to think what nobody has yet thought concerning that which everybody sees.

— *Arthur Schopenhauer*

A virtuoso is not someone who never makes an error, but someone who detects and recovers from the error.

— *James Reason*

To kill an error is as good a service as, and sometimes even better than, the establishing of a new fact.

— *Charles Darwin*

Unless someone like you cares a whole awful lot, nothing is going to get better. It's not.

— *Dr Seuss*